LIMBIC AND AUTONOMIC NERVOUS SYSTEMS RESEARCH

CONTRIBUTORS

Jasper Brener
Department of Psychology
University of Hull
Yorkshire, England

Thomas Budzynski
University of Colorado School of Medicine
Denver, Colorado

Douglas K. Candland
Department of Psychology
Bucknell University
Lewisburg, Pennsylvania

David H. Cohen
Department of Physiology
School of Medicine
University of Virginia
Charlottesville, Virginia

James Francis
Department of Psychology
University of Miami
Coral Gables, Florida

Claude J. Gaebelein
Department of Psychiatry, Medical School
University of North Carolina
Chapel Hill, North Carolina

Myron A. Hofer
Department of Psychiatry
Albert Einstein College of Medicine
and
Montefiore Hospital
New York, New York

James E. Lawler
Department of Psychiatry, Medical School
University of North Carolina
Chapel Hill, North Carolina

Alan I. Leshner
Department of Psychology
Bucknell University
Lewisburg, Pennsylvania

Charles W. Malsbury
Rockefeller University
New York, New York

Paul A. Obrist
Department of Psychiatry, Medical School
University of North Carolina
Chapel Hill, North Carolina

Bruce A. Pappas
Department of Psychology
Carleton University
Ottawa, Canada

Donald W. Pfaff
Rockefeller University
New York, New York

Larry D. Sampson
Department of Psychology
University of Miami
Coral Gables, Florida

Evelyn Satinoff
Departments of Psychology and Physiology
University of Illinois
Champaign, Illinois

Neil Schneiderman
Department of Psychology
University of Miami
Coral Gables, Florida

James S. Schwaber
Department of Psychology
University of Miami
Coral Gables, Florida

M. B. Sterman
Neuropsychology Laboratory
Veterans Administration Hospital
Sepulveda, California
and
Department of Anatomy
University of California
Los Angeles, California

Johann Stoyva
University of Colorado School of Medicine
Denver, Colorado

Bernice M. Wenzel
Departments of Physiology and Psychiatry
and
Brain Research Institute
University of California
Los Angeles, California

CONTRIBUTORS

Jasper Brener
Department of Psychology
University of Hull
Yorkshire, England

Thomas Budzynski
University of Colorado School of Medicine
Denver, Colorado

Douglas K. Candland
Department of Psychology
Bucknell University
Lewisburg, Pennsylvania

David H. Cohen
Department of Physiology
School of Medicine
University of Virginia
Charlottesville, Virginia

James Francis
Department of Psychology
University of Miami
Coral Gables, Florida

Claude J. Gaebelein
Department of Psychiatry, Medical School
University of North Carolina
Chapel Hill, North Carolina

Myron A. Hofer
Department of Psychiatry
Albert Einstein College of Medicine
and
Montefiore Hospital
New York, New York

James E. Lawler
Department of Psychiatry, Medical School
University of North Carolina
Chapel Hill, North Carolina

A. I. Leshner
Department of Psychology
Bucknell University
Lewisburg, Pennsylvania

James W. Malsbury
Rockefeller University
New York, New York

Paul A. Obrist
Department of Psychiatry, Medical School
University of North Carolina
Chapel Hill, North Carolina

Bruce A. Pappas
Department of Psychology
Carleton University
Ottawa, Canada

Donald W. Pfaff
Rockefeller University
New York, New York

Larry D. Sampson
Department of Psychology
University of Miami
Coral Gables, Florida

Evelyn Satinoff
Departments of Psychology and Physiology
University of Illinois
Champaign, Illinois

Neil Schneiderman
Department of Psychology
University of Miami
Coral Gables, Florida

James S. Schwaber
Department of Psychology
University of Miami
Coral Gables, Florida

M. B. Sterman
Neuropsychology Laboratory
Veterans Administration Hospital
Sepulveda, California
and
Department of Anatomy
University of California
Los Angeles, California

Johann Stoyva
University of Colorado School of Medicine
Denver, Colorado

Bernice M. Wenzel
Departments of Physiology and Psychiatry
and
Brain Research Institute
University of California
Los Angeles, California

LIMBIC AND AUTONOMIC
NERVOUS SYSTEMS
RESEARCH

LIMBIC AND AUTONOMIC NERVOUS SYSTEMS RESEARCH

Leo V. DiCara
Department of Psychiatry
Mental Health Research Institute
The University of Michigan
Ann Arbor, Michigan

PLENUM PRESS • NEW YORK AND LONDON

Library of Congress Cataloging in Publication Data

DiCara, Leo, 1937-
  Limbic and autonomic nervous systems research.

  Includes bibliographies.
  1. Limbic system. 2. Nervous system, Autonomic. I. Title. [DNLM: 1.
Autonomic nervous system—Physiology. 2. Limbic system—Physiology. WL307
D454L]
QP368.D5   599'.01'88   74-17327
ISBN 0-306-30786-3

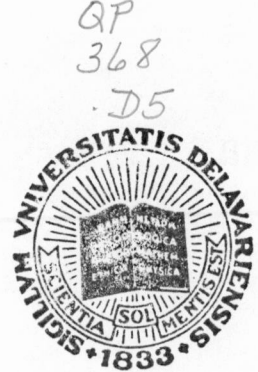

© 1974 Plenum Press, New York
A Division of Plenum Publishing Corporation
227 West 17th Street, New York, N.Y. 10011

United Kingdom edition published by Plenum Press, London
A Division of Plenum Publishing Company, Ltd.
4a Lower John Street, London W1R 3PD, England

Printed in the United States of America

Preface

The present volume has been written primarily for the advanced student and the mature investigator. The book will be of value to the student because it includes representative research problems on a variety of topics, and significant for the mature investigator, because it can help bring him up to date on specific topics in limbic and autonomic nervous system research, an area which has undergone spectacular growth, particularly during the last ten years. The twelve chapters deal with subject matter that falls loosely into four major subtopics—basic sensory and regulatory mechanisms, emotional processes, cardiovascular processes and learning, and low arousal states—but each chapter represents recent research in one particular area, and stands as a self-contained unit.

I am indebted to the many authors and publishers for their aid in granting permission to reproduce quotations, tables, and figures from their works. Specific acknowledgments are made in the text.

Leo V. DiCara

Ann Arbor

Contents

Emotional Processes

Chapter 3

Neural and Hormonal Determinants of Mating Behavior in Adult Male
Rats. A Review

Charles W. Malsbury and Donald W. Pfaff

Chapter 4

A Model of Agonistic Behavior: Endocrine and Autonomic Correlates

Douglas K. Candland and Alan I. Leshner

Chapter 5

Immunological and Chemical Sympathectomy in the Neonatal Rodent: Effects on Emotional Behavior

Bruce A. Pappas

Cardiovascular Processes and Learning

Chapter 8

CNS Integration of Learned Cardiovascular Behavior

Neil Schneiderman, James Francis, Larry D. Sampson, and
   James S. Schwaber

Low Arousal States

LIMBIC AND AUTONOMIC NERVOUS SYSTEMS RESEARCH

CHAPTER 1

The Olfactory System and Behavior

Bernice M. Wenzel

Departments of Physiology and Psychiatry
and
Brain Research Institute
University of California
Los Angeles, California

1. Introduction

In 1933, Herrick proposed that "At all stages of cortical elaboration an important function of the olfactory cortex, in addition to participation in its own specific way in cortical association, is to serve as a nonspecific activator for all cortical activities" (p. 14). Among these activities he included overt behavior, learning, memory, and affective reactions. This theme from Herrick, so reminiscent of Sherrington's description of the distance receptors as "the great inaugurators of reaction" (1906, p. 350), serves as the keynote for this article. The concern here is not with the physiology of olfaction as a specific sensory system, but rather with the contribution of the primary and secondary portions of the olfactory system to such patterns of behavior as Herrick mentioned, patterns that are not typically classified as olfactory. The terms olfactory system or direct olfactory system (Girgis, 1970) will be used to refer collectively to the olfactory mucosa in the nasal cavity; the fibers of the olfactory nerves, which originate in the mucosa; the olfactory bulb, where the mucosal fibers make synaptic contact with the second fibers in the pathway; and the secondary fibers, the courses of which are discussed below.

Chemical sensitivity is probably the oldest response of animals to the environment. Olfaction, the distance sense, became increasingly important as animal forms became more complex, until it finally dominated the early vertebrate forebrain. This olfactory dominance was markedly persistent. Herrick suggested that it reached its culmination in lower animals just as the neopallium, the great mammalian forebrain development, was about to assume dominance. He further proposed that the cerebral cortex developed only when the extension of other sensory systems into the vicinity of the olfactory cortex created the possibility for extensive new associations. Because of the paucity of spatial localization conveyed by the olfactory system, he argued that it could not be primarily concerned with precise environmental details. With such a long history of extensive and fundamental involvement in animal behavior, however, its many established relationships were not likely to be completely lost.

2. Background

2.1. Rhinencephalon

In Herrick's day, the structures considered to be directly innervated from the olfactory bulbs, hence to be concerned directly with olfactory functions, were collected under the term "rhinencephalon," which loomed somewhat larger anatomically than it does today. Kölliker (1896) characterized as the rhinencephalon those cerebral structures that were clearly distinguishable from the neopallium, including the septum, the hippocampus, the amygdala, and the cingulum, in addition to the immediate olfactory areas of the prepiriform cortex and the olfactory tubercle. Brodal (1947) was the first to remove a major component, the hippocampus, from inclusion in the term. Once begun, the partitioning of the old smell brain then continued with what Adey (1970) called "almost Calvinistic zeal." This period was climaxed by the definitive review by Pribram and Kruger (1954) in which the much weakened rhinencephalon was ultimately divided into three systems. One of these constituted the direct olfactory system; it contains those structures that receive fibers from the olfactory bulb by way of the lateral olfactory tract (olfactory tubercle, diagonal band, prepiriform cortex, and corticomedial amygdalar nucleus). The structures in the second system connect directly with those in the first but not with the olfactory bulb (subcallosal and frontotemporal juxtallocortex, septal nuclei, basolateral amygdalar nuclei), and those in the third are completely distinct from the others (hippocampus, entorhinal cortex, retrosplenial cortex, cingulate cortex). These differentiations were made on the basis of both anatomical and physiological evidence then available, and contributed greatly to ridding investigators finally of the idea that olfactory perception is the work of all structures that had so long been labeled rhinencephalic.

The first influential paper in this separation of function was that of Papez (1937), who proposed that emotional behavior was the major concern of much of the rhinencephalon. The so-called Papez circuit included the hypothalamus, mammillary body, anterior thalamic nuclei, cingulate gyrus, hippocampus, and fornix. Further connections of the hypothalamus that he considered established and important were those with the septal region and olfactory tubercle via the medial forebrain bundle, and with the amygdala through the stria terminalis. This hypothesis has had a profound effect in shaping a vast amount of subsequent research in behavioral neurophysiology under the limbic system's banner while Herrick's idea of significant olfactory involvement in a variety of behaviors was ignored.

A recent suggestion by Riss *et al.* (1969) that the olfactory system actually evolved from the limbic system intimately unites the two systems. On the basis of comparative vertebrate anatomy, they propose that the limbic system, by way of the nervus terminalis, first developed sensitivity to the internal chemical environment and that exteroception to chemical stimuli emerged later, eventually acquiring its own specialized neural structures. Such an hypothesis could account for the extensive olfacto–limbic interconnections described below and predicts the close relationship observed between the olfactory system and certain physiological functions.

2.2. The Direct Olfactory System and Its Connections

The purpose of this article is not to review in detail the anatomical and physiological evidence concerning the distribution of olfactory fibers, but only to support the contention that the network is not a tightly restricted pathway even in those forms, such as the monkey, in which relative bulb size has diminished (Fig. 1) (Heimer, 1969).

2.2.1. Anatomical Evidence

Because of the development of new techniques for tracing fiber pathways and identifying synaptic relationships, the olfactory system's precise outlines have been vigorously reexamined in the last decade. Secondary fibers in the lateral olfactory tract in mammals were found to extend not only to the anterior olfactory nucleus, the olfactory tubercle, and the prepiriform cortex (Scalia, 1968), but also to the entorhinal area, with the exception of the spheno-occipital ganglion (Kerr and Dennis, 1972; Price and Powell, 1971), and to the corticomedial amygdala (Cowan *et al.*, 1965; Girgis, 1969). Tertiary fibers have been identified as coursing between the two anterior olfactory nuclei by way of the anterior limb of the anterior commissure (Lohman and Lammers, 1967; Price and Powell, 1971), to the

anterior rudiment of the hippocampus from an unknown site (Price and Powell, 1971), to the nuclei gemini of the hypothalamus, to the mediodorsal
nucleus of the thalamus (Scott and Leonard, 1971), and to the midbrain reticular formation (Ferrer, 1969; Millhouse, 1969; Scott and Leonard, 1971;
Valverde, 1965). Other secondary and tertiary connections, such as with the
extrapyramidal system (Heimer and Wilson, 1975), are still being determined. It is now clear that a wealth of interconnections with limbic structures can be effected. In addition, many of the sites send fibers back to the
olfactory bulbs directly or in relays (Price and Powell, 1970; Rieke, 1971).

   An important consideration in discussing the olfactory system is the
distinction between the main olfactory bulb, supplied by the olfactory nerve
from receptors in the olfactory mucosa, and the accessory bulb, situated
dorsocaudally on the main bulb and innervated by the vomeronasal nerve
from receptors in the vomeronasal organ, located in an outpouch of the
nasal cavity. Accessory bulbs and their associated structures occur in
gymnophiones, anurans, most reptiles, and many mammals (Nieuwenhuys,
1967). It is absent in birds. According to recent work, some of the descriptions of olfactory projections have probably failed to distinguish between

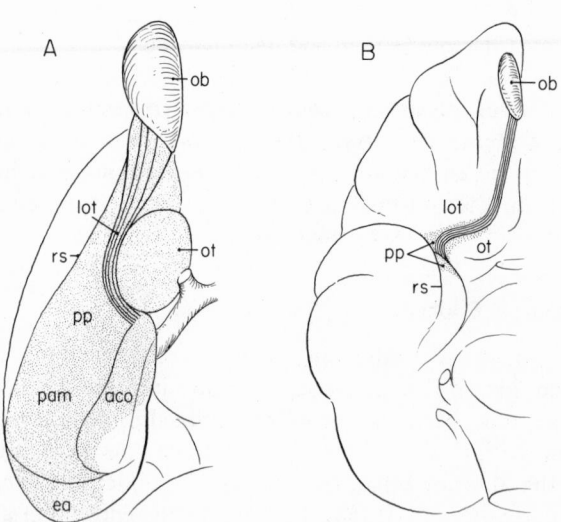

FIG. 1.   Ventral view of the brain of (A) the rat and (B) the rhesus monkey. The stippled areas
represent the olfactory bulb and the projection field of bulbar fibers, and show the species difference in the relative sizes of the olfactory system and the whole brain. aco: cortical amygdaloid
nucleus, ea: entorhinal area, lot: lateral olfactory tract, ob: olfactory bulb, ot: olfactory tubercle,
pam: periamygdaloid cortex, pp: prepiriform cortex, rs: rhinal sulcus. (From Heimer, 1969).

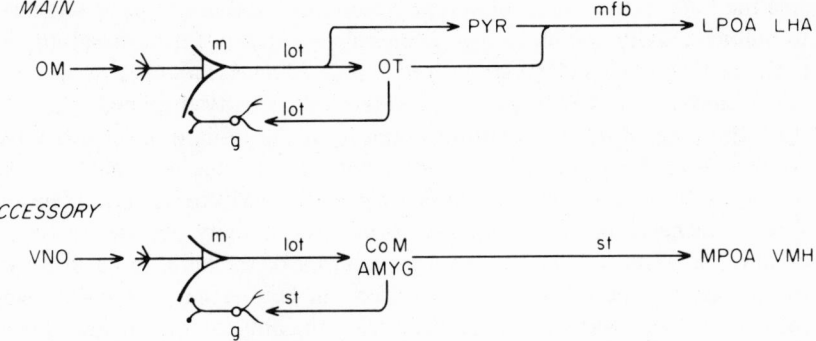

FIG. 2. A schematic comparison of the connections of the main and accessory olfactory bulbs. Accessory: accessory olfactory bulb, g: granule cell, CoM AMYG: corticomedial group of amygdaloid nuclei, lot: lateral olfactory tract, LHA: lateral hypothalamic area, LPOA: lateral preoptic area, m: mitral cell, Main: main olfactory bulb, mfb: medial forebrain bundle, MPOA: medial preoptic area, OM: olfactory mucosa, OT: olfactory tubercle, PYR: pyriform cortex, st: stria terminalis, VMH: ventromedial hypothalamic nucleus, VNO: vomeronasal organ. (From Raisman, 1972).

the main and accessory bulbs as separate origins of secondary pathways. It seems clear, for instance, that the medial and cortical amygdaloid nuclei of the rabbit receive many fibers from the accessory bulb while the main bulb projects only minimally to an anterolateral strip of the cortical nucleus (Winans and Scalia, 1970). Raisman (1972) proposes the concept of a dual olfactory system on the basis of similarly distinct projection patterns in the rat as diagrammed in Fig. 2. The importance of these observations for the purpose of the present discussion lies in the fact that most of the literature to be reviewed is based on work with rats as subjects and virtually none of it mentions the accessory bulb. Inasmuch as ablation of the main bulb often includes the accessory bulb, there may be little functional significance in the lack of distinction. Nonetheless, investigators should be alert to it and specify this aspect of their lesions more precisely when using an animal with a vomeronasal organ.

2.2.2. Physiological and Neurochemical Evidence

In addition to studies of patterns of fiber degeneration following specific lesions, recent electrophysiological evidence strengthens the growing conviction that the olfactory system has the potential for exerting widespread influence. The well-known burst activity of the olfactory bulb [Adrian's (1950) induced waves] has been recorded from many areas out-

side the bulb in the brains of several vertebrates and found to be secondary
to bulbar activity, which in turn is completely dependent on nasal air flow
in the resting animal (Graystone *et al.*, 1970; Mechelse and Lieuwens, 1969;
Riblet and Tuttle, 1970). In the cat, the burst activity disappears not only
from the prepiriform cortex after ablation of the ipsilateral olfactory bulb
(Becker and Freeman, 1968), but anywhere outside the bulb as well
following transection of the "olfactory stalk" (Mechelse and Lieuwens,
1969). Mechelse and Lieuwens found the burst activity outside the bulb to
be lower in amplitude and frequency than that of the bulb, to occur only in
the presence of bulb bursts, and to drop out before that of the bulb when
the cat went to sleep. It was recorded from the amygdaloid nucleus, the anterior amygdaloid area, the prethalamic areas, the anterior ventral nucleus,
the hypothalamus and fornix adjacent to prethalamic areas, the entopedun-
cular area and adjacent hypothalamus, the medial geniculate nucleus, and
the midbrain reticular formation. It was never recorded from the
ventrolateral, ventral posterior, lateral posterior, dorsomedial, or anterior
thalamic nuclei.

Neurons in several sites are also affected by bulbar activity resulting
either from odorous or direct electrical stimulation. Diencephalic units
respond with relatively short latencies in the lateral hypothalamus (Scott
and Pfaffmann, 1967; Sollertinskaia, 1972); in the medial thalamus and
along the projection pathways of the medial forebrain bundle and stria
medullaris (Komisaruk and Beyer, 1972); and in hypothalamic projection
sites described in anatomical work by Scott and Leonard (1971), viz., along
a group of presumed secondary fibers running caudally near the optic tract
and ventral border of the cerebral peduncle. There were no responses in the
surrounding regions. Extensive distribution of response units in the
amygdala, including cortical, basal, and medial nuclei, was reported by
Cain and Bindra (1972). They also found some responses in the hippocampus. Effects have been reported as far caudally as the midbrain reticular formation (Motokizawa and Furuya, 1973; Pfaff and Pfaffmann,
1969). Even motor pathways are affected by bulbar stimulation, at least in
the chloralose-anesthetized cat in which pyramidal and extrapyramidal discharges are suppressed by an electrical stimulus applied to the olfactory
bulb (S. Bernstein *et al.*, 1969).

Another type of evidence, still rather gross at present, comes from
analyses of biogenic amines in different brain segments following olfactory
bulb ablation (Pohorecky *et al.*, 1969; Pohorecky and Chalmers, 1971). In
rats, removal of the olfactory bulb is followed by lower norepinephrine
levels in the telencephalon and higher levels in the brainstem. These
changes become measurable by three weeks, and persist for at least a
month and a half after operation. All the results, including data for levels

of tyrosine hydroxylase and tryptophan, are compatible with an interpretation of degenerated adrenergic fibers in the telencephalon. The effects on the brainstem, however, cannot be so interpreted and are presumably trans-synaptic and dependent on an unknown mechanism. It is worth noting that the increase in norepinephrine in the brainstem is greater if the rats are housed under more crowded conditions than normal; the level in the telencephalon is unaffected by housing conditions. No change was found in serotonin levels in either the telencephalon or brainstem (Pohorecky and Chalmers, 1971). The possibility of species differences in all of these effects must be considered. Neither bilateral bulbectomy in male hamsters nor unilateral bulbectomy in female hamsters altered norepinephrine levels in the telencephalon or brainstem (Murphy and Pohorecky, 1973).

It seems fair to say, therefore, that olfaction is now being restored to a significant role in forebrain function as zealously as it was being obliterated not long ago. We have not merely returned to where we started from, however, for the present evaluation is based on far more durable data than was the earlier one and will probably resist challenge.

2.3. Olfactory Lesions and Nonolfactory Behavior

Early in this century there was some interest in the relationship between olfaction and behavior, but it was entirely directed toward the significance of specific olfactory cues in guiding complex learned responses. J. B. Watson reported in 1907 that rats made anosmic by olfactory bulbectomy were normal in every aspect of maze learning. He further reported that they recovered more slowly from the effects of the operation than did those rats that had undergone removal of their eyes, and they were "more irritable and pugnacious than usual and showed a disposition to strike their heads against the sides of their cages" (p. 51). This behavioral pattern had disappeared by four weeks after surgery and Watson attributed it to irritation from contraction of the collodion with which the wounds had been coated. Liggett and Liggett (1927) reported that after a similar experiment their bulbectomized albino rats were more active than the controls, were very irritable, and required individual housing. "They frequently bit each other's tails, ears, noses, and feet and on several occasions killed and devoured their cagemates" (p. 535). The postoperative course of this behavior was not defined further. Possible causes were suggested: (1) the loss of olfaction, (2) the removal of inhibitory tendencies, and (3) irritation from the incision. In a further experiment Liggett (1928) described his bulbectomized rats as making many stereotyped errors as compared with his normal control group and as being more active although not in a normal exploratory way, but tending more toward rapid compulsive running. He mentioned that "Possibly the olfactory lobes have functions other than that of receiving olfactory stimuli" (p. 52). Soon after, Lindley (1930) confirmed the tendency of bulbectomized rats to make stereotyped errors but made no mention of other striking behavioral differences such as irritability. On this point he concluded, "Although the olfactory lobes may have other functions than that which the name indicates, up to the present time no evidence supporting such a possibility has been brought forth" (p. 263). There the matter rested for over 20 years. Two different behavioral alterations had been observed consequent to removal of the olfactory bulbs. Both of these changes were to be confirmed in later experiments but, meanwhile, their investigation had to wait while the relationship of the olfactory system to the other components of the rhinencephalon–limbic system was examined and reexamined.

3.   Effects of Lesions in the Direct Olfactory System

Recent interest in the behavioral significance of the olfactory system has developed along two lines. One is concerned with the role played by odors in the control of such basic biological activities as reproduction and food intake (Whitten and Bronson, 1970). Although these studies are not the focus of this discussion, they must be credited with publicizing the olfactory system and stimulating new anatomical and physiological work. The other line of research stems directly from Herrick. It asks how the olfactory system in general, as distinct from specific odorous stimuli, influences such behavioral processes as attention and arousal, learning and memory, and emotion and motivation. All of the work described involves bilateral lesions in the direct olfactory system and consequently is subject to all of the perils of the ablation method. Investigators grope for appropriate behavioral terms with which to describe their experimental subjects, just like those doing behavioral research on the limbic system, making it difficult to compare results.

In this research, how to distinguish between the olfactory and nonolfactory functions of the system is a fundamental question. Some of the experiments have been conducted in the context of understanding how odor cues contribute to certain patterns of behavior. The word "anosmia" is likely to be used in the titles of research reports and the experimental animals are described as anosmic. Such usage implies a direct olfactory function. However, the emphasis here is on nonolfactory function and the concept of anosmia is considered inappropriate because it leads the reader to think in terms of olfactory perception. Experimenters from Liggett and Liggett (1927) to the present time have argued that smells play only a contributory role, if any, in these behavioral changes. This argument is supported by research findings described below in which the behavior under study varies from interanimal encounters to response situations in which odors appear to have no direct relevance, and as a species is used that is considered microsmatic on the basis of its relatively small olfactory system and its style of life, viz., the pigeon.

3.1. Orienting and Habituation

Aside from the incidental comments of Liggett (1928) and Lindley (1930) about stereotyped errors of bulbectomized rats, the first paper to deal specifically with the effect of the olfactory system in behavior was that of Wenzel and Salzman (1968). They observed the effects of olfactory bulbectomy or olfactory nerve section on pigeons' performance of a complex visual discrimination task. This work grew out of demonstrations that the pigeon has a functional olfactory system (Michelsen, 1959; Wenzel, 1967; Sieck and Wenzel, 1969), and the assumption that little use is made of it for direct olfactory purposes. It was hypothesized, therefore, that its preservation might reflect, at least in part, a nonolfactory contribution to such aspects of behavior as were mentioned by Herrick. Performance measures were taken during magazine training, shaping of the key–peck response, and acquisition of visual discrimination, its reversal, and extinction. The discrimination task required the bird to peck on a left or right response key according to the color displayed simultaneously on both keys. On a given trial, both keys were either red or green. If they were red, the correct response for half of each group was to peck on the left key; if they were green, responses on the right key were reinforced. Two control groups were included, one of sham-operated birds and another of birds that had undergone bilateral removal of an amount of tissue from the lateral surface of the forebrain that was considered approximately equivalent to the size of both olfactory bulbs. The two groups with olfactory lesions performed essentially the same, as did the two control groups. The experimental groups differed from the control groups in what might be called aspects of adaptation to the task and not in learning ability or performance. They were slower in reaching the criteria for magazine training and for response shaping, but not for discrimination training. There was no suggestion of increased irritability or difficulty in handling. Indeed, if there was any change in emotionality it seemed to be more in the opposite direction, toward timidity. The experimental birds defecated more often in the experimental box and tended to freeze at the end opposite to the magazine in the early sessions. Not only were the effects difficult to interpret in terms of simple anosmia, but such an interpretation would have led to the surprising conclusion that odorous stimuli are very important to pigeons in such a restricted environment.

The next experiments (Wenzel et al., 1969) were designed to provide further information about the effects of olfactory lesions on adaptive behavior. Four groups like those above were tested in three situations. In one the birds' reactions in response to the sound made by the food hopper each time it was presented in a standard conditioning box were studied. The hopper was empty and no light came on above it. The subjects were observed by means of closed-circuit television. About a month after these evaluations were completed, all the birds were tested in an automatic shaping procedure. Finally, several weeks later, orientation of their heart-rate responses to a 10-s light stimulus was measured. Heart beats were recorded in nine sessions of 30 stimulus presentations each. At the end of the ninth session, two tone stimuli were also presented. The lesioned birds differed from the control group in all three procedures, but there were no important differences between the nerve-sectioned and bulb-ablated groups. They made withdrawal, rather than approach, responses to the sound of the food magazine and emitted fewer responses in the shaping procedure (Fig. 3). Their normal heart-rate acceleration in response to the onset of light not only failed to show habituation with repeated stimuli, but actually increased in the later sessions. All groups responded equally, with even greater

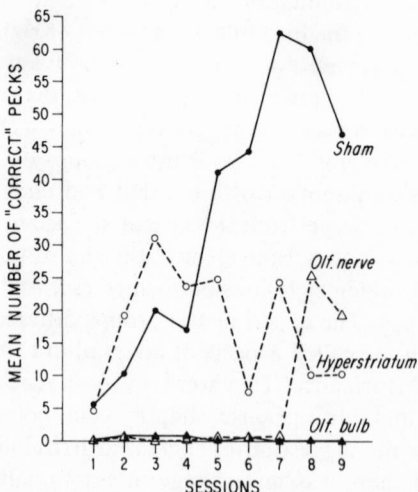

FIG. 3. Group mean numbers of pecks on the lighted key by pigeons during sessions in which hopper presentation did not immediately follow the first peck. (From Wenzel et al., 1969).

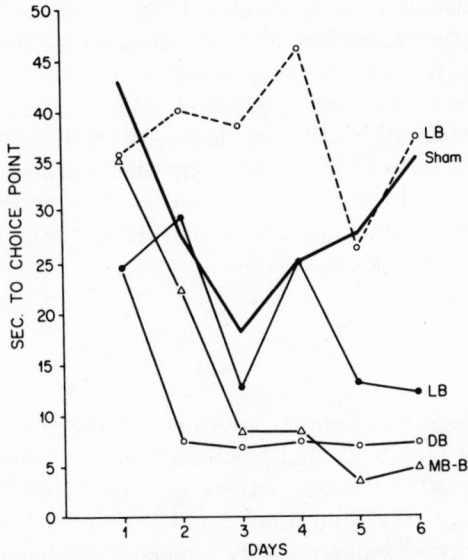

FIG. 4.   Mean running time to Y-maze choice point on successive days. All trials were omitted in which the choice point was not reached within a 3-min limit. The solid LB curve omits the data from one rat that was consistently much slower than all others in that group; the dotted curve includes all LB rats. LB: olfactory nerve section and minimal damage to the tips of the olfactory bulbs, MB-B: bilateral bulbectomy anterior to anterior olfactory nucleus; accessory bulb may be partially or totally intact, DB: total bilateral removal of olfactory bulb and peduncle, SHAM: surgical control group. (From Sieck, 1973).

acceleration in heart rate, to the final tone stimuli, thus showing that there were no differences in responsiveness to a novel stimulus at this time, but only to the repeated stimulus.

A similar effect on the heart-rate response was found by D. S. Phillips and G. K. Martin (1971) using Sprague–Dawley rats and tone stimuli. Their three groups of bulbectomized, sham-operated, and unoperated rats all showed the same initial deceleration response on the first 10 trials. During trials 11 to 20, however, the two control groups showed no change from resting level during stimulus presentations, while the bulbectomized group continued to show deceleration. There were no differences in resting level. In a later experiment (D. S. Phillips and Martin, 1972), these results were confirmed and extended to a nerve-sectioned group that was prepared by raising the olfactory bulbs slightly and severing the fia olfactoria.

Sieck's results (Sieck, 1973; Sieck and Gordon, 1972) with rats partially confirm the above. Although the bulbectomized animals ate food pellets from a magazine as promptly as did the controls and made their first bar-pressing responses sooner, they showed less habituation in running speed in a Y-maze used for exploration (Fig. 4) and greater response to a sudden tone on the second day of testing than on the first. The latter was measured by motor activity in a sensitive detection chamber. Control groups of sham-operated and of frontal-lesioned rats showed an opposite trend. The animals with olfactory lesions were less active than sham-operated controls between stimulus presentations during the second session, a difference that could also be interpreted as showing less habituation on their part. As the novelty of the tone diminished for the control rats, their exploratory behavior became less inhibited.

3.2. Activity

If olfactory-lesioned animals are slow to habituate, does this imply a possible increase in activity and reactivity? On this point the evidence is somewhat equivocal. Increased activity was mentioned by Liggett (1928; Liggett and Liggett, 1927), but Lindley (1930) described his rats as equal to controls. No effects of bulbectomy were reported for female or male rats in running wheels or in either home cages or exploration cages equipped with detection devices (Douglas *et al.*, 1969; Sieck, 1972). Not only were activity levels the same for experimental and control groups but cyclic patterns were also indistinguishable. Lower activity levels and no cyclicity were found, however, for another group of bulbectomized female rats in activity wheels (Marks *et al.*, 1971). Postweanling female mice that had received bilateral, centrally placed bulbar lesions at 5 days of age were less active than controls in a constant-temperature test area (McClelland and Cowley, 1972).

Exploratory activity, admittedly a complex measure reflecting interaction among exploratory tendencies, emotional influences, and level of motor output, has been measured in various ways. Ambulation in the open field is uniformly reported as higher for bulbectomized rats, both hooded and albino, than for control groups subjected to sham operation and septal, amygdalar, and frontal lesions (Richman *et al.*, 1972; Sieck, 1972; Sieck and Baumbach, 1973; Sieck and Gordon, 1972; Sieck *et al.*, 1973; Ueki *et al.*, 1972a). Food deprivation does not alter this relationship (Sieck and Baumbach, 1973). Exploratory activity has also been measured in a T-maze (Klein and Brown, 1969), in a Y-maze (Sieck, 1973), and in a runway with different sound levels (Sieck *et al.*, 1973). Again the data are in agreement that albino and hooded bulbectomized rats explore more than the control animals. The basic purpose of Klein and Brown was to measure the effect of anosmia on spontaneous alternation, but they noted as well that the bulbectomized animals continued to explore the maze as if they had failed to habituate to it. In the Y-maze (Sieck, 1973), the rats with more than minimal damage to the olfactory bulbs ran faster and froze less in the start section than a group of sham operates and one with section of the fila olfactoria including slight damage to the anterior tips of the bulbs (Fig. 4). No activity differences have been noted for pigeons (Wenzel, unpublished observations) but one report on mice (Richardson and Scudder, 1970), in which many natural activity patterns were evaluated in a group environment called the Mouse City, described an increase in activity, primarily in the bulbectomized animals, as a "popcorn" effect. It was observed that activity of one lesioned mouse seemed to stimulate activity in another, and so on through the group like popcorn cracking. In a study of gonadal function, bulbectomized male and female mice were said to be unusually active for several days after the operation (Whitten, 1956). The effect of olfactory lesions on activity in rodents, therefore, is generally facilitatory. The lack of a clear effect in pigeons must be studied more carefully.

3.3. Avoidance Learning

Because of the types of changes in affective and exploratory post-lesion behavior described above, some influence of olfactory lesions on avoidance learning would be expected. Several reports, the first appearing in 1965 (Ueki and Sugano), have confirmed this expectation. The emerging pattern consists of faster escape and avoidance learning after such lesions for both rats and pigeons, and poorer performance in learning passive avoidance responses. In two experiments, Hutton et al. (1974) found that nerve-sectioned pigeons improved in the performance of two-way active avoidance learning. One experiment used a combination of discriminated and nondiscriminated procedures in that movement from one compartment to the other delayed onset of the next trial for 30 s. If there was no movement between compartments for 30 s, a red light went on for 10 s, at which time shock was added to the grid floor. The red light and shock remained on until the bird fluttered through a V-shaped opening to the other compartment. Daily training sessions lasted 30 min. Under these conditions, the lesioned birds made more avoidance responses to the light than the combined sham-operated and unoperated control groups, which did not differ between themselves (Fig. 5). In a second experiment using only the discriminated procedure, similarly lesioned groups also performed at a higher level. There were no differences in extinction in either experiment.

More extensive experiments on rats have produced comparable results. Brown and Remley (1971) studied the effects of destruction of the septal area or the olfactory bulbs on escape from different types of aversive

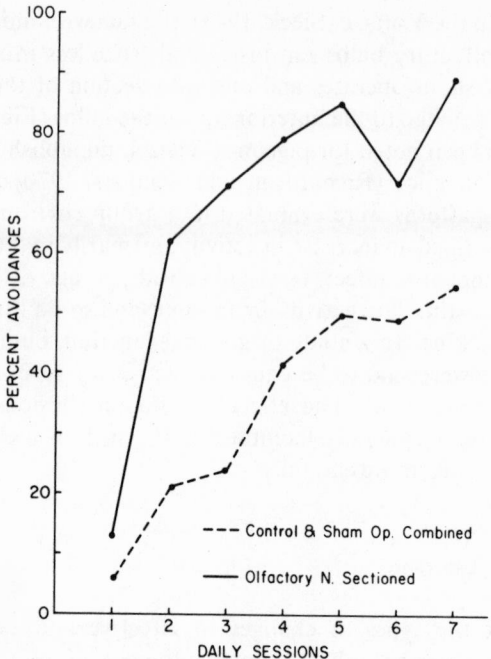

FIG. 5. Percent avoidance responses of pigeons in two-way active avoidance. The olfactory nerves had been sectioned in the birds in the experimental group. (Modified from Hutton *et al.*, 1974).

stimuli in a two-way shuttle box. The rats with septal lesions tended to be faster than control animals in acquisition and slower in extinction regardless of stimuli whereas the bulbectomized rats were faster in two of the four situations, viz., when the aversive stimulus was a heat lamp or when it was a complex consisting of the heat lamp, a buzzer, and foot shock. They tended to reach extinction more rapidly than animals with septal lesions. The authors interpreted their results as indicating hyper-reactivity following a septal lesion but felt that the results after bulbectomy were hard to interpret. In succeeding experiments (Brown *et al.*, 1971; Marks *et al.*, 1971), both active and passive avoidance learning was studied following ablation of the olfactory bulbs. Response latency of the lesioned rats in one-way shock avoidance was greater than that of normals on the early trials, a difference attributed to their inadequate orientation toward the escape door on those trials. There were no differences in extinction. Other groups of bulbectomized rats were slower than normals in reaching the criterion for passive avoidance using an electrified food cup and showed shorter latency in running to quinine when water-deprived.

In the most systematic series of experiments on this topic, Sieck (1972; 1973; Sieck and Gordon, 1972) has found a consistent trend toward better performance in active avoidance and poorer performance in passive avoidance following bulbectomy. Active avoidance in these experiments was always movement between the compartments in the same two-way shuttle-box situation with a buzzer as the conditioned stimulus (CS) and footshock as the unconditioned stimulus (US); passive avoidance was a step-down task. The extent of ablation was deliberately varied in later experiments, and Sieck noted that rats with more extensive lesions were more likely to perform poorly in passive avoidance tasks. In active avoidance, the data are entirely consistent in showing faster learning following any amount of bulbar damage. Additional confirmatory evidence was obtained in a study of food illness aversion (Hankins et al., 1973) in which the rats' olfactory systems were damaged either by bulbectomy or by irrigation of the nasal cavity with zinc sulfate, which destroys the olfactory receptor cells temporarily (Alberts and Galef, 1971; Mulvaney and Heist, 1971; Schultz, 1960). It was found that the bulbectomized subjects were slow in acquiring conditioned suppression; there was no difference between the sham-operated controls and the sulfate-treated group.

Thomas (1973) compared bulbectomized and septally damaged rats in several learning tasks. His data confirm the faster learning of two-way active avoidance after bulbectomy as well as after septal damage, but showed no effect of bulb removal on passive avoidance. His latter task might be called step-across by analogy with Sieck's step-down test. The rats were placed in one compartment of a shuttle box and shocked when they entered the other. Latency in entering the second compartment in a later session was the measure of avoidance. It is hard to see why the same results should not have been obtained in these two experiments. Thomas' septal animals showed a clear deficiency. One-way avoidance was learned more slowly by both bulbectomized and septal rats using the same apparatus, confirming the results of Marks et al. (1971).

Slower acquisition of a classically conditioned response with shock as the unconditioned stimulus has also been found with rats (D. S. Phillips and Martin, 1972). Conditioning of heart-rate deceleration with a tone, the CS, and shock through the recording electrodes, the US, proceeded more slowly in the bulbectomized group than in a nerve-sectioned group, which was slower in turn than an unoperated control group.

The generally opposite effects of olfactory system damage on active and passive avoidance argue against an explanation in terms of altered shock thresholds. Two attempts to measure the threshold in bulbectomized rats have been somewhat inconclusive (Bugbee and Eichelman, 1972; Sieck et al., 1973). The results are probably confounded by other behavioral changes in these animals. The generality of the deficiency in passive avoidance and its independence of electric shock are supported by the observation that bulbectomized rats explore freely around a confined cat, in dramatic contrast to the control rats whose behavior is greatly inhibited (Mollenauer *et al.*, 1974). The possible role of odor cues in this situation has not yet been identified.

3.4   Appetitive Learning

A few scattered observations are also available on other types of learning, most involving food or water reinforcement and, hence, deprived subjects. In reversal training with water reinforcement, bulbectomy had no effect on original learning or any of three reversals (Thomas, 1973). In some disagreement with Wenzel and Salzman's results on visual discrimination learning in pigeons, D. S. Phillips (1970) found that bulbectomized rats showed no improvement in acquiring a learning set of visual pattern discrimination (Fig. 6). The procedure for the experimental group and for

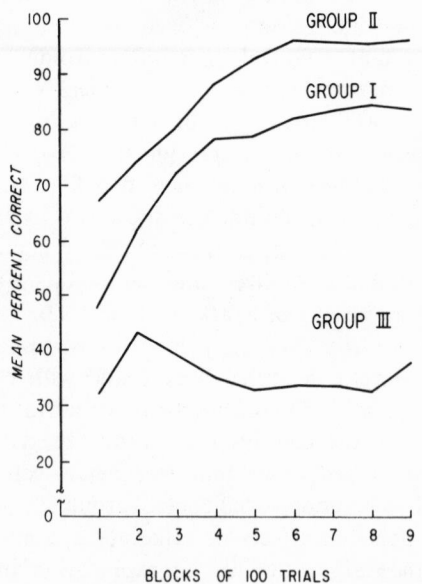

FIG. 6.   Mean percent correct responses of rats on 9 test problems in visual discrimination. Group I: unoperated, conflicting olfactory and visual cues; Group II: unoperated, congruent olfactory and visual cues; Group III: bilaterally bulbectomized, conflicting olfactory and visual cues. (From D. S. Phillips, 1970).

one unoperated control group involved the presentation of conflicting visual and olfactory cues; the two cues were consistent for a second unoperated control group. The correct choice was indicated by the visual cue in all cases. No explanation for their deficient performance could be found in any aspect of the bulbectomized rats' behavior other than a slight decrease in arousal during the first 10 to 14 days of testing. After that, they appeared normal but continued to perform at a low level.

With regard to operant responses, the data from rats disagree with those from pigeons. Both Marks *et al.* (1971) and Sieck (1973) report no difficulty in magazine training or shaping of the experimental animals. They also found a tendency for those animals with olfactory damage to respond at a higher rate than the controls. This was especially noticeable during extinction experiments on rats with the most extensive lesions; in Sieck's study they responded at a high rate and became agitated under these conditions. In contrast, female hamsters emitted fewer bar-pressing responses for nest paper after bulbectomy than before and could not be reshaped for paper reinforcement or for sucrose pellets. Magazine training with sucrose was successful, however. Another group trained to respond for sucrose pellets before bulbectomy eventually ceased responding after the operation although the pellets earned were eaten (Goodman and Firestone, 1973).

3.5 Aggression

The most accepted claim for participation of the olfactory system in general behavior regulation is that the olfactory bulbs exert an inhibitory influence on aggression in rats. The complex concept of aggression has been subdivided by Moyer (1968, 1971) into seven classes of behavior that he proposes to be largely independent of one another and to depend on at least partially distinct neural pathways. The labels he has suggested are predatory, intermale, fear-induced, irritable, territorial, maternal, and instrumental. He has pointed out that any of the neural circuits at any given time can be both inactive and insensitive, sensitized but inactive, or spontaneously active (1971). The experiments discussed below involve several of his categories, viz., intermale, irritable, predatory, and perhaps fear-induced.

3.5.1 Interanimal Aggression

The release of aggression by bulbectomy was first described for its own sake by Karli and Vergnes in 1963 (also Vergnes and Karli, 1963). It had been foreshadowed as early as Watson's report and had undoubtedly been observed without specific mention in other experiments that were directed at primary olfactory behavior. Karli had previously described a standardized pattern of mouse-killing behavior (predatory and/or irritable aggression) in wild Norway rats (1956), and had then gone on to examine this pattern in other rat strains and to identify the controlling brain pathway. After finding that amygdalectomy or amygdalar stimulation abolished the behavior in natural killers, he discovered that extensive lesions of the frontal pole induced killing behavior in rats that were not spontaneous killers. This effect was finally localized in the functioning of the olfactory bulbs. Additional work has identified associated changes in electrical activity of the dorsal hippocampus (Karli *et al.*, 1969).

Inevitably, the story has become increasingly complicated and it is not yet clear how to sort out the contributing factors of species, strain, sex, housing conditions, previous experience, method of testing, and lesion extent. In following up Karli's experiments, Ropartz (1968) found that male mice selected to be the most aggressive attackers of other male mice (intermale aggression) showed no aggression whatsoever after bulbectomy. Ropartz discounted anosmia as the sole explanation because this could not account for a failure of the bulbectomized mice to counterattack when they were paired with an intact highly aggressive mouse. He concluded that "... part of the olfactory system ... removed acts as a 'facilitation' or 'arousal' mechanism, and not only as a releasing one" (p. 99). Here, then, were two experiments on two different species with conflicting results; on the one hand was Karli's report that interspecific aggression of rats on mice was abolished by amygdalectomy and facilitated by bulbectomy, and on the other hand was Ropartz's observation of abolition of intraspecific aggression in mice by bulbectomy. Both agreed, however, that the olfactory bulb was contributing something more than transmission of olfactory information.

Subsequent research in various laboratories has tended toward general confirmation of both of these somewhat divergent results. Shock-induced intermale fighting was sharply reduced in bulbectomized mice compared with controls, and the operated animals never bit their opponents (Fortuna and Gandelman, 1972). Haug (1971) found the same postoperative absence of intermale aggression in Webster Swiss mice that Ropartz reported and showed, in addition, that testosterone failed to restore aggressive tendencies. In a more extensive experiment (Rowe and Edwards, 1971), castrated adult male Webster Swiss mice, selected as preoperative nonfighters, showed no fighting after bilateral bulbectomy followed by daily injections of testosterone except under one test condition. Fighting ensued if two castrated, bulbectomized, testosterone-injected males of comparable weight were paired in the presence of one gram of lab chow two days after a regimen of food deprivation had begun. No fighting was seen if such a male was paired with an adult male castrate with intact olfactory bulbs or with an intact male only 25 to 30 days old. Inasmuch as neither of the latter two partners tended to attack the experimental animal, Ropartz's observations about the failure of bulbectomized mice to counterattack could not be confirmed in this experiment. It has been reported in hamsters, however (Murphy and Schneider, 1970). Rowe and Edwards felt that the lack of aggression in bulbectomized mice is not attributable to an alteration in pituitary–gonadal function but that ". . . bulbectomy results in a general deficit in most forms of social behavior in mice" (p. 891) and that different neural mechanisms are presumably involved in different behavioral patterns. In support of this contention, Edwards *et al.* (1972) reported that male mice made anosmic by zinc sulfate irrigation of the nasal cavity fought less often and with longer latencies than preoperatively but did continue to fight. They proposed, therefore, that odor perception might facilitate such aggression but is not critical. Aggression among male gerbils in crowded home cages increased after bulbectomy but not after surgical deafferentation (Hull *et al.*, 1974). Individually housed male hamsters, on the other hand, showed little interest in a strange male if they had been treated with zinc sulfate or deprived of olfactory input by a combination of unilateral bulbectomy and clipping of the contralateral nostril (Devor and Murphy, 1973). In this experiment, odor cues were essential for normal social responses.

Facilitating effects of bulbectomy on mouse-killing by rats have been reported in several experiments under varying conditions. Bugbee and Eichelman (1972) compared the effects of bulbectomy, enucleation, or loss of vibrissae and found that only bulbectomy was followed by an increase in mouse-killing by male rats. In a study by Malick (1970), 54% of bulbectomized rats killed mice as compared to 38% of rats with lesions in the ventromedial nucleus of the hypothalamus, 12% of those with lesions in the septal area, and 8% of unoperated controls. Malick selected his subjects because they responded aggressively to a pencil and to a glove fixed on the end of a rod that was inserted provocatively into their cages (irritable and/or fear-induced aggression); in contrast, Karli chose subjects for bulbectomy by their failure to exhibit interspecific aggression before operation. Bandler and Chi (1972) compared the effect of bulbectomy on the aggression of male Long–Evans rats toward frogs, albino mice, and albino rats. Ten of twenty-four preoperative nonkillers of mice became killers after bulbectomy, and this change was uncorrelated with their behavior toward another rat. Aggression in the latter instance was greatly reduced in some subjects and dramatically facilitated in others. All of the rats had killed frogs before operation, but this response declined afterward, partly because they became less efficient; this happened also with rats that had been good preoperative mouse-killers. Conversely, preoperative nonkillers that became killers were very efficient in completing their kills with a quick cervical bite. Cain and Paxinos (1974) found not only that 25% of preoperative nonkillers were converted to mouse-killers by bulbectomy, but also that postoperative killing was positively correlated with irritability. In an experiment on odor cues in killing of rat pups by mouse-killing rats, Myer (1964) had noted that the mouse-killing behavior waned after bulbectomy in some animals, possibly because his rats were not allowed to eat the mice they killed. A pattern of gradually increasing aggression toward mice or a stimulus rod has also been reported after bulbectomy (Ueki *et al.,* 1972a). A comparison group of septally lesioned rats showed no mouse-killing behavior.

The purpose of another set of experiments (Spector and Hull, 1972) was to compare the effect of deafferentation of the olfactory bulb with that of bulbectomy. Male Holtzman rats were selected for preoperative failure to kill mice and were then subjected to bulbectomy or to section of the fila olfactoria by a direct approach to the olfactory cavity. None of the latter group killed postoperatively but most of the bulbectomized rats killed after operation. Their method of killing was described as inefficient, with bite marks all over the bodies. The authors concluded that ". . . removal of the bulbs also releases aggression from an inhibitory control" (Spector and Hull, 1972, p. 356) that is unaffected by removing only the peripheral bulbar afferents. A comparable difference was seen when zinc sulfate treatment was compared with bulbectomy. In the latter case, 53% of the female rats killed after operation as compared with 10% of the peripherally damaged animals (Alberts and Friedman, 1972).

H. Bernstein and Moyer (1970) found no postoperative increase in mouse-killing in male hooded rats unless the rats were housed in isolation, as they were in all of the experiments above. The bulbectomized rats, however, did bite a glove thrust into the cage more often than before operation and this score was positively correlated with mouse-killing behavior. An important procedural difference in this experiment was that a rat was scored as a nonkiller if the mouse was still alive after 30 min whereas other experimenters have typically left the mouse with the rat indefinitely and noted that the initial postoperative kill sometimes took as long as three days while subsequent killing was very much more rapid. It can be concluded that interspecific aggression in rats is generally facilitated by bulbectomy, but the frequency and response topography are still uncertain. Malick was so convinced of the effectiveness of bulbectomy in inducing a stable pattern of aggression that he recommended this model for pharmacological studies of antiaggressive agents. Of some relevance is

Myer's (1971) conclusion that mouse-killing is a natural response of Long–Evans rats, both male and female, although the threshold is higher in females. He believes that it is emitted at different frequencies as a result of differential histories of reinforcement and habituation.

3.5.2 Irritable Aggression

Many experimenters have found that irritable aggression in rats is increased by bulbectomy. All but one of the experimenters who have studied it directly have found striking augmentation, and others have mentioned it as a by-product of experiments that were directed at other topics. The single reported negative instance (Thorne and Linder, 1971) showed no differences in emotionality, measured in situations involving presentation of a pencil, capture, and the like, between bulbectomized and sham-operated albino rats of both sexes.

In all replications with male hooded rats, Sieck (1972; 1973; Sieck and Baumbach, 1973; Sieck and Gordon, 1972; Sieck et al., 1973) noted that his bulbectomized groups were harder to handle than any other group except bulbectomized females or rats with fresh septal lesions. His other groups included males with sham operations, frontal pole ablations, or cochlear destruction. Bugbee and Eichelman (1972) found the same results in comparing bulbectomy with enucleation or removal of vibrissae in males. However, Richman et al. (1972) reported vicious behavior in only 2 of 28 bulbectomized males during research on various aspects of behavior. Douglas et al. (1969) had described increased emotionality in 9 of 14 hooded female rats after bulbectomy but found no effects in males (unpublished data reported in D. S. Phillips, 1970). Of the 9 affected females, 6 were characterized as mainly fearful and 3 as aggressive and vicious. About two-thirds of Alberts and Friedman's (1972) bulbectomized females were rated as more emotional after operation than before, with the greatest difference occurring in reactivity to handling. Only 20% of the animals treated with zinc sulfate or saline solutions had higher postoperative scores. In two experiments on learning (Marks et al., 1971; Seago et al., 1968) using female albino rats, biting, viciousness, and hyperactivity were common after bulbectomy but were rarely seen in control animals. A similar effect was observed after unilateral bulbectomy in female albinos if the animals were kept in constant light for the first 26 postoperative days or were kept in isolation with normal lighting (Pohorecky and Chalmers, 1971). Because any effect of a unilateral lesion is extremely unusual, this report should be especially noted. Watson (1907) had noted photic sensitivity in his bilaterally bulbectomized rats; he described their stuffing cotton into the wire on the side of the cage from which the light came.

The effect of bulbectomy on Malick's (1970) subjects was far more durable than the effects of septal or ventromedial hypothalamic lesions. He chose the rats that scored highest in aggressiveness in initial postoperative testing under prolonged observation. Eight weeks after operation, the three surgical groups responded to provoked attack by the glove in the proportions 60%, 20%, and 15%, respectively. This behavior disappeared completely in every group after bilateral amygdaloid lesions. The results of Ueki et al. (1972a, 1972b) agree with these observations. Increased mouse-killing in their bulbectomized male rats persisted for at least 60 days after surgery, which was as long as they tested. A total reactivity score, based on reactions to pinching the tail, handling, lightly touching the back, and presenting a rod, also remained elevated. After septal lesions, however, the score rose briefly and declined by the second postoperative week.

In somewhat related work, Gandelman et al. (1971a,b) observed essentially 100% incidence of cannibalism of pups among female mice, either virgin or multiparous, if bulbectomy was done before parturition or introduction of the pups. If surgery was delayed until after delivery, cannibalism dropped proportionately until it reached 0% on Day 14. In later work Schlein et al. (1972) showed that both hormonal and nonhormonal factors were influential. Virgin mice that were given experience with pups and pregnant mice in which parturition was prevented by Caesarian section both failed to cannibalize after subsequent bulbectomy. Gandelman (1973) has also found that cannibalism of pups by 22-day old male mice increased from 0% to 54% following bulbectomy, the same incidence recorded for intact 75-day-old males. Injections of testosterone in intact juvenile males did not increase cannibalism at 22 days. No comments were made about ease of handling in these experiments, but others (Thompson and Edwards, 1972) found no differences between bilaterally bulbectomized and sham-operated or unilaterally bulbectomized female mice. Fleming and Rosenblatt (1974a,b) concluded that altered limbic functioning, rather than olfaction itself, was the essential factor in cannibalism by female rats. This conclusion was based on the fact that cannibalism did not occur after zinc sulfate treatment of the nasal cavity as compared with a high incidence after bulbectomy. This treatment, as compared with bulbectomy, merely reduced cannibalism in mice, however (Vandenbergh, 1973).

Ueki and Sugano reported very briefly in 1965 that bulbectomized rats were markedly aggressive toward any object in their vicinity, that this behavior persisted long after operation, and that such animals would be very useful in screening tranquilizers. This suggestion was soon followed in work (Kumadaki et al., 1967) that showed that both hyperemotionality to tactile stimulation and rapid mouse-killing were notably relieved by chlordiazepoxide, which did not simultaneously depress activity as the other emotionally effective drugs did (reserpine, chlorpromazine, chlorprothixene, benzperidol, phenobarbital, and meprobamate). Antidepressant drugs (imipramine, desmethylimipramine, and amitriptyline) reduced activity but had no effect on the emotional responses. Later work by Ueki *et al.* (1972b), however, found that imipramine also reduced emotional hyperreactivity in bulbectomized rats, with the effect especially evident in mouse-killing. This selectivity was not shown by the neuroleptics and tranquilizers they tested.

Reports of increased irritability after bulbectomy in rats are so frequent that one wonders at the absence of comments about such tendencies in other experiments that presumably involved the same lesion. Do these represent negative instances or were the experimental conditions set up so that irritability would not be observed even though a tendency might be present? It is hoped that all experimenters will be alert to this question in the future. It is equally true that individual differences loom large in the positive accounts. Cain's (1974a) data showing that damage to the anterior olfactory nucleus is critical for the development of extreme irritability helps to explain at least some of the variability.

No one has proposed that the olfactory system is critically involved in the entire array of aggression. On the other hand, there is no evidence as yet to show that it does not contribute in some way to all types, at least in rats. Many of the limbic and hypothalamic structures supposedly composing the circuits that have been proposed for the various types of aggression receive bulbar projection fibers or tertiary olfactory fibers. It would seem reasonable, therefore, for the olfactory system to influence all of them, possibly to varying extents.

It is important to know whether we can generalize about other animals on the basis of data concerning rats and mice. No evidence of irritable aggression has been seen in pigeons after bulbectomy (Hutton and Wenzel, 1974; Papi *et al.*, 1972; Wenzel and Salzman, 1968; Wenzel *et al.*, 1969), and there are no reports of such work with monkeys. Human clinical literature is similarly uninformative on this point. Limited evidence on the hamster agrees regarding an effect but disagrees about its direction. One report (Murphy and Schneider, 1970) describes bulbectomized males as "apathetic and unemotional" toward females and without territorial or other social behavior in general. They proposed that "The loss of mating behavior must therefore be viewed as one aspect of a more general syndrome" (p. 303). Sexual behavior was not restored by testosterone. Similar effects were noted in later work (Devor and Murphy, 1973) with male hamsters that were unilaterally bulbectomized and had the contralateral nostril clipped shut, or had been treated with zinc sulfate. Mating behavior was restored if the nostril clip was transferred to the side ipsilateral to bulbectomy, as well as after recovery from the zinc sulfate treatment. It was concluded, therefore, that odor perception was essential. Female hamsters became more difficult to handle after bilateral bulbectomy (Carter, 1973), but this effect wore off by the third postoperative week (Goodman and Firestone, 1973). Pronounced changes in social behavior were noted in female hamsters (Leonard, 1972) after unilateral or bilateral bulbectomy at 10 days of age. These animals appeared relatively normal until after mating, whereupon scent marking and defensive and aggressive behavior disappeared in contrast to controls who displayed such patterns during lactation. On the basis of the similarity between the unilaterally and bilaterally bulbectomized animals, anosmia was rejected as an explanation, in favor of a nonspecific contribution. This rare instance of a large unilateral effect may have occurred because of the age at operation. Extreme hyperactivity of both males and females has been noted (Doty *et al.*, 1971), and the authors speculated as to whether the concomitant loss of sexual responses might have resulted from general disorientation or changes in emotionality or activity.

3.6   Effects on Physiological Functions

Another set of observations should be mentioned as further evidence for the widespread nonspecific involvement of the olfactory system. Riss *et al.* (1969) have stressed especially the relationship between olfactory function and that of the preoptic zone of the hypothalamus. The examples given here were selected because the effects appear not to depend specifically on odors.

3.6.1   Endocrine Activity

It has been known for some time (Whitten, 1956) that removal of the olfactory bulbs from virgin female mice at 6–7 weeks of age leads to smaller ovaries at maturity than those of control mice. Corpora lutea are absent or atrophic and the vagina is typically closed. When such mice were paired with normal males for 12 days, no copulation plugs were found. The possible strain dependence of this effect is suggested by Vandenbergh's (1973) report that 50% of his bulbectomized female mice conceived. No structural changes occurred in the testes of bulbectomized virgin males but after five nights of pairing with normal females only one plug was found whereas the usual result is virtually 100%. Lack of preoperative sexual experience might have contributed to these results but obviously could not have been the main factor. Thompson and Edwards (1972) have shown that bilateral bulbectomy reduces sexual receptivity in both virgin and experienced female mice. Some effect of previous sexual experience was indicated by the lowered receptivity in virgins after removal of only one olfactory bulb. Their experiment also controlled for effects of bulbectomy on pituitary–gonadal function by using spayed mice and hormonal replacement. Peripheral anosmia impairs receptivity less than bulbectomy (Edwards and Burge, 1973). Another experiment showed the effect of the rate of bulbectomy on the sexual behavior of experienced male mice (Rowe and Smith, 1973). If both bulbs were ablated in the same operation, sexual behavior was severely affected; successive unilateral bulbectomies separated by 30 days had no effect, however. Anosmia alone, therefore, appeared to be an insufficient explanation, as has also been shown with peripheral anosmia produced by zinc sulfate (Edwards and Burge, 1973). In hamsters and rats, male sexual behavior is variably affected by peripheral treatment with zinc sulfate or procaine hydrochloride. Powers and Winans (1973) found no changes but others report different degrees of loss, typically of very brief duration (Cain and Paxinos, 1974; Devor and Murphy, 1973; Doty and Anisko, 1973; Larsson, 1971; Lisk et al., 1972). There is complete agreement that bulbectomy permanently prevents sexual responses in males (Bermant and Taylor, 1969; Boty et al., 1971; Larsson, 1969; Murphy and Schneider, 1970).

Research on immature and mature female rabbits (Franck, 1966a,b) has shown that bulbectomy is followed by extensive changes in both the genital tract and sexual behavior. If the rabbits are six weeks old at operation, the sexual organs do not develop and at maturity virtually all the females reject males completely. One-third of them actually behaved more like males than females. When the lesion was made on adult females, one year later the ovaries were smaller and the uterine horns appeared both grossly and microscopically like those of a castrate. The behavior three-months postoperatively included occasional acceptance of a male by some females, consistent indifference, and active refusal of males accompanied by "android" behavior. Laparotomies after 15 days of testing showed ruptured follicles in four cases of females that had accepted a male. Of these, two exhibited pseudopregnancy and the other two became pregnant but did not reach term. When these animals were tested a year later, they refused males obstinately. Franck raised the question of indirect significance of the rhinencephalon, as he called it, on gonadal function and sexual behavior.

A similar effect on rats' ovaries has been reported together with alterations in the adenohypophysis and the thyroid gland (Balboni, 1967). In the pituitary, both thyrotrophic and gonadotrophic cells were altered. Thyroid function increased 60 days postoperatively but by 120 days the gland had become hypoactive. Increased thyroid uptake in rats one month after bulbectomy has also been reported (Digiesi, 1967). No later measurements were made on these animals.

Adrenal function can be affected by electrical stimulation of the olfactory mucosa (Orlandi and Serra, 1970) or bulb, as well as by ablation of the bulbs (Loyber *et al.,* 1972). Human plasma cortisol levels increased to a peak about 20 min after stimulation of the mucosa for 10 min. Levels reached corresponded to those seen in association with psychological stress. From their work with rats, Loyber *et al.* concluded that bulbar stimulation or removal affects adrenal function indirectly through ACTH as well as directly through the spinal cord. Levels of serum albumin and alpha globulin are altered under these conditions, as are concentrations of adrenal ascorbic acid and plasma corticosterone. After bulbectomy, adrenocortical changes occur and there is also an increase in medullary connective tissue.

An effect of bilateral bulbectomy on insulin function in rats has also been seen (Perassi *et al.,* 1972); blood sugar levels were restored more slowly after hypoglycemia in bulbectomized animals than in normal controls or those with lesions in the cerebral cortex.

3.6.2 Water Intake

Interest in patterns of water intake following bulbectomy was generated by a report of the presence of osmoreceptors in the olfactory bulb of the dog (Sundsten and Sawyer, 1959). Increased water intake and urinary output in rats after bulbectomy were attributed in one case (Novakova and Dlouha, 1960) to reduced antidiuretic activity and in another (Digiesi, 1967) to simple anosmia. Both interpretations may well be possible. Supporting evidence was presented for each and the total effect could reflect their combined influence. At best the limited literature available at present suggests an insensitivity to sodium overload in bulbectomized rats (Chiaraviglio, 1969; Vance, 1967a,c), but this effect is far from well established (Vance, 1967b; Wilcove and Vance, 1972). There is no mention in any of these papers of other behavioral characteristics of bulbectomized animals.

3.6.3 Temperature Regulation

Three isolated reports raise the question of altered temperature regulation after bulbectomy. Brown and Remley's (1971) bulbectomized rats escaped from radiant heat faster than rats with septal lesions and sham-operated and unoperated control animals. No such difference occurred when a buzzer was also sounded at each end of the two-compartment test box, but it reappeared when footshock was added to the stimulus complex. It has also been reported (Edwards and Roberts, 1972) that bulbectomized female mice do not huddle in sleep nor when placed in the refrigerator. These two findings are consistent with the interpretation of a lowered set point, but Edwards and Roberts also found that the bulbectomized mice made appropriate behavioral responses when no interaction with other mice was involved. They concluded that the deficit was in general social behavior rather than in thermoregulation. On the other hand, bulbectomized female mice do very little nest building (Vandenbergh, 1973; Zarrow *et al.*, 1971), even when kept at 7° C for two days. Obviously, much more information is needed.

3.6.4 Early Development

There is evidence that bulbectomy soon after birth affects the development of rat pups; such animals gain weight more slowly than littermates with occipital control operations, and their eyes opened 2 days earlier. Both of these differences could have been the result of anosmia, in the first instance interfering with nursing and in the second inducing a compensatory mechanism (Schönfelder and Schwartze, 1971).

4. Interpretation

A reasoned reading of the literature on olfactory lesions leads to the conclusion that the olfactory system is an active participant in a variety of functions already identified with limbic and hypothalamic structures, and that it is doing something more than processing signals of odorous stimuli. Reduced input from the olfactory system affects many aspects of brain function. How the system exerts its normal effects is an exciting question on which little evidence now exists. The anatomical, physiological, and neurochemical data reviewed in Section 2 show a variety of possibilities and point to important directions for future research.

4.1 Anosmia

Loss of odor sensation probably contributes something to the postoperative effects on some behavior patterns, at least in macrosmatic species, but there are several arguments against an interpretation dependent on anosmia alone.

1. One of the most compelling is the difficulty in explaining how anosmia could account for the many behavioral changes observed. The loss of olfactory sensation seems largely irrelevant to the behavior of a mouse that will not defend itself when attacked or a pigeon that is slow to initiate key pecking.

2. Some experiments have included control groups with peripheral lesions in other sensory systems and have found no effects comparable to
those seen in olfactory-lesioned groups. These controls included blinding by
enucleation (Bugbee and Eichelman, 1972; Klein and Brown, 1969; Lindley,
1930; Richardson and Scudder, 1970; Watson, 1907) and glossopharyngealectomy (Scudder and Richardson, 1969).

3. Attempts have been made to induce peripheral anosmia with no
more than minimal direct damage to the anterior tips of the olfactory bulbs
in an effort to evaluate the relative contributions of sensory loss alone and
loss of brain tissue as well. Three methods have been used with rats, viz.,
severing the fila olfactoria by passing a cutting instrument around the tips
of the bulbs, destroying of the olfactory cavity by a direct surgical approach,
and irrigating the entire nasal cavity with zinc sulfate or anesthetic agents.
The latter method has also been applied to mice and hamsters. Its pitfalls are
many and it does not appear to be the method of choice (Sieck and Baumbach, 1974), especially in the case of zinc sulfate. In the pigeon, the olfactory
nerve fibers are collected into two discrete bundles and complete nerve
section has been done by means of a direct approach to the area between the
olfactory cavity and the anterior limit of the brain. In all the experiments on
rats, the results strongly suggest that minimal olfactory damage is followed
by less dramatic changes in behavior than larger lesions that destroy secondary neurons directly. No such differences have been seen with pigeons. It
must be kept in mind that transneuronal cell degeneration in the olfactory
bulb is well documented (Estable-Puig and de Estable, 1969; Pinching and
Powell, 1971), although the effect appears to be greatly delayed in the rat as
compared with the rabbit. Some bulbar damage is possible, therefore, even
without direct intervention. The alternative way of removing sensory input
by eliminating all environmental sources is virtually hopeless because of the
constant odors arising from the animal itself. Even though a reasonable level
of adaptation to these odors might be assumed, they inevitably vary in
intensity and frequency so that adaptation would be far from constant. A
good possibility for the pigeon or any species that has a distinct olfactory
nerve bundle might be the use of a thermal neural lesion, which would be reversible and could be maintained for long or short periods. The opposite
strategy, filling the environment with a single strong odor to minimize or
obliterate all other distinctive odors, has never been reported. Ropartz
(1968) compared the effect of bulbectomy on mice's aggression with that of
thoroughly perfuming one partner in each encounter. In the latter case,
fights occurred in 82% of the encounters as compared with 0% in bulbectomized mice. The frequency between normal mice was 98%. Fortuna and

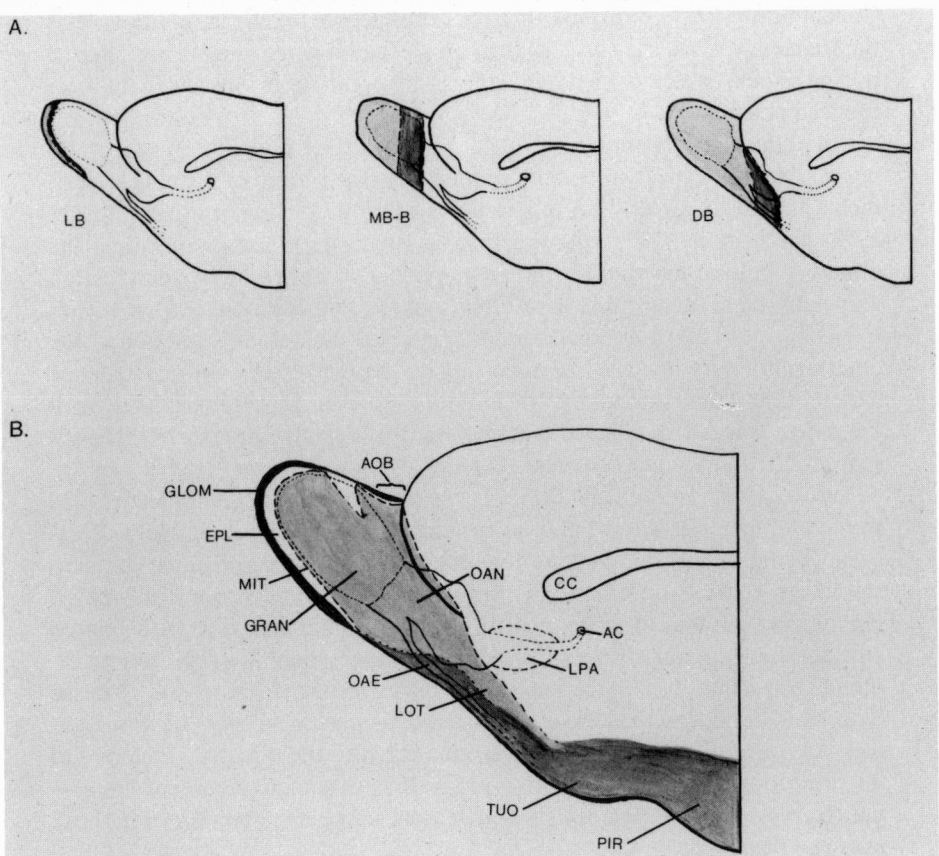

FIG. 7. (A) Scale drawings of rat brain in mid-sagittal plane showing lesion extent of the three surgical groups. Lightly shaded areas indicate the least and darkly shaded areas the greatest lesion extent. Locations of some major olfactory structures are indicated. (B) A transparent view of the anterior forebrain of the rat in mid-sagittal section. Outlines of major olfactory nuclei and tracts are drawn to scale. The lightly shaded area represents approximate origins and visible course of the lateral olfactory tract (LOT). The darkly shaded area is the approximate location of cortical LOT terminations and some secondary olfactory centers. Included in it are parts of the olfactory tubercle (TUO), prepiriform cortex, periamygdaloid and piriform cortices (PIR). AOB: accessory olfactory bulb, GLOM: glomerular layer, EPL: external plexiform layer, MIT: mitral layer, GRAN: granular layer, OAE: anterior olfactory nucleus pars externa, LOT: lateral olfactory tract, TUO: olfactory tubercle, PIR: piriform cortex, LPA: lateral parolfactory area (nucleus accumbens, part of anterior olfactory nucleus), AC: anterior commissure, CC: corpus callosum, OAN: anterior olfactory nucleus (anterior end fuses with granular layer). (From Sieck, 1973).

Gandelman (1972) confirmed this relationship but found, in addition, that the frequency of fighting rose sharply in perfumed pairs when it was elicited by footshock, which stimulated almost no fighting in unscented bulbectomized pairs.

4. Unilateral lesions have little, if any, effect and the effects of bilateral damage appear to be both graded and distinctive. In the only experiments that bear directly on this issue, Sieck (1973; Sieck and Baumbach, 1973; Sieck et al., 1973) showed that rats with deep lesions including the olfactory bulb and peduncle change more than rats with bulbar destruction alone or with section of the nerve fibers and only slight damage to the bulbar tips (Fig. 7). In another experiment the extent of bilateral destruction of the anterior olfactory nucleus was positively correlated with a passive avoidance deficit while lateral olfactory tract lesions were negatively correlated with the rate of active avoidance acquisition (Sieck and Gordon, 1973). It is regrettable that many of the reports cited above include no detailed account of lesion extent. Statements typically are limited to the fact that the bulbs were completely destroyed and no frontal damage occurred, without specifying the posterior limit of the olfactory damage. Indeed, in some cases no statement whatsoever is made about verification of the lesions. Occasionally, it is pointed out that lesion extents differed somewhat and were uncorrelated with the range in behavioral effects. At this stage, then, it is too early to attempt a systematic comparison of results in terms of lesion size. Precise placements and descriptions of lesions should be supplied by all investigators. In order to understand the relations between the olfactory system and its projection sites, we must also make the distinction between vomeronasal–accessory bulb and olfactory mucosa–main bulb subdivisions in those species so equipped.

From the opposite perspective, the importance of the results described here to experimenters studying the specific effects of anosmia can hardly be overemphasized. The interpretation of results in such experiments must be done cautiously in order to separate the sensory and nonsensory effects. The production of anosmia by bulbectomy alone is contraindicated.

4.2. Limbic Functions

Broadly interpreted, Herrick's suggestion that the olfactory system is significantly involved in a wide range of behaviors has been supported. It appears to participate less in cortical activities, however, than in activities in which the limbic system is now considered to play a leading role—in short, the proposals of Herrick and of Papez converge at this point.

The principal contribution of the work reviewed here is its demonstration of an intimate functional link between the direct olfactory system and limbic and hypothalamic areas. The types of responses affected by olfactory lesions, and the direction of the effects, are very similar to those reported after lesion of other subcortical and diencephalic structures (Cain, 1974b). Such overlapping effects have already been noted for limbic sites, e.g., similar passive avoidance deficits were observed after septal (Thomas, 1972), hippocampal (McCleary, 1966), and amygdaloid (Pellegrino, 1968) lesions. The point has often been made that the central nervous system is not necessarily organized in terms of the behavioral categories exemplified by standard laboratory testing procedures, and that the concept of individual localization apparently leaves much to be desired. Further support for this point has certainly been provided here, but an alternative mode of organization has not been clearly suggested. Future experiments must include carefully selected control tasks in order to clarify the nature of the central regulation over behavior being exerted by limbic structures. Attention must also be paid to the animal's natural behavior; reports should include such details as the relation between testing time and circadian influences. For example, all of Sieck's tests were performed under dim red light during the 12-hour dark phase, but few other researchers have followed this procedure. From attention to such details should come valuable clues for the correct analysis.

As might be expected from the lesion data, it has also been shown that self-stimulation through an electrode in the olfactory bulb is sustained at parameters essentially the same as those that are most effective for electrodes in the lateral hypothalamus (Phillips and Mogenson, 1969) and that the rate increases when amyl acetate or peppermint, presumably pleasant odors, permeate the odor space and decreases when quinoline, an unpleasant odor, is present (A. G. Phillips, 1970). The effects of the odors are seen when the stimulus parameters are below their optimal levels and not at maximal rates. Not surprisingly, lever-pressing rates sustained by stimulation through lateral hypothalamic electrodes are reduced following bulbectomy, application of KCl to the bulbs, injection of procaine or norepinephrine into the nostrils, or plugging the nostrils, but not after zinc sulfate irrigation of the nasal cavity (M. I. Phillips, 1972). Herrick's argument that the widely distributed olfactory system contributes to the activation or sensitizing of the entire nervous system should be recalled.

Just as dissociable functions have been identified for different portions of the septum (Fried, 1972), so the various components of the olfactory pathway may well make separable contributions (e.g., Sieck et al., 1974). Information about the localization of a sensory, as compared with a limbic, role might be obtained by carefully tracing the anatomical connections of the axons from the olfactory bulb in different species selected to represent a wide range of olfactory control over behavior. Except for aqueous mammals, who lack olfactory receptors and bulbs, all vertebrates appear to have central pathways that originate in the olfactory bulbs. The ultimate destinations of these fibers, however, are very poorly understood in forms other than the rat. If this information were available and could be compared with the importance of olfactory information to each species, then the outlines of a dual system might emerge. The structures involved in processing olfactory information should be relatively persistent and prominent in those forms that rely heavily on odor cues, and much less prominent in those that do not. The remaining structures of what is now thought of as an olfactory (sensory) pathway, if relatively persistent and prominent in both microsomatic and macrosmatic forms, should represent the limbic portion. The importance of this portion in influencing general behavior could help to account for the preservation of an olfactory system in animals that are not strongly influenced by odors.

The question of species-specific effects is urgent at this stage of investigation. The reminder that the information now available constitutes, at best, the olfacto-limbic-hypothalamic neurobehavior of the rat must be strongly emphasized. Cannot the possibility be considered that we are dealing with a behavioral complex that has been assembled in various ways to produce different species-specific patterns of behavior under natural conditions and, hence, different postoperative changes? The human penchant for verbal labeling may be contributing to our conceptual difficulty. Involvement with the maintenance of life and the preservation of the species (MacLean, 1959) and, thus, with motivation seems undeniable. It may be that such functions are multiply represented and that this group of structures operates in a more holistic way. Information about a variety of natural behavior patterns, as opposed to more artificial laboratory tasks, is much needed for different species (Sieck *et al.*, 1973). A great deal of thoughtfully conceived experimentation and imaginative theorizing will eventually solve this puzzle of complex behavior patterns, in which the olfactory system appears to play such an important role.

5. Summary

The direct olfactory system, defined as the olfactory mucosae, nerves, bulbs, and secondary fibers originating in the mitral cell layer of the bulbs, has been the subject of recent investigations concerning its possible role in behaviors seemingly unrelated to odor perception. Occasional incidental reports of irritability and hyperreactivity in rats that had undergone bilateral removal of the olfactory bulbs to make them anosmic have appeared since 1907. Herrick proposed in 1933 that the olfactory system, by virtue of its ubiquity, extensive development, and fundamental importance throughout vertebrate ancestry, played an energizing and sensitizing role for the entire nervous system. Research of the last half-decade, primarily with rats, has shown that the olfactory system is indeed involved in functions now assigned to limbic and hypothalamic structures. Bulbectomized animals are slower to habituate, more likely to show hyperactivity or reactivity and irritability, more proficient in acquisition of active avoidance responses but deficient in passive avoidance, and slower to extinguish appetitive responses. In addition, changes have been noted in various types of aggressive behavior. Various endocrine organs, including the gonads, thyroid, and pituitary–adrenal axis, and physiological functions such as water balance, and possibly temperature regulation, may be affected. Direct or single-synaptic connections between the olfactory bulb and many limbic and diencephalic structures, and even as far caudal as the midbrain reticular formation, have been described or functionally implied. Catecholamine concentrations in the forebrain and brainstem are altered after removal of the olfactory bulbs. What is not yet known is how these connections function to mediate the observed effects, how broadly representative of vertebrate species the results obtained really are, and how to characterize the behavioral mix apparently controlled by the olfacto–limbic–hypothalamic circuitry.

6. References

Adey, W. R., 1970, Higher olfactory centres, in: *Taste and Smell in Vertebrates*, (G. E. W. Wolstenholme and J. Knight, eds.), pp. 357–378, Churchill, London.

Adrian, E. D., 1950, The electrical activity of the mammalian olfactory bulb, *EEG Clin. Neurophysiol. 2*:377.

Alberts, J. R., and Friedman, M. I., 1972, Olfactory bulb removal but not anosmia increases emotionality and mouse killing, *Nature 238*:454.

Alberts, J. R., and Galef, B. G., Jr., 1971, Acute anosmia in the rat: A behavioral test of a peripherally-induced olfactory deficit, *Physiol. Behav. 6*:619.

Balboni, G.-C., 1967, Sur les modifications d'adénohypophyse, de la thryoïde et de l'ovaire après ablation des bulbes olfactifs, *Bull. Assoc. Anat.* (Paris) *137*:160.

Bandler, R. J., Jr., and Chi, C. C., 1972, Effects of olfactory bulb removal on aggression: A reevaluation, *Physiol. Behav. 8*:207.

Becker, C. J., and Freeman, W. J., 1968, Prepyriform electrical activity after loss of peripheral or central input, or both, *Physiol. Behav. 3*:597.

Bermant, G., and Taylor, L., 1969, Interactive effects of experience and olfactory bulb lesions in male rat copulation, *Physiol. Behav. 4*:13.

Bernstein, H., and Moyer, K. E., 1970, Aggressive behavior in the rat: effects of isolation and olfactory bulb lesions, *Brain Res. 20*:75.

Bernstein, S., Lamarche, M., and Buser, P., 1969, Suppressive effect of the olfactory bulb on pyramidal and extrapyramidal discharges in the cat, *Arch. Sci. Biol. 53:*73.

Brodal, A., 1947, The hippocampus and the sense of smell, *Brain 70:*179.

Brown, G. E., and Remley, N. R., 1971, The effects of septal and olfactory bulb lesions on stimulus reactivity, *Physiol. Behav. 6:*497.

Brown, G. E., Harrell, E., and Remley, N. R., 1971, Passive avoidance in septal and anosmic rats using quinine as the aversive stimulus, *Physiol. Behav. 6:*543.

Bugbee, N. M., and Eichelman, B. S., Jr., 1972, Sensory alterations and aggressive behavior in the rat, *Physiol. Behav. 8:*981.

Cain, D. P., 1974a, Olfactory bulbectomy: neural structures involved in irritability and aggression in the male rat, *J. Comp. Physiol. Psychol. 86:*213.

Cain, D. P., 1974b, The role of the olfactory bulb in limbic mechanisms, *Psychol. Bull.,* in press.

Cain, D. P., and Bindra, D., 1972, Responses of amygdala single units to odors in the rat, *Exp. Neurol. 35:*98.

Cain, D. P., and Paxinos, G., 1974, Olfactory bulbectomy and mucosal damage: effects on copulation, irritability, and interspecific aggression in male rats, *J. Comp. Physiol. Psychol. 86:*202.

Carter, C. S., 1973, Olfaction and sexual receptivity in the female golden hamster, *Physiol. Behav. 10:*47.

Chiaraviglio, E., 1969, The effect of lesions in the septal area and olfactory bulbs on sodium chloride intake, *Physiol. Behav. 4:*693.

Cowan, W. M., Raisman, G., and Powell, T. P. S., 1965, The connexions of the amygdala, *J. Neurol. Neurosurg. Psychiat. 28:*137.

Devor, M., and Murphy, M. R., 1973, The effect of peripheral olfactory blockade on the social behavior of the male golden hamster, *Behav. Biol. 9:*31.

Digiesi, V., 1967, Olfaction et fonctions métaboliques de la vie végétative, *Acta Neuroveg.* (Wein) *30:*30.

Doty, R. L. and Anisko, J. J., 1973, Procaine hydrochloride olfactory block eliminates mounting in the male golden hamster, *Physiol. Behav. 10:*395.

Doty, R. L., Carter, C. S., and Clemens, L. G., 1971, Olfactory control of sexual behavior in the male and early-androgenized female hamster, *Horm. Behav. 2:*325.

Douglas, R. J., Isaacson, R. L., and Moss, R. L., 1969, Olfactory lesions, emotionality and activity, *Physiol. Behav. 4:*379.

Edwards, D. A., and Burge, K. G., 1973, Olfactory control of the sexual behavior of male and female mice, *Physiol. Behav. 11:*867.

Edwards, D. A., and Roberts, R. L., 1972, Olfactory bulb removal produces a selective deficit in behavioral thermoregulation, *Physiol. Behav. 9:*747.

Edwards, D. A., Thompson, M. L., and Burge, K. G., 1972, Olfactory bulb removal vs. peripherally induced anosmia: Differential effects on the aggressive behavior of male mice, *Behav. Biol. 7:*823.

Estable-Puig, J., and de Estable, R., 1969, Acute ultrastructural changes in the rat olfactory glomeruli after peripheral de-afferentation, *Exp. Neurol. 24:*592.

Ferrer, N. G., 1969, Efferent projections of the anterior olfactory nucleus, *J. Comp. Neurol. 137:*309.

Fleming, A. S., and Rosenblatt, J. S., 1974a, Olfactory regulation of maternal behavior in rats: I. Effects of olfactory bulb removal in experienced and inexperienced lactating and cycling females, *J. Comp. Physiol. Psychol. 86:*221.

Fleming, A. S., and Rosenblatt, J. S., 1974b, Olfactory regulation of maternal behavior in rats: II. Effects of peripherally induced anosmia and lesions of the lateral olfactory tract in pup-induced virgins, *J. Comp. Physiol. Psychol. 86:*233.

Fortuna, M., and Gandelman, R., 1972, Elimination of pain-induced aggression in male mice following olfactory bulb removal, *Physiol. Behav. 9:*397.

Franck, H., 1966a, Effets de l'ablation des bulbes olfactifs sur la physiologie génitale chez la Lapine adulte, *C. R. Soc. Biol. 160:*863.

Franck, H., 1966b, Ablation des bulbes olfactifs chez la Lapine impubère. Répercussions sur le tractus génital et le comportement sexuel, *C. R. Soc. Biol. 160:*389.

Fried, P. A., 1972, Septum and behavior: a review, *Psychol. Bull. 78:*292.

Gandelman, R., 1973, The development of cannibalism in male Rockland–Swiss mice and the influence of olfactory bulb removal, *Devel. Psychobiol. 6:*159.

Gandelman, R., Zarrow, M. X., and Denenberg, V. H., 1971a, Stimulus control of cannibalism and maternal behavior in anosmic mice, *Physiol. Behav. 7:*583.

Gandelman, R., Zarrow, M. X., Denenberg, V. H., and Myers, M., 1971b, Olfactory bulb removal eliminates maternal behavior in the mouse, *Science 171:*210.

Girgis, M., 1969, The amygdala and the sense of smell, *Acta Anat. 72:*502.

Girgis, M., 1970, The rhinencephalon, *Acta Anat. 76:*157.

Goodman, E. D., and Firestone, M. I., 1973, Olfactory bulb lesions: nest reinforcement and handling reactivity in hamsters, *Physiol. Behav. 10:*1.

Graystone, P., Low, B., Rogers, J., and McLennan, H., 1970, The induced wave activity of the olfactory bulbs of toads, iguanas and snakes, *Comp. Biochem. Physiol. 37:*493.

Hankins, W. G., Garcia, J., and Rusiniak, K. W., 1973, Dissociation of odor and taste in baitshyness, *Behav. Biol. 8:*407.

Haug, M., 1971, Comportement agressif des Souris males anosmiques traitées avec un androgène de synthèse, *C. R. Acad. Sci. 272:*3188.

Heimer, L., 1969, The secondary olfactory connections in mammals, reptiles and sharks, *Ann. N.Y. Acad. Sci. 167:*129.

Heimer, L., and Wilson, R. D., 1975, The allocortical projections to the basal ganglia in the rat, in: *The Golgi Centennial Symposium Proceedings* (M. Santini, ed.), in press, Raven Press, New York.

Herrick, C. J., 1933, The functions of the olfactory parts of the cerebral cortex, *Proc. Nat. Acad. Sci. 19:*7.

Hull, E. M., Hamilton, K. L., Engwall, D. B., and Rosselli, L., 1974, Effects of olfactory bulbectomy and peripheral deafferentation on reactions to crowding in gerbils (*Meriones unguiculatus*), *J. Comp. Physiol. Psychol. 86:*247.

Hutton, R. S., Wenzel, B. M., Baker, T., and Homuth, M., 1974, Two-way avoidance learning in pigeons after olfactory nerve section, *Physiol. Behav. 13:*57–62.

Karli, P., 1956, The Norway rat's killing response to the white mouse. An experimental analysis, *Behaviour 10:*81.

Karli, P., and Vergnes, M., 1963, Déclenchement du comportement d'agression interspécifique Rat–Souris par des lésions expérimentales de la bandelette olfactive latérale et du cortex prépyriforme, *C. R. Soc. Biol. 157:*372.

Karli, P., Vergnes, M., and Didiergeorges, F., 1969, Rat–mouse interspecific aggressive behaviour and its manipulation by brain ablation and by brain stimulation, in: *Aggressive Behaviour*, (S. Garattini, and E. B. Sigg, eds.), pp. 47–55, Wiley Interscience Division, New York.

Kerr, D. B., and Dennis, B. J., 1972, Collateral projection of the lateral olfactory tract to entorhinal cortical areas in the cat, *Brain Res. 36:*399.

Klein, D., and Brown, T. S., 1969, Exploratory behavior and spontaneous alternation in blind and anosmic rats, *J. Comp. Physiol. Psychol. 68:*107.

Kölliker, A., 1896, *Handbuch der Gewebelehre des Menschen,* Vol. 2, Engelmann, Leipzig.

Komisaruk, B. R., and Beyer, C., 1972, Responses of diencephalic neurons to olfactory bulb stimulation, odor, and arousal, *Brain Res. 36:*153.

Kumadaki, N., Hitomi, M., and Kumada, S., 1967, Effect of psychotherapeutic drugs on hyperemotionality of rats in which the olfactory bulb was removed, *Japan. J. Pharm.* *17:*659.

Larsson, K., 1969, Failure of gonadal and gonadotrophic hormones to compensate for an impaired sexual function in anosmic male rats, *Physiol. Behav.* *4:*733.

Larsson, K., 1971, Impaired mating performances in male rats after anosmia induced peripherally or centrally, *Brain. Behav. Evol.* *4:*463.

Leonard, C. M., 1972, Effects of neonatal (Day 10) olfactory bulb lesions on social behavior of female golden hamsters (*Mesocricetus auratus*), *J. Comp. Physiol. Psychol.* *80:*208.

Liggett, J. R., 1928, An experimental study of the olfactory sensitivity of the white rat, *Genet. Psychol. Monog.* *3:*1.

Liggett, J. R., and Liggett, M. W., 1927, On the modifications of the learning rate of the white rat following the removal of the olfactory lobes, *J. Genet. Psychol.* *34:*525.

Lindley, S. B., 1930, The maze-learning ability of anosmic and blind anosmic rats, *J. Genet. Psychol.* *37:*245.

Lisk, R. D., Zeiss, J., and Ciaccio, L. A., 1972, The influence of olfaction on sexual behavior in the male golden hamster (Mesocricetus auratus), *J. Exp. Zool.* *181:*69.

Lohman, A. H. M., and Lammers, H. J., 1967, On the structure and fibre connections of the olfactory centres in mammals, in: "Sensory Mechanisms," (Y. Zotterman, ed.), *Prog. Brain Res.* *23:*65.

Loyber, I., Perassi, N. I., Palma, J. A., and Lecuona, F. A., 1972, Effects on serum proteins of stimulation of olfactory bulbs in spinal rats, *Exp. Neurol.* *34:*535.

MacLean, P. D., 1959, The limbic system with respect to two basic life principles, in: *The Central Nervous System and Behavior,* (M. A. B. Brazier, ed.), pp. 31–118, Josiah Macy, Jr. Foundation, N. Y.

Malick, J. B., 1970, A behavioral comparison of three lesion-induced models of aggression in the rat, *Physiol. Behav.* *5:*679.

Marks, H. E., Remley, N. R., Seago, J. D., and Hastings, D. W., 1971, Effects of bilateral lesions of the olfactory bulbs of rats on measures of learning and motivation, *Physiol. Behav.* *7:*1.

McCleary, R. A., 1966, Response-modulating functions of the limbic system: Initiation and suppression, in: *Progress in Physiological Psychology,* (E. Stellar and J. M. Sprague, eds.) pp. 209–272, Academic Press, New York.

McClelland, R. J., and Cowley, J. J., 1972, The effects of lesions of the olfactory bulbs on the growth and behavior of mice, *Physiol. Behav.* *9:*319.

Mechelse, K., and Lieuwens, W. H. G., 1969, Vigilance and rhinencephalic burst activity, *Psychiat. Neurol. Neurochir.* *72:*97.

Michelsen, W. J., 1959, Procedure for studying olfactory discrimination in pigeons, *Science* *130:*630.

Millhouse, O. E., 1969, A Golgi study of the descending medial forebrain bundle, *Brain Res.* *15:*341.

Mollenauer, S., Plotnik, R., and Snyder, E., 1974, Effects of olfactory bulb removal on fear responses and passive avoidance in the rat, *Physiol. Behav.* *12:*141.

Motokizawa, F., and Furuya, N., 1973, Neural pathway associated with the EEG arousal response by olfactory stimulation, *EEG Clin Neurophysiol.* *35:*83.

Moyer, K. E., 1968, Kinds of aggression and their physiological basis, *Comm. Behav. Biol.* *2:*65.

Moyer, K. E., 1971, A preliminary physiological model of aggressive behavior, in: *The Physiology of Aggression and Defeat,* (B. E. Eleftheriou and J. P. Scott, eds.), pp. 223–263, Plenum, New York.

Mulvaney, B. D., and Heist, H. E., 1971, Regeneration of rabbit olfactory epithilium, *Amer. J. Anat. 131:*241–251.

Murphy, M. R., and Pohorecky, L. A., 1973, Effects of olfactory bulb removal on brain norepinephrine in golden hamsters, *Pharmacol. Biochem. Behav. 1:*231.

Murphy, M. R., and Schneider, G. E., 1970, Olfactory bulb removal eliminates mating behavior in the male golden hamster, *Science 167:*302.

Myer, J. S., 1964, Stimulus control of mouse-killing in rats, *J. Comp. Physiol. Psychol. 58:*112.

Myer, J. S., 1971, Experience and the stability of mouse killing by rats, *J. Comp. Physiol. Psychol. 75:*264.

Nieuwenhuys, R., 1967, Comparative anatomy of olfactory centres and tracts, in "Sensory Mechanisms," (Y. Zotterman, ed.), *Prog. Brain Res. 23:*1.

Novakova, V., and Dlouha, H., 1960, Effect of severing the olfactory bulbs on the intake and excretion of water in the rat, *Nature 186:*638.

Orlandi, F., and Serra, D., 1970, La risposta diencefalica alla electtrostimolazione del nervo olfattivo, *Folia Endocr. 23:*114.

Papez, J. W., 1937, A proposed mechanism of emotion, *Arch. Neurol. Psychiat. 38:*725.

Papi, F., Fiore, L., Fiaschi, V., and Benvenuti, S., 1972, Olfaction and homing in pigeons, *Monitore Zool. Ital. 6:*85.

Pellegrino, L., 1968, Amygdaloid lesions and behavioral inhibition in the rat, *J. Comp. Physiol. Psychol. 65:*483.

Perassi, N. I., Loyber, I., and Palma, J. A., 1972, Insulin sensitivity and glucose tolerance in rats without olfactory bulbs, *Neuroendocrinol. 9:*83.

Pfaff, D. W., and Pfaffmann, C., 1969, Olfactory and hormonal influences on the basal forebrain of the male rat, *Brain Res. 15:*137.

Phillips, A. G., 1970, Enhancement and inhibition of olfactory bulb self-stimulation by odors, *Physiol. Behav. 5:*1127.

Phillips, A. G., and Mogenson, G. J., 1969, Self-stimulation of the olfactory bulb, *Physiol. Behav. 4:*195.

Phillips, D. S., 1970, Effects of olfactory bulb ablation on visual discrimination, *Physiol. Behav. 5:*13.

Phillips, D. S., and Martin, G. K., 1971, Effects of olfactory bulb ablation upon heart rate, *Physiol. Behav. 7:*535.

Phillips, D. S., and Martin, G. K., 1972, Heart rate conditioning of anosmic rats, *Physiol. Behav. 8:*33.

Phillips, M. I., 1972, Olfactory bulb removal blocks self-stimulation. Paper delivered at annual meeting of American Psychological Association, Honolulu.

Pinching, A. J., and Powell, T. P. S., 1971, Ultrastructural features of transneuronal cell degeneration in the olfactory system, *J. Cell. Sci. 8:*253.

Pohorecky, L. A., and Chalmers, J. P., 1971, Effects of olfactory bulb lesions on brain monoamines, *Life Sci.* Pt. 1 *10:*985.

Pohorecky, L. A., Larin, F., and Wurtman, R. J., 1969, Mechanism of changes in brain norepinephrine levels following olfactory bulb lesions, *Life Sci. 8:*1309.

Powers, J. B., and Winans, S. S., 1973, Sexual behavior in peripherally anosmic male hamsters, *Physiol. Behav. 10:*361.

Pribram, K. H., and Kruger, L., 1954, Functions of the "olfactory brain," *Ann. N.Y. Acad. Sci. 58:*109.

Price, J. L., and Powell, T. P. S., 1970, An experimental study of the site of origin and the course of the centrifugal fibres to the olfactory bulb in the rat, *J. Anat. 107:*215.

Price, J. L., and Powell, T. P. S., 1971, Certain observations on the olfactory pathway, *J. Anat. 110:*105.

Raisman, G., 1972, An experimental study of the projection of the amygdala to the accessory olfactory bulb and its relationship to the concept of a dual olfactory system, *Exp. Brain Res. 14:*395.

Riblet, L. A., and Tuttle, W. W., 1970, Investigation of the amygdaloid and olfactory electrographic response in the cat after toxic dosage of lidocaine, *EEG Clin. Neurophysiol. 28:*601.

Richardson, D., and Scudder, C. L., 1970, Effect of olfactory bulbectomy and enucleation on behavior of the mouse, *Psychonom. Sci. 19:*277.

Richman, C. L., Gulkin, R., and Knoblock, K., 1972, Effects of bulbectomization, strain, and gentling on emotionality and exploratory behavior in rats, *Physiol. Behav. 8:*447.

Rieke, G. K., 1971, The corticomedial amygdalo-bulbar centrifugal systems in olfaction in the rat. Unpublished doctoral dissertation, Louisiana State University Medical Center, New Orleans.

Riss, W., Halpern, M., and Scalia, F., 1969, Anatomical aspects of the evolution of the limbic and olfactory systems and their potential significance for behavior, *Ann. N.Y. Acad. Sci. 159:*1096.

Ropartz, P., 1968, The relation between olfactory stimulation and aggressive behavior in mice, *Anim. Behav. 16:*97.

Rowe, F. A., and Edwards, D. A., 1971, Olfactory bulb removal: Influences on the aggressive behaviors of male mice, *Physiol. Behav. 7:*889.

Rowe, F. A., and Smith, W. E., 1973, Simultaneous and successive olfactory bulb removal: influences on the mating behavior of male mice, *Physiol. Behav. 10:*443.

Scalia, F., 1968, A review of recent experimental studies on the distribution of olfactory tracts in mammals, *Brain Behav. Evol. 1:*101.

Schlein, P. A., Zarrow, M. X., Cohen, H. A., Denenberg, V. H., and Johnson, N. P., 1972, The differential effect of anosmia on maternal behaviour in the virgin and primiparous rat, *J. Reprod. Fert. 30:*139.

Schönfelder, J., and Schwartze, P., 1971, Beiträge zur steuerung der Bursttätigkeit des Bulbus olfactorius, *Acta Biol. Med. Germ. 27:*103.

Schultz, E. W., 1960, Repair of the olfactory mucosa with special reference to regeneration of olfactory cells (sensory neurons), *Amer. J. Pathol. 37:*1.

Scott, J. W., and Leonard, C. M., 1971, The olfactory connections of the lateral hypothalamus in the rat, mouse and hamster, *J. Comp. Neurol. 141:*331.

Scott, J. W., and Pfaffmann, C., 1967, Olfactory input to the hypothalamus: electrophysiological evidence, *Science 158:*1592.

Scudder, C. L., and Richardson, D., 1969, On the behavioral effects of bilateral glossopharyngealectomy in mice, *Psychonom. Sci. 16:*141.

Seago, J. D., Ludvigson, H. W., and Remley, N. R., 1968, Effects of anosmia on apparent double alternation in the rat, *J. Comp. Physiol. Psychol. 71:*435.

Sherrington, C. S., 1906, *The Integrative Action of the Nervous System,* Yale University Press, New Haven.

Sieck, M. H., 1972, The role of the olfactory system in avoidance learning and activity, *Physiol. Behav. 8:*705.

Sieck, M. H., 1973, Selective olfactory system lesions in rats and changes in appetitive and aversive behavior, *Physiol. Behav. 10:*731.

Sieck, M. H., and Baumbach, H. D., 1973, The effects of olfactory system lesions and food deprivation on spontaneous behavior patterns of male hooded rats, *Physiol. Behav. 11:*381.

Sieck, M. H., and Baumbach, H. D., 1974, Differential effects of peripheral and central anosmia producing techniques on spontaneous behavior patterns, *Physiol. Behav.* in press.

Sieck, M. H., and Gordon, B., 1972, Selective olfactory bulb lesions: reactivity changes and avoidance learning in rats, *Physiol. Behav. 9:*545.

Sieck, M. H., and Gordon, B., 1973, Anterior olfactory nucleus or lateral olfactory tract destruction in rats and changes in aversive and appetitive behavior, *Physiol. Behav. 10:*1051.

Sieck, M. H., and Wenzel, B. M., 1969, Electrical activity of the olfactory bulb of the pigeon, *EEG Clin. Neurophysiol. 26:*62.

Sieck, M. H., Turner, J. F., Gordon, B. L., and Struble, R. G., 1973, Some quantitative measures of activity and reactivity in rats after selective olfactory lesions, *Physiol. Behav. 11:*71.

Sieck, M. H., Baumbach, H. D., Gordon, B. L., and Turner, J. F., 1974, Changes in spontaneous, odor modulated and shock induced behavior patterns following discrete olfactory system lesions, *Physiol. Behav.* in press.

Sollertinskaia, T. N., 1972, Electrophysiological data on the projections of the olfactory system in the hypothalamus of turtles, *Fiziol. ZH SSSR 58:*17.

Spector, S. A., and Hull, E. M., 1972, Anosmia and mouse-killing by rats: a nonolfactory role for the olfactory bulbs, *J. Comp. Physiol. Psychol. 80:*354.

Sundsten, J. W., and Sawyer, C. H., 1959, Electroencephalographic evidence of osmosensitive elements in olfactory bulb of dog brain, *Proc. Soc. Exp. Biol. Med. 101:*524.

Thomas, J. B., 1972, Non-appetitive passive avoidance in rats with septal lesions, *Physiol. Behav. 8:*1087.

Thomas, J. B., 1973, Some behavioral effects of olfactory bulb damage in the rat, *J. Comp. Physiol. Psychol. 83:*140.

Thompson, M. L., and Edwards, D. A., 1972, Olfactory bulb ablation and hormonally induced mating in spayed female mice, *Physiol. Behav. 8:*1141.

Thorne, R. M., and Linder, L. H., 1971, No change in emotionality of rats following bulbectomy, *Psychon. Sci. 24:*207.

Ueki, S., and Sugano, H., 1965, Effect of olfactory bulb lesion on behavior. Abstracts of Papers, 23rd Int. Cong. Physiol. Sci., Tokyo, Japan, Abstract #1095.

Ueki, S., Nurimoto, S., and Ogawa, N., 1972a, Characteristics in emotional behavior of the rat with bilateral olfactory bulb ablations, *Folio Psychiat. Neurol. Jap. 26:*227.

Ueki, S., Nurimoto, S., and Ogawa, N., 1972b, Effects of psychotropic drugs on emotional behavior in rats with limbic lesions, with special reference to olfactory bulb ablations, *Fol. Psychiat. Neurol. Jap. 26:*245.

Valverde, F., 1965, *Studies on the Piriform Lobe,* Harvard University Press, Cambridge, Mass.

Vance, W. B., 1967a, Olfactory bulb resection and water intake in the white rat, *Psychon. Sci. 8:*131.

Vance, W. B., 1967b, Water intake of hyposalemic anosmic rats, *Psychon. Sci. 9:*297.

Vance, W. B., 1967c, Sodium thirst in nephrectomized and nephrectomized-anosmic rats, *Psychon. Sci. 9:*301.

Vandenbergh, J. G., 1973, Effects of central and peripheral anosmia on reproduction of female mice, *Physiol. Behav. 10:*257.

Vergnes, M., and Karli, P., 1963, Déclenchement du comportement d'agression interspécifique Rat–Souris par ablation bilatérale des bulbes olfactifs. Action de l'hydrozine sur cette agressivité provoquée, *C. R. Soc. Biol. 157:*1061.

Watson, J. B., 1907, Kinaesthetic and organic sensations: their role in the reactions of the white rat to the maze, *Psychol. Rev. Monogr. Suppl.* Vol. 8, No. 33, 142 pp.

Wenzel, B. M., 1967, Olfactory perception in birds, in: *Olfaction and Taste II,* (T. Hayashi, ed.), pp. 203–217, Pergamon, New York.

Wenzel, B. M., and Salzman, A., 1968, Olfactory bulb ablation or nerve section and pigeons' behavior in non-olfactory learning, *Exp. Neurol. 22:*472.

Wenzel, B. M., Albritton, P. F., Salzman, A., and Oberjat, T. E., 1969, Behavioral changes in pigeons following olfactory nerve section or bulb ablation, in: *Olfaction and Taste III,* (C. Pfaffmann, ed.), pp. 278–287, Rockefeller University Press, New York.

Whitten, W. K., 1956, The effect of removal of the olfactory bulbs on the gonads of mice, *J. Endocrinol. 14:*160.

Whitten, W. K., and Bronson, F. H., 1970, The role of pheromones in mammalian reproduction, in: *Communication by Chemical Signals,* (J. W. Johnston, Jr., D. G. Moulton, and A. Turk, eds.), pp. 309–326, Appleton-Century-Crofts, New York.

Wilcove, W. G., and Vance, W. B., 1972, The effects of olfactory and frontal pole lesions on the drinking response to hypertonic loading in rats, *Psychon. Sci. 27:*295.

Winans, S. S., and Scalia, F., 1970, Amygdaloid nucleus: new afferent input from the vomeronasal organ, *Science 170:*330.

Zarrow, M. X., Gandelman, R., and Denenberg, V. H., 1971, Lack of nest building and maternal behavior in the mouse following olfactory bulb removal, *Horm. Behav. 2:*227.

CHAPTER 2

Neural Integration of Thermoregulatory Responses*

Evelyn Satinoff

Departments of Psychology and Physiology
University of Illinois
Champaign, Illinois

1. Introduction

Temperature regulation, along with several other fields, is experiencing a quiet revolution in which the hypothalamus is losing its preeminent position as the major center of integrative control. This chapter considers whether the revolution can succeed or, indeed, if it has already. It examines the historical evidence which led to the hypothalamus being regarded as the only thermostat of the brain. It then discusses the current evidence for altering that view — evidence that other parts of the brain have been shown to be both thermosensitive and able to initiate thermoregulatory responses whether or not the hypothalamus is present.

Let us first define what is meant in this context by integration. "The end result of reflex action is always one of some functional meaning for the organism, and reflex actions occurring one after the other are coordinated in sequences of some purposeful character. Such coordination of neural activity into spatial and sequential patterns that serve a useful end is the essence of the integrative action of the nervous system" (Mountcastle, 1956). This idea of patterns that serve a useful end implies not only the activation of all appropriate responses, but also inhibition of inappropriate ones—in other words, a mixture of allied facilitation and antagonistic suppression. The definition might also require that the responses occur promptly in the presence of an appropriate stimulus—in other words, at normal activation thresholds.

* I thank Drs. Joseph Eisenman, R. D. Luce, and Philip Teitelbaum for their many helpful criticisms of the manuscript.

There are really two kinds of integration. Mountcastle was defining one that I will call "response integration." This is the integration of several separate reflexes into a coordinated individual response. For instance, normal panting in a dog involves the mouth opening, the tongue extending and moving back and forth rhythmically, and the respiratory rate increasing and staying at a high level. All of these separate components are integrated to produce smooth panting. The other type I will call "pattern integration." This means that a particular stimulus, such as heat, can elicit all the responses designed to increase heat loss and decrease heat production at the same time. Thus, when it is hot a dog will pant, salivate, vasodilate, decrease thyroid activity, and sprawl on its side, all at the same time. If given an opportunity to escape from the heat, it will do so.

One can seriously question whether complex thermoregulatory response patterns are integrated *at all*. Rather, according to an alternative view, each response in a particular pattern is actually independent of every other response in that pattern, and the reason they are generally seen together is that the activating stimulus is specific to thermoregulation and is sufficiently widespread to excite them all at the same time. The fact, then, that coordinated responses are elicited by heating or cooling the rostral hypothalamus, for instance, would be a result of the accidental confluence of all the individual receptor–effector pathways in that part of the brain. The evidence for this view comes mainly from behavioral experiments and will be considered in that section.

2. Hypothalamus

2.1. Its Importance in Temperature Regulation

Ott (1884) in the United States and Richet (1884) in France first recognized that the hypothalamus plays an essential role in normal thermoregulation. Using the ablation technique Isenschmid and Schnitzler (1914) fully substantiated this localization, and their observations have been repeatedly verified. The localization was further supported by the observation that as successive levels of the brain stem were transected, animals were essentially poikilothermic unless the hypothalamus remained connected to the rest of the brain below, in which case they were able to maintain their body temperatures under wide external temperature ranges [see Bligh (1966) for an excellent review]. Once lesions and transections established where to look, the powerful technique of thermal stimulation was used to analyze the nature of the regulation. Magoun *et al.* (1938) first showed that local radio-frequency heating of discrete hypothalamic areas in anesthetized cats evoked the heat loss responses of increased respiration, panting, and sweating from the toe pads. These reactions were most marked when the heating electrodes were in the anterior hypothalamus and the preoptic area just rostral to it, but they could still be elicited by more caudal stimulation. These results were confirmed in monkeys (Beaton *et al.*, 1941) and interpreted as identifying a reactive region in the anterior hypothalamus containing elements excited by rising temperature which in turn activated heat loss mechanisms.

Andersson *et al.* (1956) demonstrated that electrical stimulation of the preoptic/anterior hypothalamic area (PO/AH) of goats led to vigorous panting, cutaneous vasodilation, and a drop in rectal temperatures. Fusco *et al.* (1961) found the same heat loss responses, plus appropriate changes in oxygen consumption, during hot water perfusion of the PO/AH in dogs, and showed that these responses were modified by the peripheral temperature. When the air was warm, heating the hypothalamus caused vigorous panting and vasodilation, whereas, in cold air, it simply inhibited shivering. Andersson *et al.* (1962a) further showed for goats that preoptic heating blocked the thyroid response to cold, and Morishima and Gale (1972) later demonstrated for baboons that heating this area caused cutaneous vasodilation and a fall in heart rate, blood pressure, and excretion of urinary catecholamines. These studies, taken together, show that local electrical stimulation or heating of the PO/AH causes respiratory, cardiovascular, somatic, and endocrine responses designed to decrease heat production and increase heat loss. Cooling this area in a variety of species leads to the antagonistic responses of shivering, cutaneous vasoconstriction, increased oxygen consumption, elevation of heart rate and blood pressure, thyroid activation, and increases in urinary catecholamines (Andersson *et al.*, 1962b; Hammel *et al.*, 1960; Morishima and Gale, 1972; Sundsten, 1967).

All of these experiments gradually built up the view that the PO/AH was the main thermostat of the brain and contained a high percentage of thermosensitive units, that is, cells which alter their firing rates with changes in their temperature. In 1963 such units were identified by Nakayama *et al.* who recorded single unit activity in this area in anesthetized cats during local heating and cooling. They found that about 20% of the 1000 neurons tested increased their firing rate when local temperature was increased over a range of 32–41°C. These units had Q_{10}'s of 5–15. (This means that the units fired from 5 to 15 times their initial discharge rate as a result of a 10°C increase in temperature. Thermally insensitive neurons have Q_{10}'s of 1–2; that is, for a 10°C change in temperature they, at most, double their firing rate.) Soon after, Hardy *et al.* (1964) reported the existence of cool-sensitive cells in the preoptic area, that is, cells which increase their firing rates with decreases in their temperature (negative Q_{10} units). The posterior hypothalamus also contains thermosensitive cells, but relatively many fewer (Edinger and Eisenman, 1970).

Eisenman and Jackson (1967) distinguished between two classes of temperature-sensitive neurons. One type, highly localized to the preoptic and septal areas, exhibits a smooth, continuous increase in firing rate with increases in brain temperature. These cells, with $Q_{10} > 2$, are relatively insensitive to barbiturates, and the authors classified them as primary thermodetectors. The other type, more widely distributed in the hypothalamus, has discontinuous response curves; their activity does not change until their temperature exceeds some threshold value (Fig. 1). Cool-sensitive cells increase their firing rate when brain temperature falls below a certain point, warm-sensitive cells when the temperature rises above some value. The firing rates of these cells are depressed by barbiturates, suggesting that they are synaptically activated. Eisenman and Jackson proposed that these cells are interneurons concerned with motor outflow.

Both types of hypothalamic neurons, continuous and discontinuous, play a role in summating temperature signals from the rest of the brain and

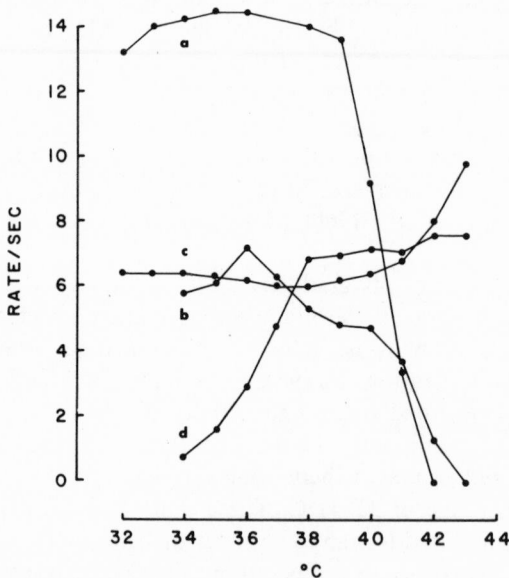

FIG. 1.   Responses of units showing discontinuous slopes. a and b: cool-sensitive units, c and d: warm-sensitive. [From Eisenman and Jackson (1967).]

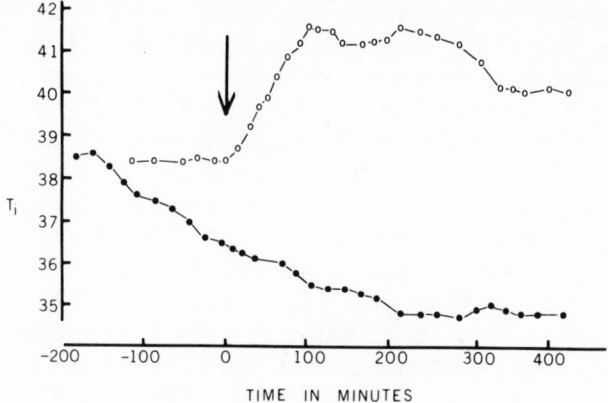

FIG. 2. Colonic temperatures in low mesencephalic cat 111 (O — O) (249th postoperative day) and hypothalamic cat 3 (●— ●) (109th postoperative day) before and after injection of 0.02 ml of typhoid vaccine. Cat 111 was taken off thermal control 160 minutes before the injection and was thereafter at an ambient temperature which varied between 27.0 and 29.5°C. T_i: internal temperature. [From Bard *et al.* (1970).]

body. There are units which have altered firing rates in response to changes in their own temperature only, to changes in skin temperature only (Wit and Wang, 1968), to changes in both (Hellon, 1970), or to thermal changes in the midbrain (Nakayama and Hardy, 1969) or spinal cord (Guieu and Hardy, 1970a). Clearly thermal stability rests on a high degree of complexity in the types and interactions of thermosensitive cells within the hypothalamus.

Because thermosensitive cells responsible for regulating the balance between heat production and heat loss are concentrated in the hypothalamus, and because fever must result from a shift in that balance, Bard *et al.* (1970) inferred that animals without a hypothalamus would not be able to develop a fever in response to pyrogen injection. [Bacterial pyrogens are assumed to cause fever by stimulating the release of a substance from the white blood cells. This substance, leukocytic or endogenous pyrogen, is then presumed to travel via the blood to the hypothalamus where it affects the firing rate of thermosensitive units.] In fact, pontile and mesencephalic cats did not become febrile after injections of typhoid vaccine, a common pyrogenic agent (Bard *et al.*, 1970). Their hypothalamic cat developed a normal fever (Fig 2). After injecting the pyrogen, Bard *et al.* obtained enough endogenous pyrogen from the blood of the decerebrate cats to produce a fever when it was injected into normal animals. They concluded from these experiments that there are no subhypothalamic mechanisms in cats able to mediate pyrogenic fever. [Chambers *et al.* (1949) reported that pontile and medullary cats, but not midbrain animals, showed febrile responses to pyrogen. They concluded that a mechanism capable of evoking a fever existed in the medulla or the spinal cord or both. This point will be discussed further in the section on the medulla. Rosendorff and Mooney (1971) later showed that leucocytic pyrogen injected into the midbrain sometimes produced fever, but with a longer latency and lower peak than if it had been injected into the PO/AH.]

Villablanca and Myers (1965) found that cats became febrile only when the pyrogen was microinjected into the PO/AH. Other hypothalamic and subcortical structures were insensitive and did not lead to any rise in temperature. Cooper *et al.* (1967) verified this specific site of action in rabbits.

The evidence that pyrogens caused fever by acting on cells in the hypothalamus raised the question of how these cells increase an animal's temperature. In 1963, Feldberg and Myers published a neurochemical theory of this mechanism. They proposed that one biogenic amine, serotonin, is selectively released in the PO/AH when thermogenesis is called for and a different amine, norepinephrine, is released when cooling is needed. All variations around the set point (the reference, or equilibrium temperature, normally 37°C) are related to changes in the balance of the two opposing amines (Myers, 1969). This theory has been responsible for a great deal of work on many species in different laboratories. Although the general theory of chemical mediation of temperature regulation has been confirmed many times, it is still not completely clear which particular amines are involved and how they act in different species. [See Lomax (1970) for a fine review of the evidence concerning this issue.]

In summary, when the hypothalamus is left connected to the rest of the brain below, animals can maintain normal body temperatures in thermally extreme environments. In response to hypothalamic heating or cooling, well-coordinated, long-lasting, low-threshold responses appear. The animals are able to develop fevers in response to bacterial pyrogens. In addition to being sensitive to its own temperature, the hypothalamus receives temperature signals from the rest of the brain and body. The result is an output which leads to coordinated, appropriate changes in cardiovascular activity, respiratory evaporative heat loss, shivering and nonshivering thermogenesis, and adrenal and thyroid output. The cells responsible for all of these responses lie in the anterior portion of the hypothalamus. Their firing rates appear to be governed by the balance of transmitter substances which shift as changes in heat production and heat loss are required to maintain thermal equilibrium.

2.2. Hypothalamic Separation between Heat Loss and Heat Production

2.2.1. Is There a Functional Separation between the Two Mechanisms?

In an excellent review of this subject, Cabanac (1970) listed several compelling reasons to believe that heat loss and heat production mechanisms are largely functionally independent. For instance, dogs will shiver and pant at the same time when their hypothalamic temperature is rapidly cycled by alternate perfusion of cold and warm water (Hardy, 1961). Also, drugs can have differential effects on the two mechanisms. Chlorpromazine and reserpine shifted the threshold curve for shivering in dogs and had little or no effect on the panting curve (Cabanac, 1970). Lastly, the basis for a functional separation has been established with the discoveries of individual warm- and cool-sensitive neurons.

2.2.2. Is There an Anatomical Separation?

If there is a functional separation between heat production and heat loss mechanisms, there are obviously anatomically separate cells which achieve it. The question is whether they are grouped in geographically separate, nonintermeshed structures. In 1913, Hans Meyer suggested that two reciprocally innervated centers existed, one for heat, the other for cold. In the 1930's and 40's, Ranson (1940) and his co-workers, working within this dual-center framework, divided the hypothalamus into an anterior heat loss portion and a posterior heat production part. This distinction was made mainly on the basis of lesion studies demonstrating that cats with lesions in the lateral part of the rostral hypothalamus could not prevent hypothermia in a warm room, but could maintain normal body temperature in the cold (Clark *et al.*, 1939a; Teague and Ranson, 1936). Because cats with lesions in the lateral part of the caudal hypothalamus could not maintain their temperatures in either warm or cold environments, (Clark *et al.*, 1939a), the heat loss pathway was postulated to descend to the posterior part of the diencephalon (Fig. 3). This division was supported by the work of Magoun *et al.* (1938) and Beaton *et al.* (1941), who showed that the heat loss responses of panting in cats and sweating in monkeys were activated during diathermic PO/AH heating.

This anterior/posterior division for temperature regulation does not stand out so sharply upon close examination,* as Clark (1960) argued in a

---

* Ranson himself was aware of this. In discussing the neural mechanisms which protect the body against chilling he wrote, "Very large lesions anywhere in the hypothalamus cause a loss of the capacity to keep the body temperature up to normal, and this loss is more pronounced when the lesions are caudally placed" (Ranson and Magoun, 1939, p. 154). Generally, however, he opted for more specific localization, and this is the view that prevailed for a long time.

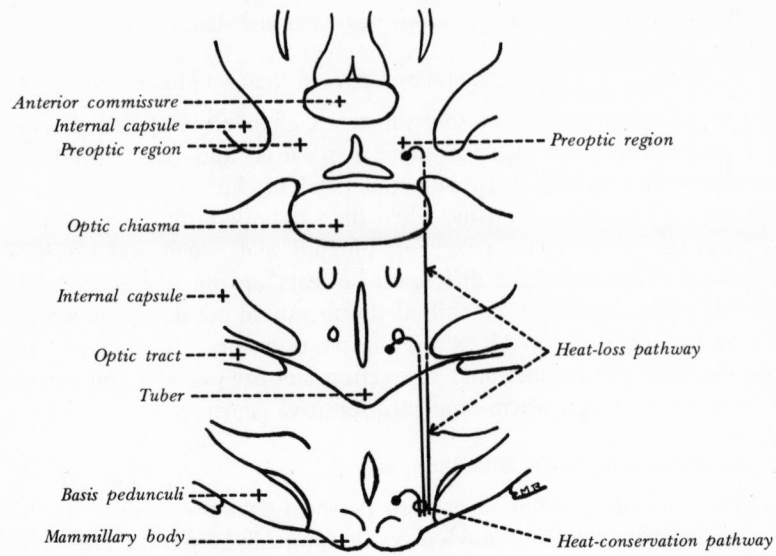

Anterior commissure
Internal capsule
Preoptic region
Preoptic region

Optic chiasma

Internal capsule
Optic tract
Tuber
Heat-loss pathway

Basis pedunculi
Mammillary body
Heat-conservation pathway

FIG. 3. Diagrammatic representation of the mechanism for temperature regulation, superimposed upon schematic drawings of three transverse sections through the preoptic region and hypothalamus. [From Ranson and Clark (1959).]

critical discussion of the problem. Many of Teague and Ranson's cats with PO/AH lesions showed deficits in the heat and also became hypothermic in the cold. The literature now includes many reports of animals with preoptic lesions which cannot maintain their body temperatures in cold environments, including rats (Cytawa and Teitelbaum, 1967; Carlisle, 1969; Satinoff and Rutstein, 1970), ground squirrels (Satinoff, 1967), cats (McCrum, 1953; Squires and Jacobson, 1968), and goats (Andersson et al., 1965). Moreover, Hammel et al. (1960) demonstrated elegantly that cooling the PO/AH in dogs leads to increased heat production, shivering, and a rise in temperature. These results have been confirmed in many other species including rats (Satinoff, 1964), cats (Sundsten, 1967), goats (Andersson et al., 1962), oxen (Calvert et al., 1972) rhesus monkeys (Hayward and Baker, 1968), and baboons (Gale and Jobin, 1967). Thermally stimulating the posterior hypothalamus leads to no such changes (Adair and Hardy, 1971; Freeman and Davis, 1959). As cited earlier, recent experiments using neural transmitter substances injected directly into the PO/AH in a variety of species have shown that this area is sensitive to transmitters that cause both increases and decreases in body temperature (Hellon, 1972). The posterior hypothalamus is not sensitive to such injections (Myers, 1970).

Since the posterior hypothalamus contains very few thermosensitive cells (Edinger and Eisenman, 1970), it may play primarily a motor role in physiological heat production. A major center for shivering has been localized there (Hemingway, 1963), and Birzis and Hemingway (1957) correlated the activity of neurons in the posterior hypothalamus with the onset and cessation of shivering in cats. The firing rates of these cells, which they showed were effector neurons, decreased when shivering was inhibited by warming the skin even though there was no rise in core temperature.

Where do these results leave Meyer's and later Ranson's dual-center hypothesis? If it is taken in its strict sense — that there are anatomically distinct integrating centers, one in the PO/AH regulating heat loss only and the other in the posterior hypothalamus regulating heat production only — then it is not tenable. Thermal sensitivity and integration of both of these responses seem to be primarily preoptic functions. The posterior hypothalamus seems to play mainly a motor role in physiological heat production.

However, this may not be its only role in temperature regulation. Recently Myers and his associates have suggested the intriguing idea that the mechanism for controlling body temperature around a given set point depends on a constant, inborn balance between sodium and calcium ions within the posterior hypothalamus which provides the reference input to the preoptic thermostat (Myers and Yaksh, 1971; Myers and Veale, 1970). If this is the case, then this area is also an essential part of the nonmotor thermoregulatory control system. In addition, the posterior hypothalamus, and the median forebrain bundle that courses through it, may have an important role in behavioral temperature regulation, as will be discussed in a later section.

3. Levels of Nervous Control of Reflexive Thermoregulation

3.1. Introduction

The previous section discussed evidence that led to the view that the hypothalamus, particularly the PO/AH, was the only thermostat of the brain. The most important evidence for this view is that animals with transections below the hypothalamus are poikilothermic, whereas, with the hypothalamus connected to the rest of the brain below they have effective temperature regulation. Three subsidiary lines of evidence are: (1) that hypothalamic thermal stimulation produces coordinated thermoregulatory responses; (2) that hypothalamic lesions eliminate those responses; and (3) that thermosensitive cells are concentrated there. For many years, Keller and Thauer have been the principal opponents to this view; Keller pointed out that heat loss responses can be obtained in decerebrate dogs, and Thauer argued that the spinal cord is thermosensitive. In the last few years there has been increasing interest in the thermoregulatory capacities of subhypothalamic structures. The evidence is now incontrovertible that other areas of the brain contain thermosensitive units which can induce heat loss and heat production responses in the absence of the hypothalamus. This naturally reduces the importance of the hypothalamus, making it only one of a number of areas of the brain capable of integrating thermoregulatory responses. I will next review the evidence that there are extrahypothalamic thermoregulatory centers.

3.2. Spinal Cord

3.2.1. Can Spinal Animals Thermoregulate?

For many years it was held that animals with transections of the spinal cord at high cervical levels are completely unable to regulate their body temperature. In 1924, Sherrington demonstrated that spinal dogs do not shiver below the level of the transection even when they are plunged into ice water, nor was any improvement seen even long after the effects of spinal shock had worn off. The dogs were able to pant in the heat, but this did not prevent a large rise in body temperature, probably caused by the severe failure to adjust vascular responses appropriately. Guttman *et al.* (1958) confirmed this result in spinal men: in the cold they do not shiver in the limbs innervated below the transection; nor do such men sweat in the heat. When their core temperatures are increased, such men increase their respiratory rates, but it is totally ineffective in lowering their temperature. Most other experiments on spinal animals have resulted in the same conclusion. [See Ranson (1940) for review.] In addition, there have been many demonstrations that decerebrate preparations have little or no temperature control, so it seemed reasonable to assume that the spinal cord was incapable of initiating any heat loss or heat production responses in the absence of supraspinal influences.

The earliest dissenting voice was Thauer's (1935), who reported that although spinal rabbits become hypothermic when exposed to a mildly cool environment they gradually recover their ability to regulate their temperature. If this recovered ability is indeed nervous, it would prove that the presence of the spinal cord alone enables rabbits to thermoregulate adequately in the absence of higher structures (most notably the hypothalamus) previously thought critical to such regulation.

Thauer's work was not followed up for many years. Recently, however, there has been renewed interest in the question of whether the isolated spinal cord is sufficient to elicit heat loss or production responses when areas below the level of spinal transection are heated or cooled. For the heat loss response of panting the answer is clearly no, because the motor centers for panting are located in the medulla and pons. However, sweating below the level of complete spinal cord lesions has been induced in paraplegic men by exposing them to warm air temperatures. Sweating first appeared on the feet and was then successively induced on the calf, trunk, and upper extremities, which is the same pattern seen in normal subjects (Seckendorf and Randall, 1961). Because the sweating was so sparse that only very sensitive techniques could measure it, Randall (1963) believed that the cutaneous thermoreceptors could not elicit normally profuse sweating without the hypothalamus, which, he suggested, facilitates the excitatory state of the spinal sweat centers. In any case, this experiment clearly demonstrated that many of the efferent sudomotor pathways and sweat glands remain functional below the level of spinal transection.

Several investigators have recently reported that they could obtain shivering in spinal rabbits and dogs during either spinal or whole-body cooling (Simon *et al.*, 1966; Kosaka *et al.*, 1967; Kosaka and Simon, 1968a,b; Thauer, 1970). There are several differences between the shivering of spinal and intact animals. The activation temperatures are much lower in spinal animals than in intact ones. Shivering in most normal animals is visible, but in spinal preparations it must generally be identified from the EMG. True phasic shivering bursts occurred in twelve of fourteen normal rabbits, but in only one of fifteen spinal animals.

Because the intensity and pattern of cold-induced tremor is so different in spinal animals, all of the above experimenters agree that the shivering mechanism is altered by supraspinal influences. The question remains whether this cold-induced tremor is indeed true shivering. Koizumi *et al.* (1959) have shown that cooling increases the amplitude and duration of spinal reflexes and that more motoneurons are recruited as hypothermia progresses. As Thauer (1970) pointed out, the increased excitability of spinal motoneurons is caused to a large extent by the direct effect of temperature on the membrane potential of these motoneurons, so the increased tremor seen in spinal animals may be due in part to this membrane thermosensitivity.

Is the cold-induced tremor of any thermoregulatory significance? To answer this question one has to determine whether spinal animals cool more slowly than other spinal preparations in which the tremors have been abolished by, for instance, anesthesia, curare, or ganglionic blocking agents, but these experiments have not yet been done.

In summary, spinal preparations, uninfluenced by any higher structures, can sweat and shiver, although these responses are fragmentary and inefficient and their thresholds of activation are much higher than those of intact animals.

We are still left with the problem of how Thauer's rabbits regained their ability to maintain their temperature in a cool environment. The standard method of testing spinal animals had been to house them in incubators and then subject them to high or low air temperatures for several hours. Sherrington tested his dogs in this way as did Clark (1940) who found that cervically sectioned cats could not maintain their body temperatures when transferred from a 30° to a 20°C room. Thauer did not maintain his rabbits this way. Generally, he lowered the temperature of the incubator gradually over a week's duration until it reached the room temperature of 20°C, where it remained. When Clark tested some of his cats in this manner, gradually accustoming them to a 22°C environment and then subjecting them to 18°C, he found that their body temperatures dropped less rapidly than other cats that had been living continuously in a 30°C incubator. When the former group was transferred back to the incubator, they became hyperthermic relative to the spinal cats who had remained there, and it took 3 to 4 days for their temperatures to return to normal. These experiments demonstrated that cervically sectioned cats were also able to adjust to slowly changing air temperatures within a narrow range. But Clark (1940) and Ranson (1940) attributed this to a metabolic, nonnervous adaptation because it was so slow—requiring days, not minutes, to reach completion. Thermal acclimatization does develop relatively slowly, and the basic mechanisms responsible for the chemical thermogenesis that underlies it reside at the cellular level (Hannon, 1963), so it is most likely that Thauer's results are best explained by a metabolic, not a nervous, mechanism.

Despite this, Thauer's inference that thermoregulatory structures could be widespread in the nervous system has proved to be correct and has stimulated research on thermosensitivity which is showing that the spinal cord has more of a role in temperature regulation than had previously been suspected.

3.2.2. Does the Spinal Cord Contain Thermosensitive Structures?

Even though the isolated spinal cord is generally unable to maintain normal body temperature, it appears to play an important role as an originator of temperature signals that can influence thermoregulatory responses. Jessen and his collaborators (Jessen and Mayer, 1971; Jessen and Ludwig, 1971; Jessen and Simon, 1971) have shown that spinal cooling in unanesthetized dogs causes shivering and increases oxygen consumption, whereas heating leads to panting. Generally, the cord has to be warmed to higher temperatures to elicit panting or cooled to lower ones to elicit shivering than is needed when the thermal stimulation is hypothalamic. Nonetheless, the responses were remarkably similar. When the two areas were heated simultaneously, the effects summed, confirming earlier results of Guieu and Hardy (1970b) in anesthetized rabbits. The increase in heat production produced by cooling one of the two areas could be counteracted by heating the other one, but the panting elicited by heating one area was not offset by cooling the other area. Guieu and Hardy's earlier work, using rabbits, does not completely confirm this identity of function. Although spinal cooling did not alter the polypnea produced by preoptic heating, preoptic cooling completely inhibited the panting induced by spinal heating. In other words, when opposing temperature changes were imposed, the observed responses were always those appropriate to the stimulation of the preoptic area. These authors concluded that thermal panting is controlled by temperatures in the spinal cord, PO/AH, and other deep-body receptors, but the PO/AH monitors and integrates its own and other thermal signals.

At present no way is known to reconcile Jessen and Simon's view that the function of spinal and hypothalamic thermosensitive units are equivalent in controlling the whole animal's thermoregulation with Guieu and Hardy's view that they are arranged hierarchically with the spinal cord dominated by the preoptic region. The results of Kosaka et al. (1969) are in agreement with the latter interpretation. Panting of rabbits in response to spinal heating was unchanged after decortication and was abolished after midbrain transection. The authors suggested that the integration of panting probably takes place in the hypothalamus. Whatever the final outcome, it is clear that Thauer and the workers who came after him have demonstrated that the spinal cord does play an important role in thermoregulation.

To examine the possibility that the thermosensitive elements might not be in the spinal cord itself, but rather in the meninges or other tissues of the vertebral canal, Meurer et al. (1967) transected the dorsal roots of the lumbosacral cord. Then they warmed the intact thoracic cord (to localize the cooling to the denervated part) and cooled the deafferented part. The experimental procedure and results are shown in Fig. 4. In such a rhizotomized preparation cooling the deafferented part of the cord evoked a shiveringlike tremor in the hind limbs. This experiment leaves no doubt that thermosensitive structures exist in the spinal cord itself.

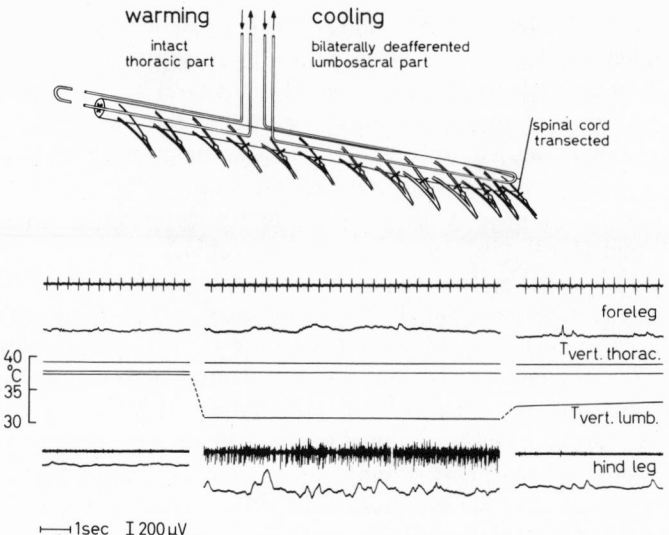

FIG. 4. Shivering in a lightly anesthetized dog with bilateral transection of the dorsal spinal roots from L 1 to the end of the spinal cord before, during, and after local cooling of the deafferented lumbosacral part of the spinal cord with one thermode, while the intact thoracic part was warmed with a second thermode. Air temperature: 30°C. Upper part of the figure: scheme of the experiment. Lower part of the figure: tracings 1 and 2: EMG and mechanogram of a foreleg, 3: peridural temperature in the thoracic region of the vertebral canal, 4: rectal temperature, 5: peridural temperature in the lumbosacral region of the vertebral canal, 6 and 7: EMG and mechanogram of a hindleg. [From Meurer *et al.* (1967).]

3.3. Medulla and Pons

3.3.1. Transections

Even when the brain transection or ablation leaves both the medulla and pons connected to the spinal cord, temperature maintenance is still so poor that the animals must be considered as essentially poikilothermic. Bazett and Penfield (1922) reported that decerebrate cats have no power of temperature control whatsoever in the cold, and they have to be rigorously maintained in an incubator or warm water bath. These cats never shiver in the cold. Although their respiratory rate increases when they are overheated, the rate is never that of a normal cat in the same circumstances.

The best studies of chronic decerebrate animals are those of Bard and his associates (Bard and Macht, 1958; Bard *et al.*, 1970) whose animals remained in good condition for many months. During exposure to cold, their pontile and low mesencephalic cats all piloerected and exhibited clonic, jerky movements of the extremities which stopped upon rewarming. In a heated chamber, all of these cats showed cutaneous vasodilation and panting. However, panting occurred only when rectal temperatures reached levels of 41–44°C. In addition, panting occurred only if the cats' mouths were forced open, and it was never at normally high rates. Keller (1933) reported similar results. His semiacute pontile cats never shivered in the cold or increased their respiratory rate to normal levels in the heat. However, when the transections spared either lateral or medial pathways, heat production mechanisms were not greatly impaired and some animals were even hyperthermic at room temperature (Keller, 1938). Keller (1933) also noted slight shivering in dogs with only the medulla attached to the spinal cord, an observation whose importance will become apparent at the end of the next section.

Connor and Crawford (1969) confirmed the hypothermia and lack of shivering in cats with complete midpontine transections. They also reported a higher body temperature at neutral environments in cats after radio-frequency lesions had destroyed the medial pons, while sparing the lateral portion. This sustained hyperthermia was initially caused by shivering and later by increased muscle tonus, since it could be abolished by injecting gallamine, a neuromuscular blocking agent. The authors point out that the reticular pathways mediating shivering in cats are more widely distributed in the lateral portion of the pons (Birzis and Hemingway, 1956). In other words, with the whole pons disconnected from any descending influence, there is no shivering or increased tonus. When the shivering pathways are still connected to the brain above, but the medial pons is gone, the animals are in a state of excessive tonus. This implies that the lateral shivering pathway is facilitated from more rostral brain areas and is inhibited by the medial pons. However, the hypertonus seen after medial reticular lesions may not be thermoregulatory in nature any more than is the extensor rigidity exhibited by decerebrate preparations. If it is truly a thermoregulatory response, implying that the cats are regulating around a higher set point, then it should abate if, for instance, the animals are heat stressed such that their body temperature will exceed that higher set point unless they bring heat loss responses into play.

3.3.2. Medullary Heating and Cooling

In anesthetized and decerebrate cats cardiovascular and respiratory responses have been reported during medullary heating and cooling (Holmes *et al.*, 1960; Chai *et al.*, 1965; Tabatabai, 1972a,b). This implies that some portions of the medulla are thermally sensitive, but they may have little to do with normal autonomic thermoregulation. As Tabatabai

(1972a) points out, heat affects tissue in many ways, including changing membrane polarization and causing local vasodilation which alters the concentrations of local metabolites. Thus, if heating or cooling is done near cardiovascular or respiratory centers, it would be possible to find respiratory or cardiovascular changes which may not be primarily thermoregulatory.

However, Chai and Lin (1972) recently made the important observation that thermal stimulation of the medulla of unanesthetized monkeys produces many elements of thermoregulation. Cooling causes vasoconstriction, shivering of the jaws, slower respiration, tachycardia, restlessness, and a slight increase in body temperature. Heating, besides leading to respiratory acceleration and hypotension, leads to cutaneous vasodilation, drowsiness, and a slight decrease in body temperature. [It also causes retching or emesis or both in most cats, supporting Tabatabai's argument for nonspecific effects of heating.]

Recently Lipton (1973) found that medullary cooling in conscious rats leads to shivering and a rise in body temperature, whereas heating causes a fall. These changes are in the same direction as those seen after PO/AH thermal stimulation. There are, however, several differences between medullary and preoptic stimulation. Shivering is much more easily elicited with medullary cooling, for instance. Furthermore, rectal temperatures are more variable during medullary stimulation. The general medullary/rectal temperature relation is unchanged after preoptic lesions. Lipton concluded that medullary thermosensitivity is independent of the hypothalamus and can exert a secondary, less precise control over body temperature. Chai and Wang (1970) reached a conclusion compatible with Lipton's when they postulated that the thermosensitive elements in the medulla are important only during extreme temperature changes.

There is an apparent paradox here. Spinal animals shiver [although the pattern and intensity differ from normals]. Decerebrate animals do not shiver, yet the medulla is capable of initiating shivering. One would expect that leaving more brain should lead to a more effective response rather than eliminating it altogether. This paradox has been beautifully resolved by an experiment of Chambers et al. (1974). Cooling the spinal cord of unanesthetized cats produced corresponding shivering, cutaneous vasoconstriction and piloerection with little change in rectal temperature. High-level decerebration abolished these effects and rectal temperatures declined as long as the cooling was continued. Lowering the level of decerebration to the caudal pons or medulla reinstated the responses to spinal cooling. Cooling the spinal cord of chronic spinal cats below the level of transection (T6) also produced thermoregulatory responses in the hind limbs, although of smaller intensity and without piloerection (Fig. 5). High-

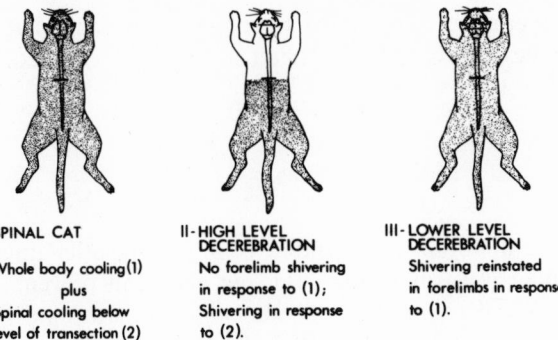

I - SPINAL CAT	II - HIGH LEVEL DECEREBRATION	III - LOWER LEVEL DECEREBRATION
Whole body cooling (1) plus Spinal cooling below level of transection (2) led to Whole body shivering.	No forelimb shivering in response to (1); Shivering in response to (2).	Shivering reinstated in forelimbs in response to (1).

FIG. 5. Effects of spinal and whole body cooling on shivering in unanesthetized cats. I: Spinal transection at T6, II: High decerebration at the level of the superior colliculus, III: II plus lower-level decerebration from below the inferior colliculus dorsally to the trapezoid body ventrally. Shivering was observed in shaded areas. (Diagram designed by Evan Snyder.)

level decerebration abolished shivering in the forelimbs during whole-body cooling while permitting shivering below T6 during spinal cord cooling. Lowering the level of decerebration to the lower pons or medulla reinstated shivering in the forelimbs.

These data suggest that the spinal cord and medulla facilitate thermoregulatory responses to cold. Normally they are tonically inhibited by the midbrain above, and this is why high level decerebrates are poikilothermic. When the medullary and spinal centers are released from this inhibition, they can and do initiate thermoregulatory responses to cold. Assuming that thermoregulatory responses are controlled by alternating levels of inhibition and facilitation explains why leaving more of the brain intact can produce more drastic results.

One recurrent observation remains puzzling. Local medullary or spinal cooling of decerebrate animals is much more effective in eliciting thermoregulatory responses than cooling the whole body. At the onset of cooling the whole body, this observation is easily explained by assuming that the cutaneous thermoreceptors project to nervous tissue above the level of decerebration. But this difference persists even when the core temperature, and therefore the temperature of the spinal cord or medulla, has reached the temperatures used when these areas are cooled locally. Possibly the time taken to reach the low temperature makes a difference. Local cooling lowers temperature almost immediately whereas cooling the whole body takes many minutes or hours to reach the same level. The firing rates of thermosensitive neurons may depend not only on their absolute temperature, but on the time taken to reach that temperature. Such a hypothesis is, however, difficult to fit into current concepts of thermodetector function.

3.4. Midbrain

When the midbrain is separated from the hypothalamus above, animals cannot keep warm in the cold, but they can prevent severe hyperthermia in a warm room. This phenomenon has been amply described by Keller and his associates (Keller, 1963; Keller and McClaskey, 1964). None of Keller's completely transected dogs ever shivered or was able to maintain its body temperature in a 3°C air temperature. However, if any tissue remained between the midbrain and the hypothalamus, fragmentary control of body temperature was evident. After a month or so, the rate of decline in rectal temperatures was slower than initially and slight shivering was observed.

We can interpret these results within the framework of Chambers *et al.* (1974). If the medulla facilitates shivering and the midbrain inhibits the medulla, then the hypothalamus might inhibit the midbrain inhibition. Thus, as long as some hypothalamic tissue is left intact, it can attenuate the midbrain inhibitory influence on the medulla.*

These totally decerebrate dogs, who were completely unable to regulate in the cold, nevertheless tolerated warm environments. They exhibited what Keller called a "raised heat-dissipation threshold"; that is, panting was delayed until core temperature reached a higher level than normal threshold, but once panting appeared it was completely effective in preventing a further rise in temperature.

Keller's results were completely confirmed by Bard *et al.* (1970). In the cold, their high midbrain cats piloerected and showed the clonic, jerking movements described earlier. At very low body temperatures, fine, rapid tremors appeared, but these tremors had no thermoregulatory effectiveness (Bard and Macht, 1958). None of the cats ever vasoconstricted. In the heat,

---

* This concept of successive levels of inhibitory and facilitatory control of thermoregulatory responses may illustrate a fundamental principle of response integration, that is, that these levels affect reflexes which may be mediated by much lower parts of the neuraxis. Ruch (1960) has summarized evidence based on transection experiments in cats demonstrating at least four levels in the control of the micturition reflex: 1) cortical inhibition, 2) posterior hypothalamic facilitation, 3) mesencephalic inhibition, and 4) pontine facilitation. The same principle obtains for nervous influence over the galvanic skin reflex (Ingram, 1960). This Jacksonian concept of alternating levels of CNS function can explain how a few simple reflexes may be incorporated into many different action patterns, with higher-level complexity superimposed on lower mechanisms to smooth and control them. However, a discussion of the details of such an organization is not within the scope of this chapter.

the respiratory rate increased slightly at lower body temperatures than in low mesencephalic animals. Spontaneous panting appeared at rectal temperatures between 42–43°C and all the cats vasodilated cutaneously. Thus both Keller and then Bard and Macht found that decerebrate cats and dogs become hypothermic in the cold, but are able to prevent severe hyperthermia in hot environments.

Keller (1932) reported an interesting difference in the determination of vasomotor tone between intact and midbrain cats. When the core temperatures of normal cats were raised, the ear vessels dilated maximally and remained dilated, even when the cats were removed from the hot incubator, until rectal temperatures had returned to normal. In midbrain preparations, overheating also dilated the ear vessels, but they constricted quickly when the animals were returned to room air, even while the core temperatures remained elevated. Thus it appears that ambient temperature alone determines cutaneous vasomotor state in midbrain cats, not blood temperature as in intact animals. In other words, vasodilation in midbrain cats is governed mainly by a peripheral stimulus, not an interaction of central and peripheral stimuli, as in normals.

Regulation against heat is also impaired in midbrain animals in the sense that panting, the major avenue for heat loss in dogs, is not activated until core temperatures are abnormally high. Once activated, however, it is fully effective in preventing any further rise in body temperature. This implies that, as a response to thermal stress, panting is integrated at a midbrain level but normally is facilitated by higher nervous areas. It is interesting to note that high decerebrate rats are poikilothermic not only in the cold, but in the heat as well (Woods, 1964). Why does the heat dissipation threshold not simply increase in the heat? This may be because rats do not pant. Saliva secretion and spreading is their major method for dissipating heat, analogous to panting in cats and dogs, and that response is disrupted by preoptic lesions (Hainsworth and Stricker, 1970). Rats' other avenue for losing heat, vasodilation, even if effective, might not be sufficient to prevent fatal hyperthermia in very hot environments. In less drastic situations it appears that rats with PO/AH lesions do show a raised heat dissipation threshold with respect to vasodilation. Forcing rats with PO/AH lesions to exercise on a treadmill results in vasodilation at a significantly higher core temperature than in control animals. The vasodilation, once initiated, is sufficient to prevent any further rise in core temperature with exercise (Han and Brobeck, 1961; Thompson and Stevenson, 1965). Thus it may be that decerebrate rats would show the same raised heat dissipation threshold for vasodilation as carnivores do for panting, but when they are tested in an extremely hot environment their inability to salivate masks this effect.

Animals without any hypothalamic or higher tissue seem to have two basic thermoregulation problems—vastly different thresholds of activation and poor integration of thermoregulatory responses. The stimulus required to activate any thermoregulatory response must be more intense than is needed in normal animals. This implies that one missing level of control in these animals is the facilitation of lower centers by impulses arriving from higher ones. Signals which normally activate thermal responses may only be effective against a background of general tonic excitation flowing from more rostral to more caudal areas.* In other words, when the central excitatory state is reduced, signals, to be effective, must be large enough to overcome a general neural depression. [The same high threshold is seen in the expression of emotional behavior. Bard and Macht (1958) reported that fragments of anger could be evoked in high mesencephalic cats only with very strong nociceptive stimuli.]

The most important level of control, that of proper integration of responses, also cannot be achieved without the hypothalamus. Many components of thermoregulation are present in midbrain animals. Regardless of how useful the responses are or the temperature necessary to elicit them, midbrain preparations can pant, salivate, show muscle tremor, vasoconstrict, and piloerect. But without the hypothalamus, these responses seem to occur in a mixed jumble. For instance, Bard and Macht's mesencephalic cats "shivered" at rectal temperatures of 28°C while, at the same time, salivating profusely. Bard et al. (1970) observed piloerection in the cold, but it was often seen when the animals were warm. Keller (1938) reported that high midbrain cats were cutaneously vasodilated and often panted even when they were in a cool environment or had extremely low rectal temperatures. In addition, stimuli which are normally unconnected to panting, such as bodily movement, urination, or slight tail pinching, elicited it with ease—all this in face of the fact that these animals did not pant in the heat, a normal stimulus for it, until core temperatures were abnormally high. This implies that thermal panting is facilitated from above whereas, at the level of the midbrain, nonthermal stimuli have access to and facilitate the panting mechanism.†

Such inappropriate and conflicting responses are commonly seen in af-

---

* This does not imply that all excitatory impulses originate rostrally and then descend. Probably impulses originating in the reticular activating system ascend to the telencephalon and diencephalon and then descend to facilitate effectively. If so, then localized reticular lesions could cause the same lack of tonic facilitation, but to my knowledge there is no evidence bearing on this point.

† Keller concluded that a portion of the heat dissipation outflow is temperature dependent, but not thermally activated. This brings to mind a study of cool-sensitive units in the midbrain reticular formation of rabbits. These units responded to decreases in skin temperature. Many of them, classified as interneurons by their firing characteristics, were also activated by mechanical peripheral stimulation (Nakayama and Hardy, 1969). Warm-sensitive units also exist in the midbrain (Cabanac and Hardy, 1968, 1969), and if they showed similar changes to nonthermal peripheral stimuli, they could provide a basis for Keller's results.

fective and emotional behavior. Fragments of responses appropriate to both fear and rage and to both escape and aggression, regularly were seen in cats lacking a hypothalamus (Bard and Macht, 1958). Bazett and Penfield (1922) reported the interesting case of a decerebrate cat which, after an hour in a hammock in a water bath to maintain its temperature, was found in the bath kicking at the stirrer, with all claws extended, and purring. While being removed from the bath, its head fell under water. Upon being rescued and wrapped in a towel, it immediately began to purr again.

In summary, although the midbrain is sufficient for the appearance of panting, it is only in the presence of the hypothalamus that well-coordinated, low-threshold responses occur and inappropriate responses are inhibited. In fact, this is an operational definition of an integrative center. If a transection at one level of the brain yields a combination of antagonistic responses, and the addition of a small amount of tissue at the next higher level provides for appropriate coordination of these responses, we have proof of the existence of centers of integration in that tissue.

3.5. Telencephalon

More anterior parts of the brain are also involved in thermoregulation. Andersson (1957) reported that electrical stimulation of the septal area of goats in a warm room produced the coordinated responses of shivering, peripheral vasoconstriction, sometimes piloerection, and an inhibition of panting. The shivering stopped, however, when rectal temperatures had risen about 0.5°C. Furthermore, septal stimulation was not very effective in inhibiting panting when rectal temperatures had risen 1.0–1.5°C. These results contrast strongly with the effects of stimulating the preoptic "heat loss center" of goats in the cold, which maintained panting and cutaneous vasodilation and suppressed shivering for more than two hours, thereby driving temperatures down by as much as 10°C. Andersson concluded that this difference might indicate some dominance of the preoptic heat loss center over the structural elements concerned with overcooling. Stuart *et al.* (1961) confirmed these results in cats and also noted that a greater stimulus intensity was needed in the septal area to produce less intense shivering than during hypothalamic stimulation. Eisenman and Jackson's (1967) finding of thermally responsive neurons throughout the septum of cats is consistent with these stimulation studies.

Since septal stimulation elicits heat production responses it is reasonable to anticipate that lesions will eliminate them. Cats with large bilaterally placed lesions in the septal area, fornix, and medial anterior thalamus did indeed become hypothermic, but this was always associated with other changes such as hyperglycemia, hypokinesia, coma, and spontaneous death (Bond *et al.*, 1957). On the other hand, Stuart *et al.* (1962) reported that septal lesions alone had no effect on the heat production responses of cats in the cold. These results are difficult to compare with those of Bond *et al.*, since most of Bond *et al.*'s cats died within 5 days of surgery, and none of Stuart *et al.*'s cats were tested until at least 26 days postoperatively. Stuart *et al.* might well have found heat production deficits had they tested their cats earlier. There may, indeed, have been a complete or partial loss of a particular response after incomplete ablation which may have recovered almost completely after 26 days.

Clark *et al.* (1939b) found no significant disturbances in thermoregulation when their cats with thalamic lesions were tested in hot or cold environments at least 2 weeks after surgery. Finger and Maickel (1970) confirmed these results in rats with somatosensory cortical or thalamic lesions tested 3 months postoperatively.

The cortex contains thermally sensitive neurons (Barker and Carpenter, 1970) and is also involved in thermoregulation. It appears to play an inhibitory role with respect to panting. Immediately after withdrawal of anesthesia, acutely decorticate cats at normal body temperature began to pant spontaneously. Decorticate polypneic panting can be considered as an example of a release phenomenon which occurs when lower centers are released from higher inhibitory control. In this case, as in many others, the lower centers are diencephalic because the response is abolished after hypothalamic transection (Lilienthal and Otenasek, 1937).

Pinkston *et al.* (1934) reported that chronic decorticate cats and dogs maintain their temperatures under average conditions and also in thermally extreme environments. Their responses are not completely normal; they were chronically vasodilated and failed to constrict in the cold. They did not show true rapid panting in the warm room and the increase in respiration that did occur appeared at higher than normal core temperatures. [The authors did note polypneic panting during recovery from anesthesia and attributed the later loss of the response to secondary thalamic degeneration.] Cold stimulated immediate and vigorous shivering, with a consequent rise in core temperature, as compared with the delayed and less marked reaction of intact animals. The decorticates often shivered at ordinary room temperatures, which was interpreted as a release phenomenon, brought about when the cortex, which normally inhibits the response, is removed. However, since these animals were unable to conserve heat as well as normals, their overactive shivering might have been a perfectly normal compensation for inadequate vasoconstriction. Their body temperatures at the end of their stay in the cold room were the same as when they first began to shiver, which was true of normal dogs also.

Delgado and Livingston (1948) reported findings on vasomotor tone which are consistent with the above. After chronic bilateral ablation of the posterior orbital gyrus of the frontal lobe in monkeys, the temperature of the extremities was markedly elevated. Vasoconstriction to cold was inadequate. The authors concluded that the cortical regions of autonomic representation apparently project through the more rudimentary centers of the hypothalamus and medulla and represent a level of higher control.

Blass (1969) did not find results similar to those of Pinkson *et al*. He reported that rats with frontal pole ablations maintained an elevated body temperature in cold, neutral, and warm environments. However, since the PO/AH was also damaged in his preparations, and since animals with PO/AH lesions are generally hyperthermic, it is difficult to evaluate the differences between his rats and rats with preoptic lesions alone.

Buresova (1957) reported that rats and mice subjected to spreading cortical depression cooled more rapidly than normals in the cold and died sooner in the heat. She attributed the rapid cooling to disturbances in chemical thermogenesis. Cytawa and Teitelbaum (1967) used the same technique in rats that, following PO/AH lesions, had recovered their ability to regulate in the cold. When the cortex of such recovered rats was functionally ablated by the technique of spreading depression [potassium chloride applied directly to the cortical surface, which evokes a local decrease in EEG amplitude which spreads in all directions throughout the cortex], the rats were no longer able to thermoregulate adequately, and their body temperatures dropped drastically. Normal rats' temperatures also dropped, but not so far. This experiment demonstrated a cortical involvement with the subcortical structures responsible for maintaining body temperatures in the cold.

In summary, the septal area appears to play an important role in temperature regulation. The thalamus has so far not been strongly implicated but most of the experiments on animals with thalamic lesions have been performed well after the period when recovery of function might be expected to have occurred. Decorticate cats and dogs pant less than normals in hot environments, whereas they shiver more readily and more often than normals in cold environments and maintain higher body temperatures. Cortical inactivation by spreading depression also impairs temperature regulation. The inescapable conclusion from all of these studies is that all levels of the nervous system, from spinal cord to cortex, are necessary for normal reflexive thermoregulation.

4. Behavioral Thermoregulation

4.1. Introduction

The preceding parts of this chapter were concerned with the question of how the nervous system controls reflexive, autonomic, involuntary thermoregulatory responses. We saw that there are a number of neural loci containing thermosensitive cells from which reflexive responses can be elicited. The remainder of the chapter deals with the neural control of behavioral thermoregulation, a more widely used and possibly more effective means of achieving thermal homeostasis. As Benzinger (1970) has remarked, "Shivering indicates a failure of intelligent behavior."

Because all thermoregulatory responses are aimed at the same goal, it would be reasonable to suppose that the controllers are identical. Behavioral thermoregulation as a field of study would not then be very enticing since one could assume that whenever physiological responses were activated, parallel behavioral responses would also occur if the situation permitted, and also that nonmotor damage to one system would always lead to similar losses in the other. However, these two classes of regulation appear to be functionally and anatomically separate, which implies different neural networks for each.

Furthermore, if behavioral and physiological responses are integrated separately in the brain, one may ask if there is a further fractionation — that is, is each response, regardless of its nature, integrated separately also? In other words, is there any pattern integration in the nervous system at all? I will present data on both physiological and behavioral responses which suggest that there is not.

Since the first experiments of Satinoff (1964) showing that brain cooling elicits not only reflexive, but also behavioral thermoregulation, the field has expanded rapidly. Being a relatively new topic, there is not as much information about behavioral as about autonomic responses. I will review the evidence that different levels of the brain are capable of initiating motivated thermoregulatory behavior, and then I will discuss the problem of pattern integration.

4.2. Spinal Cord

Spinal thermal stimulation may be sufficient to evoke simple behavioral responses. During thoracic spinal cooling pigeons not only fluffed their feathers (a response analogous to piloerection in furred mammals) but also changed from a standing to a crouching posture and covered their legs with their plumage, just as normal pigeons behave in the cold (Rautenberg, quoted in Thauer, 1970).

Cabanac (1972) examined the effects of spinal heating and cooling in dogs on the operant response of pressing a panel to change the air temperature. Cooling the cord had very little effect on the behavior, whereas heating led to an increase in the dog's working for cooler air. However, the cord had to be heated to a temperature close to the pain threshold before any responses were elicited. These two experiments imply that spinal thermal signals can evoke some behavioral response, but there are too few data so far to allow us to say anything about the nature or precision of this control.

4.3. Medulla and Pons

Signals from the medulla definitely influence behavioral thermoregulation. When the temperature of the rostral medulla/caudal pontine area was altered, rats used an operant response appropriately to obtain heat or cool air (Lipton, 1971). There was no change in PO/AH temperature during the medullary stimulation. In room air, the rats' rectal temperatures changed appropriately in the opposite direction from the thermal stimulus. The rats shivered when the medulla was cooled and became quiescent when it was warmed. These responses were not altered by PO/AH lesions. In behavioral experiments the time spent pressing a pedal to lower ambient temperature was proportional to medullary temperature. After PO/AH lesions, the influence of medullary temperature on this behavior was enhanced (Lipton, 1973). Lipton concluded that medullary thermosensitivity can exert a secondary control over body temperature which is independent of the hypothalamus but is normally inhibited by it; when the PO/AH is lesioned, the behavior is released from its normally inhibitory influence.

While this interpretation is interesting, it must be remembered that rats with PO/AH damage generally have higher response rates than normal in thermally extreme environments (Lipton, 1968; Carlisle, 1969; Satinoff and Rutstein, 1970). It seems appropriate, therefore, to compare the response rates of PO/AH lesioned rats during medullary cooling or warming relative to their lesioned base rates. If the results of medullary thermal stimulation are similar to those after PO/AH stimulation, rats should barpress for warm air in a neutral environment. One could then examine the effects of the lesion on response rate during medullary stimulation without the confounding effects of autonomic impairment. Besides barpressing for cool air, rats will also groom and increase their activity during medullary heating (Roberts and Mooney, 1973). These authors concluded that medullary warming could elicit several of the normal heat loss responses in this species, but not as effectively as when the hypothalamus was warmed.

4.4. Midbrain

Sometimes behavioral responses do not change when an area of the brain that is implicated in physiological thermoregulation is thermally stimulated. For instance, thermal stimulation of the midbrain reticular formation of rabbits caused changes in the firing rate of temperature-sensitive units in the PO/AH (Cabanac and Hardy, 1969) and sometimes altered their metabolic rate (Hardy, 1969). Nevertheless, Adair and Stitt (1971) found that neither heating nor cooling this region in squirrel monkeys had any effect on physiological or behavioral thermoregulatory responses. This may, of course, simply be a species difference. Adair and Stitt suggest that in intact animals signals from the midbrain are weak compared to hypothalamic signals and might exert some degree of control over thermoregulatory responses if the hypothalamus were injured. If this suggestion is correct, thermal stimulation of the midbrain reticular formation should be effective in animals with hypothalamic damage.

4.5. Hypothalamus

The hypothalamus exerts strong control over behavioral as well as physiological thermoregulatory responses. In rats, preoptic cooling at environmental temperatures of 5 and 24°C activated the reflexive responses of shivering and piloerection. In addition, when the rats were given access to a bar which turned on a heat lamp, at both ambient temperatures they pressed more when their brains were cooled than when they were not. The same temperature levels were reached whether or not heat could be obtained voluntarily (Satinoff, 1964). Conversely, hypothalamic heating led to decreases in rates of responding for heat in cold environments (Carlisle, 1966). These experiments demonstrated that manipulations of hypothalamic temperature arouse not only reflexive acts designed to promote thermal stability, but also arouse the urge to keep warm. These results have been verified in several species including pigs (Baldwin and Ingram, 1967), rats (Murgatroyd and Hardy, 1970), squirrel monkeys (Adair et al., 1970), and baboons (Gale et al., 1970). Rats will also work to cool themselves off when their hypothalamus is warmed (Corbit, 1970; Murgatroyd and Hardy, 1970). Further, Corbit (1969) showed that rats would work to restore hypothalamic as well as skin temperatures to neutral values when either had been displaced by heating or cooling.

Because preoptic thermal stimulation elicits both physiological and motivated responses, it would be reasonable to expect that damage in that area would impair both types of regulation. This is certainly the case for reflexive responses, as we have seen, but it is only true for certain, not all, motivated behaviors. Food intake and activity can be considered as behavioral thermoregulations. In the cold, normal rats eat more food and are more active. In warm environments they eat less and reduce their activity. Preoptic lesioned rats did not increase their food intake in the cold in the same proportion as did controls, nor did they increase the time spent running in a wheel, and consequently they remained slightly hypothermic (Hamilton and Brobeck, 1966). In the heat, lesioned rats ate their regular amount of food, even with body temperatures of 40°C. In contrast, when heat stressed sufficiently to produce such high temperatures, normal rats ate practically nothing (Hamilton, 1967). Furthermore, the lesioned rats maintained this higher food intake at 32°C even when they had to press a bar at high fixed ratios to receive a pellet of food. At that ambient temperature, normal rats' response rates were drastically reduced (Hamilton and Brobeck, 1964). The lesioned rats reduced their running activity in the heat in a manner similar to controls (Hamilton and Brobeck, 1966). However, since such rats are, in general, less active than controls, it may be that only a slight additional negative stimulus [warm skin or warm core, perhaps] is sufficient to reduce it even further.

In summary, although preoptic lesioned rats lowered their activity in the heat in a normal fashion, they were inadequately active in the cold and they did not show adequate changes in food intake in either hot or cool environments. These behavioral deficits were evident as long as nine months postoperatively.

When responding effects a change in the ambient temperature, however, behavioral thermoregulation is left almost intact. Lipton (1968) first showed that preoptic lesioned rats, which become severely hyperthermic in a hot environment, press a bar to turn a heat lamp off and a cooling fan on, and thereby avoid death from overheating. Later Carlisle (1969) reported that when such rats were given an opportunity to press a bar for heat in the cold, they kept the heat lamp on much longer than did normals and were able to prevent severe hypothermia. Satinoff and Rutstein (1970) verified this phenomenon. Without access to the bar, lesioned rats' temperature dropped an average of 2.4°C per hour in 8 weekly 1-hour cold stress tests (Table 1). With the bar, the rats kept the heat lamp on 32% of the time [compared with 0.05% for food-deprived controls] and maintained their temperatures within 0.7°C of normal (Table 2).

In short, preoptic thermal stimulation evokes both reflexive and motivated responses designed to restore thermal balance. Lesions in the same place damage reflexive regulation, as would be expected, and reduce changes in food intake and activity, but leave operant thermoregulatory responding almost intact.

TABLE 1. Mean Change in Body Temperature (°C) after the First, Fourth, and Eighth Placement at an Ambient Temperature of 5°C for One Hour [From Satinoff and Rutstein (1970)]

Group	ΔT_B during cold-stress tests					
	1st Test		4th Test		8th Test	
		range ↓		range ↓		range ↓
Lesions $N = 5$	−3.18	−0.5 to −6.8	−1.88	0.5 to −6.5	−2.16	−0.2 to −4.6
Controls						
Normal weight $N = 5$	1.06	−0.1 to 1.8	0.48	0.1 to 1.1	0.72	0.4 to 1.1
80% body weight $N = 5$	0.02	0.0 to 0.1	0.10	−0.5 to 0.5	0.12	0.0 to 0.5

Pressing a bar for warm or cool air provides a kind of thermal change different from that produced by eating or running. The operant (bar press) is initiated primarily by changes in peripheral temperature and the reinforcement is immediately felt cutaneously (Weiss and Laties, 1961). It is a method of altering heat loss. Changes in food intake and activity are chemical means of altering heat production which work by changing the metabolic rate. The reinforcement is initiated internally and spreads to the periphery. Perhaps animals with PO/AH lesions are not as sensitive as normals to changes in their core temperature; if so, then they will not be reinforced for changing it. Alternatively, if there is a metabolic impairment such that metabolic rate does not change normally in response to food eaten, there will again be no reinforcement.

The reinforcement obtained by barpressing for heat or cold does not depend on the integrity of either core thermodetectors or chemical thermogenesis. The animal only has to sense a deviation from optimal skin temperature, be motivated to regain thermal homeostasis, and have the ability to make the required response. I suggest that animals with preoptic lesions will perform any behavioral response where the reinforcement is immediate, physical, and peripheral; examples are nestbuilding in the cold, taking showers in the heat [this, in fact, was demonstrated by Toth (1973)], and going to the neutral part of a thermal gradient.

We have just seen part of the evidence for the statement that the neural networks involved in physiological and operant thermoregulation are different. The rest of the evidence lies in the fact that lateral hypothalamic lesions can disrupt thermoregulatory operants while leaving the reflexive regulation intact. Rats that had built nests and pressed a lever to turn on a heat lamp no longer did either after lateral hypothalamic lesions. Most such animals were, nevertheless, able to maintain their temperature adequately physiologically. These operant deficits were not necessarily accompanied by any impairment in feeding or drinking (Table 3). This is an important point. If *all* behaviors had been disrupted equally by the lesions, and had recovered at the same rate, there would be no reason for separating out temperature regulation as a special behavior system passing through the lateral hypothalamus. One could argue that the thresholds for a general motivational system had been raised, and then the observation of a higher threshold for a particular system would be trivial. But, as Table 3 shows, the rats exhibited all possible combinations of losses and time to recovery. One (XY 10) ate and drank normally from the first postoperative day, but did not work for heat for 2 months. Another (SY 9) did not drink water for 3 months, yet responded normally to obtain heat within a week. The lack of responding for heat was not caused by motor or memory impairment, because on days when the rats were given a drug which lowered their body temperature, they responded well, whereas

TABLE 2. Mean Duration of Heat-On Time and Mean Change
in Body Temperature for All Two-Hour Sessions in The Cold
with Access to the Bar and Heat Lamp[a]
[From Satinoff and Rutstein (1970)]

Group	Duration of heat-on time (sec)		Mean change in T_B (°C) for sessions with heat lamp	
Trials =	1–8	9–18	1–8	9–18
Lesions $N = 5$	2286.6	2771.5	−0.54	−0.75
Controls normal weight $N = 5$	130		0.50	
Controls kept at 80% ad libitum body weight $N = 5$	202.4		0.26	

[a] All control data are for an average of eight trials.

TABLE 3. Eating, Drinking, Nest Building, and Operant Behavior of Rats with
PO/AH Lesions
[From Satinoff and Shan (1971)]

| Animal | Adipsia aphagia Anorexia[a] | Nestbuilding | Barpressing[b] | |
			For heat	For shock
XY 15	yes (166[c], 3, 17)	no	impaired (99[c])	—
XY 10	no (0, 0, 0)	—	impaired (61)	—
SY 18	yes (27, 3, 14)	no	impaired (41)	impaired (30)
XY 8	no (0, 0, 0)	—	impaired (32[c])	—
XY 3	yes (8, 1, 8)	—	impaired (18)	—
SY 9	yes (90, 2, 14)	no	impaired (7)	impaired (15)
SY 8	yes (11, 3, 3)	no	impaired (7)	impaired (11)

[a] Numbers in parentheses indicate number of days, respectively, that the rats were
adipsic, aphagic, and anorexic.
[b] Numbers in parentheses indicate days on which barpressing rates returned to preoperative levels.
[c] No recovery seen for the duration of the experiment.

response rates returned to near-zero on nondrug days (Fig. 6) (Satinoff and
Shan, 1971).

Motivational apathy is one likely cause of the decreased responding
exhibited by rats with lateral hypothalamic lesions. Stein (1964) proposed
that the medial forebrain bundle, which courses through the lateral
hypothalamus, is part of a motivational system which facilitates operant
behavior. Other behaviors, such as feeding and drinking (Teitelbaum and
Epstein, 1962), mousekilling (Karli and Vergnes, 1964), and shock avoidance (Balinska, 1968), can also be disrupted by lateral hypothalamic lesions.

Animals with lateral hypothalamic lesions may also have sensory deficits. They may not be sensitive to peripheral thermal stimuli and that may
be why they do not press for heat in the cold until their internal tempera-

tures drop. This interpretation implies that the lateral hypothalamus is part of a pathway which relays cutaneous thermal information to other parts of the brain. However, when the damage is in the central nervous system (CNS) and not in the periphery, it becomes difficult to distinguish between sensory and motivational deficits. It would be necessary to determine if an animal that fails to respond to obtain heat can, in fact, use a change in skin temperature as a discriminative stimulus signalling whether or not a reinforcement (different from heat) were coming in an operant situation. Of course, the animal's motivation for that reinforcement would have to be intact.

These results, that rats with lateral hypothalamic lesions will not work to obtain heat, are compatible with Adair and Hardy's (1971) findings that thermal stimulation of the posterior hypothalamus in squirrel monkeys elicited only operant, not autonomic, thermoregulatory responses. The lateral and posterior hypothalamus appear to be part of the same pathway. Lesions in the posterior hypothalamus generally lead to more drastic defi-

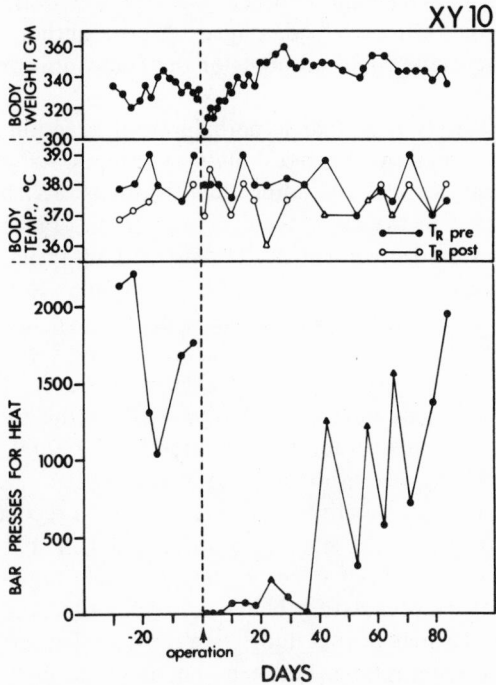

FIG. 6. Effect of lateral hypothalamic lesions on body weight, body temperature, and responding for heat at 5°C. (▲ = 1.5 ml quinine HCl (5mg/ml) given intraperitoneally immediately before the session.) [From Satinoff and Shan (1971)].

cits, like somnolence and complete, and possibly permanent, adipsia and aphagia (McGinty, 1969). Lateral lesions cause less severe effects; the rats are drowsy instead of totally somnolent, and later their adipsia and aphagia recover through stages to relatively normal drinking and eating (Wampler, 1970; Teitelbaum and Epstein, 1962). Since the medial forebrain bundle runs through both areas, it is reasonable that lesions should eliminate and stimulation should excite the same sorts of behavior.

4.6.   Telencephalon

Information on telencephalic influences on thermoregulatory behavior is sparse. Rats with frontal pole ablations performed appropriate behavioral responses in cold or hot air to maintain their core temperature about 1°C above normal (Blass, 1969, 1971). It appeared as if their set temperature had been elevated and that they were defending this new level. However, it is difficult to determine precisely the influence of the frontal poles on this behavior because other parts of the brain, including the preoptic area, were extensively damaged. As the author himself pointed out, that damage alone could account for the behavioral and physiological changes observed.

There is certainly a cortico–hypothalamic interaction with respect to operant thermoregulation. When a unilateral preoptic lesion was combined with contralateral cortical spreading depression in rats, bar pressing for heat was increased in the cold (Rudiger and Seyer, 1968). Since cortical spreading depression decreases hypothalamic activity ipsilaterally (Bures *et al.*, 1961), this result was to be expected; it is similar to making bilateral preoptic lesions which we know increase lever pressing for heat. However, in another set of similar experiments, thermosensitive locomotion in a cold and neutral shuttlebox disappeared (Rudiger and Seyer, 1965). If the lesions in this experiment were more lateral than in the previous one, this result could be explained in terms of a lateral–behavioral/medial–physiological distinction. However, no histology was reported in either paper and so these apparently contradictory results remain to be reconciled.

Olfactory bulb removal leads to a specific deficit in behavioral thermoregulation. Bulbectomized mice no longer huddle together in the cold. Other forms of thermoregulatory behavior, such as increasing food intake and going to the warmer of two floors, are normal. This specific deficit involves the neural connections between the olfactory bulb and unknown parts of the brain, because mice made anosmic by application of zinc sulfate are no different from controls (Edwards and Roberts, 1972). This experiment demonstrates very nicely that one must test animals in a variety of thermal situations and that the particular response under study must always be considered in terms of all of the animal's behavior patterns. The authors did this experiment as an additional test of their hypothesis that bulbectomy disrupts all forms of social behavior in mice. If they had only looked at huddling in the cold after bulbectomy, they might have concluded that thermoregulatory behavior was disrupted. Actually, it appears that the class of thermoregulatory behaviors is unaffected in general, and only that particular form which is also a member of the class of social behaviors is lost.

5. Integration of Complex Thermoregulatory Response Patterns

5.1. Evidence Against Integration

We have just seen that behavioral thermoregulatory responses can be elicited or impaired independently of reflexive responses. We have further seen that some behavioral responses can be more strongly impaired than others after preoptic lesions. There appears to be, therefore, very little, if any, pattern integration within these broad categories. It is now reasonable to ask whether there is any integration at all between any individual components of a complex pattern. Do thermoregulatory responses occur together for reasons other than simply that the thermal stimulus excites many independent mechanisms at the same time? The reason, then, that the preoptic area has been considered as a major integrative center may have nothing to do with integration per se, but simply may be an artifact of the functionally separate but anatomically overlapping passage of individual pathways through that part of the brain. Roberts (1970; and Roberts and Mooney, 1974) has presented convincing evidence for this view. Diathermic warming of different brain areas from the septal area to the medulla elicited one or two of the three main behavioral hyperthermic responses of rats. These responses are grooming, prone body extension, and escapelike locomotion. Fewer than 3% of the electrodes produced all three responses. Roberts concluded that no integrative center was required, that the rat's hyperthermic behavior pattern was a result of largely independent channels from thermal detector to motor effector.

Drs. Dominic Valentino, Philip Teitelbaum, and I have recently obtained results which can easily be interpreted as indicating separate channels for reflexive thermoregulatory responses. We studied the nature of the cold defense deficits and the course of recovery in rats after electrolytic lesions in the PO/AH. For a variable period after the lesions, when the animals were placed in the cold they did not shiver, increase their metabolic

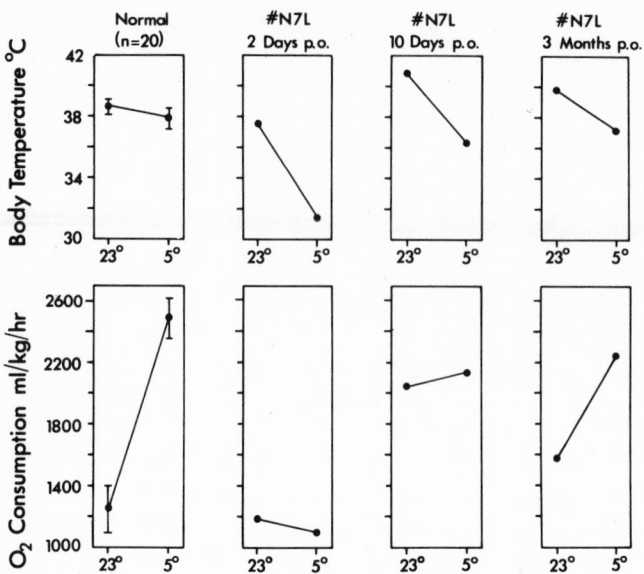

FIG. 7.   Body temperature and oxygen consumption rates for 20 normal rats (first column) and one typical rat with PO/AH lesions (next 3 columns) measured at room temperatures of 23 and 5°C.

rate, or vasoconstrict adequately. Over the course of several months, the animals eventually recovered their ability to maintain their body temperatures in the cold. All the deficits recovered gradually in an orderly sequence, but not at the same rate. Oxygen consumption was the first to appear. In fact, a few weeks postoperatively, the lesioned rats in room air had metabolic rates as high as normal rats in the cold (Fig. 7). Then, more slowly, shivering returned. At first there was no muscle activity at all. Then there was maintained muscle tonus, followed by mild, isolated shivering bursts, until finally rhythmic, violent shivering appeared (Fig. 8).* Adequate vasoconstriction recovered last.

The point is that these three responses, shivering, vasoconstriction, and increased metabolic rate, appeared to recover independently. Normal vasoconstriction appeared in some rats when they were already shivering normally, whereas in others the shivering was still weak. Shivering in the cold

* It is interesting that the recovery of shivering over the course of many months paralleled the phases of onset of shivering within a session of cold exposure in normal homeotherms (Hemingway and Stuart, 1963). It is tempting to speculate that the different control levels of the nervous system responsible for these phases in temperature control in normal animals are the same levels which are recovering differentially in time after brain damage.

was first observed in some rats while they had extremely high oxygen consumption rates in room air, but in others not until the metabolic rate had passed through this high level and was returning to normal. The different responses recovered independently of each other after PO/AH lesions. If these responses were organized in separate pathways, it could be argued that the differential recovery times were caused by more or less damage to those pathways under the electrode tip. In any case, it is not obvious how damage to a single integrative center could produce such results.

5.2. Evidence for Integration

The preceding evidence can explain how one gets coordinated behavioral and autonomic responses from heating or cooling the PO/AH without recourse to a concept of general integration. All the separate pathways run through the preoptic area and the stimulus excites each one independently. However, some concept of higher-order integration is still needed to explain why inappropriate responses are suppressed. Recall that

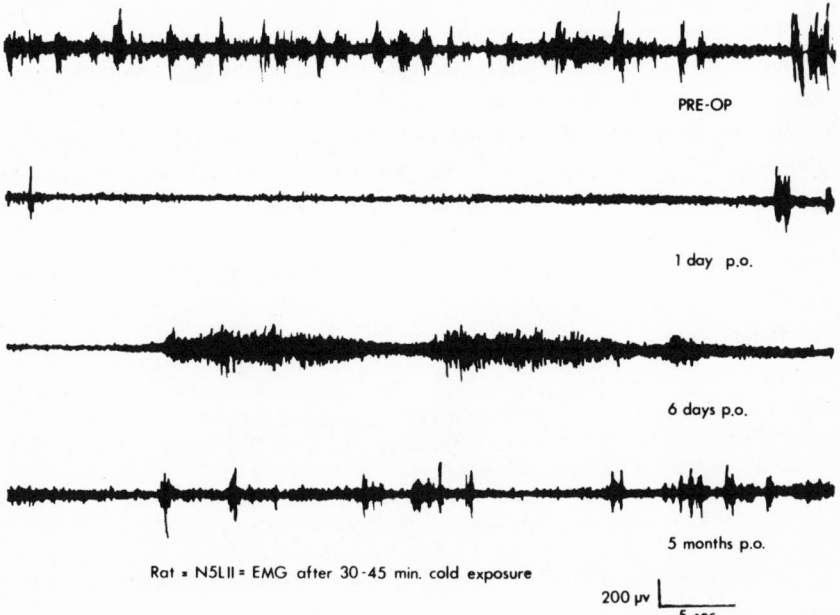

PRE-OP

1 day p.o.

6 days p.o.

5 months p.o.

Rat = N5LII = EMG after 30-45 min. cold exposure

200 μv ⌊___
       5 sec

FIG. 8. Loss of shivering immediately after PO/AH lesions and its sequential recovery over the course of several months. Even after five months shivering is not completely normal. p.o.: postoperative.

high decerebrate animals shiver at low body temperatures while also salivating profusely, a normal response to heat stress. Others pant in a cool environment (see end of section 3.4 for other examples). When the hypothalamus remains with the rest of the brain below, such inappropriate responses never occur. The hypothalamus must therefore be exerting control over lower centers concerned with thermoregulation. Such control can only be exerted by selective facilitation and inhibition and that, after all, is what integration is.

Some concept of higher-level control, involving not only the hypothalamus but the telencephalon as well, is clearly needed. Priorities change. Animals do other things besides regulate their body temperature. Some of these other behavior patterns may require responses which would be inimical to ideal temperature regulation at the moment. But ideal temperature regulation is no longer of prime importance, and thermoregulatory responses may be called into the service of another pattern entirely. A cat in a warm room may be lying sprawled on its side, vasodilated and panting. If an unfriendly dog enters the room the cat will stand up, vasoconstrict, hiss, growl, and piloerect. The warmth is still present, but a more dominant stimulus has activated responses some of which also happen to be part of the animal's pattern in the cold.

The external world contains many stimuli sometimes requiring contradictory responses. Many responses are part of different complex behavior patterns. As long as these patterns are organized in dominance hierarchies, such that the organism can instantly call into play the appropriate constellation and suppress the others, the concept of integration will be necessary.

6. References

Adair, E. R., and Hardy, J. D., 1971, Posterior hypothalamic thermal stimulation can alter behavioral, but not physiological, temperature regulation. Paper presented at International Congress of Physiology, Munich.

Adair, E., and Stitt, J. T., 1971, Behavioral temperature regulation in the squirrel monkey: Effects of midbrain temperature displacements, *J. Physiol.* (Paris) *63:*191.

Adair, E. R., Casby, J. U., and Stolwijk, J. A. J., 1970, Behavioral temperature regulation in the squirrel monkey: Changes induced by shifts in hypothalamic temperature, *J. Comp. Physiol. Psychol. 72:*17.

Andersson, B., 1957, Cold defense reactions elicited by electrical stimulation within the septal area of the brain in goats, *Acta Physiol. Scand. 41:*90.

Andersson, B., Grant, R., and Larsson, C., 1956, Central control of heat loss mechanisms in the goat, *Acta Physiol. Scand. 37:*261.

Andersson, B., Gale, C. C., and Sundsten, J. W., 1962, Effects of chronic central cooling on alimentation and thermoregulation, *Acta Physiol. Scand. 55:*177.

Andersson, B., Ekman, L., Gale, C. C., and Sundsten, J. W., 1962a, Blocking of the thyroid response to cold by local warming of the preoptic region, *Acta Physiol. Scand. 56:*94.

Andersson, B., Ekman, L., Gale, C. C., and Sundsten, J. W., 1962b, Activation of the thyroid gland by cooling of the preoptic area in the goat, *Acta Physiol. Scand. 54:*191.

Andersson, B., Gale, C., Hokfelt, B., and Larsson, B., 1965, Acute and chronic effects of preoptic lesions, *Acta Physiol. Scand. 65:*45.

Baldwin, B. A., and Ingram, D. L., 1967, The effect of heating and cooling the hypothalamus on behavioural thermoregulation in the pig, *J. Physiol.* (London) *191:*375.

Balinska, H., 1968, The hypothalamic lesions: Effects on appetitive and aversive behavior in rats, *Acta Biol. Exptl.* (Warsaw) *28:*47.

Bard, P., and Macht, M. B., 1958, The behaviour of chronically decerebrate cats, in *The Neurological Basis of Behaviour,* CIBA Foundation Symposium, Churchill, London, pp. 55–71.

Bard, P., Woods, J. W., and Bleier, R., 1970, The effects of cooling, heating and pyrogen on chronically decerebrate cats, in *Physiological and Behavioral Temperature Regulation,* J. D. Hardy, A. P. Gagge, and J. A. J. Stolwijk, eds., Thomas, Springfield, Illinois, pp. 519–545.

Barker, J. L., and Carpenter, D. O., 1970, Thermosensitivity of neurons in the sensorimotor cortex of the cat, *Science, 169:*597.

Bazett, H. C., and Penfield, W. G., 1922, A study of the Sherrington decerebrate animal in the chronic as well as the acute condition, *Brain 45:*185.

Beaton, L. E., McKinley, W. A., Berry, C. M., and Ranson, S. W., 1941, Localization of cerebral center activating heat-loss mechanisms in monkeys, *J. Neurophysiol. 4:*478.

Benzinger, T. H., 1970, Peripheral cold reception and central warm reception, sensory mechanisms of behavioral and autonomic homeostasis, in *Physiological and Behavioral Temperature Regulation,* J. D. Hardy, A. P. Gagge, and J. A. J. Stolwijk, eds., Thomas, Springfield, Illinois, pp. 831–855.

Birzis, L., and Hemingway, A., 1956, Descending brain stem connections controlling shivering in cat, *J. Neurophysiol. 19:*37.

Birzis, L., and Hemingway, A., 1957, Efferent brain discharge during shivering, *J. Neurophysiol. 20:*156.

Blass, E. M., 1969, Thermoregulatory adjustments in rats after removal of the frontal poles of the brain. *J. Comp. Physiol. Psychol. 69:*83.

Blass, E. M., 1971, Effects of frontal-pole-ablation on temperature regulation in the rat, *J. Comp. Physiol. Psychol. 74:*233.

Bligh, J., 1966, The thermosensitivity of the hypothalamus and thermoregulation in mammals, *Biol. Rev. 41:*317.

Bond, D. D., Randt, C. T., Bidder, T. G., and Rowland, V., 1957, Posterior septal, fornical, and anterior thalamic lesions in the cat, *AMA Arch. Neurol. Psychiat. 78:*143.

Bures, J., Buresova, O., Fifkova, E., Olds, J., Olds, M. E., and Travis, R. P., 1961, Spreading depression and subcortical drive centers, *Physiol. Bohemoslav. 10:*321.

Buresova, O., 1957, Disturbances in thermoregulation and metabolism as a result of prolonged EEG depression, (in Russian), *Physiol. Bohemoslov. 6:*369.

Cabanac, M., 1970, Interaction of cold and warm temperature signals in the brain stem, in *Physiological and Behavioral Temperature Regulation,* J. D. Hardy, A. P. Gagge, and J. A. J. Stolwijk, eds., Thomas, Springfield, Illinois, pp. 549–561.

Cabanac, M., 1972, Thermoregulatory behavior, in *Essays on Temperature Regulation,* J. Bligh and R. Moore, eds., North Holland, Amsterdam, pp. 19–36.

Cabanac, M., and Hardy, J. D., 1968, Spread of neuron activity from sites of local heating and cooling of the brainstem, *Proc. XXIV Intrntl Cong. Physiol. Sci. 7:*70.

Cabanac, M., and Hardy, J. D., 1969, Réponses unitaires et thermorégulatrices lors de réchauffements et refroidissements localisés de la région préoptique et du mésencéphale chez le lapin, *J. Physiol.* (Paris) *61:*331.

Calvert, D. T., Clough, D. P. Findlay, J. D., and Thompson, G. E., 1972, Hypothalamic cooling, heat production and plasma lipids in the ox, *Life Sci. 11:*223.

Carlisle, H. J., 1966, Behavioural significance of hypothalamic temperature-sensitive cells, *Nature 209:*1324.

Carlisle, H. J., 1969, The effects of preoptic and anterior hypothalamic lesions on behavioral thermoregulation in the cold, *J. Comp. Physiol. Psychol. 69:*391.

Chai, C. Y., and Lin, M. T., 1972, Effects of heating and cooling the spinal cord and medulla oblongata on thermoregulation in monkeys, *J. Physiol.* (London) *225:*297.

Chai, C. Y., and Wang, S. C., 1970, Cardiovascular and respiratory responses to cooling of the medulla oblongata of the cat, *Proc. Soc. Exp. Biol. Med. 134:*763.

Chai, C. Y., Mu, J. Y., and Brobeck, J. R., 1965, Cardiovascular and respiratory responses from local heating of medulla oblongata, *Am. J. Physiol. 209:*301.

Chambers, W. W., Koenig, H., Koenig, R., and Windle, W. F., 1949, Site of action in the central nervous system of a bacterial pyrogen, *Am. J. Physiol. 159:*209.

Chambers, W. W., Seigel, M. S., Liu, J. C., and Liu, C. N., 1974, Thermoregulatory responses of decerebrate and spinal cats, *Exptl. Neurol. 42:*282.

Clark, G., 1940, Temperature regulation in chronic cervical cats, *Am. J. Physiol. 130:*712.

Clark, G., 1960, Heat dissipation function following experimental anterior hypothalamic lesions in cats, in *Neural Aspects of Temperature Regulation,* E. G. Viereck, ed., Arctic Biology and Medicine, Transactions of the First Symposium, pp. 149–192.

Clark, G., Magoun, H. W., and Ranson, S. W., 1939a, Hypothalamic regulation of body temperature, *J. Neurophysiol. 2:*61.

Clark, G., Magoun, H. W. and Ranson, S. W., 1939b, Temperature regulation in cats with thalamic lesions, *J. Neurophysiol. 2:*202.

Connor, J. D., and Crawford, I. L., 1969, Hyperthermia in midpontine lesioned cats, *Brain Res. 15:*590.

Cooper, K. E., Cranston, W. I., and Honour, A. J., 1967, Observations on the site and mode of action of pyrogens in the rabbit brain, *J. Physiol.* (London) *191:*325.

Corbit, J. D., 1969, Behavioral regulation of hypothalamic temperature, *Science 166:*256.

Corbit, J. D., 1970, Behavioral regulation of body temperature, in *Physiological and Behavioral Temperature Regulation,* J. D. Hardy, A. P. Gagge, and J. A. J. Stolwijk, eds., Thomas, Springfield, Illinois, pp. 777–801.

Cytawa, J., and Teitelbaum, P., 1967, Spreading depression and recovery of subcortical functions, *Acta Biol. Exptl.* (Warsaw) *27:*345.

Delgado, J., and Livingston, R., 1948, Some respiratory, vascular and thermal responses to stimulation of orbital surface of frontal lobe, *J. Neurophysiol. 11:*39.

Edinger, H. M., and Eisenman, J. S., 1970, Thermosensitive neurons in tuberal and posterior hypothalamus of cats, *Am. J. Physiol. 219:*1098.

Edwards, D. A., and Roberts, R. L., 1972, Olfactory bulb removal produces a selective deficit in behavioral thermoregulation, *Physiol. Behav. 9:*747.

Eisenman, J. S., and Jackson, D. C., 1967, Thermal response patterns of septal and preoptic neurons in cats, *Exptl. Neurol. 19:*33.

Feldberg, W., and Myers, R. D., 1963, A new concept of temperature regulation by amines in the hypothalamus, *Nature 200:*1325.

Finger, S., and Maickel, R. P., 1970, Lesions of cortical and thalamic somatosensory areas and body temperature maintenance, *Brain Res. 21:*284.

Freeman, W. J., and Davis, D. D., 1959, Effects on cats of conductive hypothalamic cooling, *Am. J. Physiol. 197:*145.

Fusco, M. M., Hardy, J. D., and Hammel, H. T., 1961, Interaction of central and peripheral factors in physiological temperature regulation, *Am. J. Physiol. 200:*572.

Gale, C. C., and Jobin, M., 1967, Further studies on CNS–endocrine responses to hypothalamic cooling in unanesthetized baboons, *Fed. Proc. 26:*255.

Gale, C. C., Mathews, M., and Young, J., 1970, Behavioral thermoregulatory responses to hypothalamic cooling and warming in baboons, *Physiol. Behav. 5:*1.

Guieu, J. D., and Hardy, J. D., 1970a, Effects of heating and cooling of the spinal cord on preoptic unit activity, *J. Appl. Physiol. 29:*675.

Guieu, J. D., and Hardy, J. D., 1970b, Effects of preoptic and spinal cord temperature in control of thermal polypnea, *J. Appl. Physiol. 28:*540.

Guttmann, L., Silver, J., and Wyndham, C. H., 1958, Thermoregulation in spinal man, *J. Physiol.* (London) *142:*406.

Hainsworth, R., and Stricker, E., 1970, Salivary cooling by rats in the heat, in *Physiological and Behavioral Temperature Regulation,* J. D. Hardy, A. A. J. Gagge, and J. P. Stolwijk, eds., Thomas, Springfield, Illinois, pp. 611–626.

Hamilton, C. L., 1967, Food and temperature in *Handbook of Physiology: Alimentary Canal,* sect. 6, vol. 1, Am. Physiol. Soc., Washington, D.C., pp. 303–318.

Hamilton, C. L., and Brobeck, J. R., 1964, Food intake and temperature regulation in rats with rostral hypothalamic lesions, *Am. J. Physiol. 207:*291.

Hamilton, C. L., and Brobeck, J. R., 1966, Food intake and activity of rats with rostral hypothalamic lesions, *Proc. Soc. Exptl. Biol. Med. 122:*270.

Hammel, H. T., Hardy, J. D., and Fusco, M. M., 1960, Thermoregulatory responses to hypothalamic cooling in unanesthetized dogs, *Am. J. Physiol. 198:*481.

Han, P. W., and Brobeck, J. R., 1961, Deficits of temperature regulation in rats with hypothalamic lesions, *Am. J. Physiol. 200:*707.

Hannon, J. P., 1963, Cellular mechanisms in the metabolic acclimatization to cold, in *Temperature: Its Measurement and Control in Science and Industry, Vol. 3,* J. D. Hardy, ed., Reinhold, New York, pp. 469–484.

Hardy, J. D., 1961, Physiology of temperature regulation, *Physiol. Rev. 41:*521.

Hardy, J. D., 1969, Thermoregulatory responses to temperature changes in the midbrain of the rabbit, *Fed. Proc. 28:*713.

Hardy, J. D., Hellon, R. F., and Sutherland, K., 1964, Temperature-sensitive neurons in the dog's hypothalamus, *J. Physiol.* (London) *175:*242.

Hayward, J. N., and Baker, M. A., 1968, Diuretic and thermoregulatory responses to preoptic cooling in the monkey, *Am. J. Physiol. 214:*843.

Hellon, R. F., 1970, Hypothalamic neurons responding to changes in hypothalamic and ambient temperatures, in *Physiological and Behavioral Temperature Regulation,* J. D. Hardy, A. P. Gagge, and J. A. J. Stolwijk, eds., Thomas, Springfield, Illinois, pp. 463–471.

Hellon, R. F., 1972, Central transmitters and thermoregulation, in *Essays in Temperature Regulation,* J. Bligh and R. Moore, eds., North Holland, Amsterdam, pp. 71–85.

Hemingway, A., 1963, Shivering, *Physiol. Rev. 43:*397.

Hemingway, A., and Stuart, D. G., 1963, Shivering in man and animals, in *Temperature: Its Measurement and Control in Science and Industry, Vol. 3,* J. D. Hardy, ed., Reinhold, New York, pp. 407–427.

Holmes, R. L., Newman, P. P., and Wolstencroft, J. H., 1960, A heat sensitive region in the medulla, *J. Physiol.* (London) *152:*93.

Ingram, W. R., 1960, Central autonomic mechanisms, in *Handbook of Physiology: Neurophysiology,* sect. 1, vol. 2, Am. Physiol. Soc., Washington, D.C., pp. 951–978.

Isenschmid, R., and Schnitzler, W., 1914, Beitrag zur Lokalisation des der Wärmeregulation vorstehenden Zentral-apparates im Zwischenhirn, *Arch. Exp. Path. 76:*202.

Jessen, C., and Ludwig, O., 1971,Spinal cord and hypothalamus as core sensors of temperature in the conscious dog. II. Addition of signals, *Pflug. Arch. 324:*205.

Jessen, C., and Mayer, E. T., 1971, Spinal cord and hypothalamus as core sensors of temperature in the conscious dog. I. Equivalence of responses, *Pflug. Arch. 324:*189.

Jessen, C., and Simon, E., 1971, Spinal cord and hypothalamus as core sensors of temperature in the conscious dog. III. Identity of functions, *Pflug. Arch. 324:*217.

Karli, P., and Vergnes, M., 1964, Dissociation expérimentale du comportement d'agression interspécifique Rat-Souris et du comportement alimentaire. *Comp. Ren. Soc. Biol. 158:*650.

Keller, A. D., 1932, Autonomic discharges elicited by physiological stimuli in midbrain preparations, *Am. J. Physiol. 100:*576.

Keller, A. D., 1933, Observations of the localization in the brain-stem of mechanisms controlling body temperature, *Am. J. Med. Sci. 185:*746.

Keller, A. D., 1938, Separation in the brain stem of the mechanisms of heat loss from those of heat production, *J. Neurophysiol. 1:*543.

Keller, A. D., 1963, Temperature regulation disturbances in dogs following hypothalamic ablations, in *Temperature: Its Measurement and Control in Science and Industry, Vol. 3,* J. D. Hardy, ed., Reinhold, New York, pp. 571–584.

Keller, A. D., and McClaskey, E. B., 1964, Localization, by the brain slicing method, of the level or levels of the cephalic brainstem upon which effective heat dissipation is dependent, *Am. J. Phys. Med. 43:*181.

Koizumi, K., Brooks, C. McC., and Ushiyama, J., 1959, Hypothermia and reaction patterns of the nervous system, *Ann. N.Y. Acad. Sci. 80:*449.

Kosaka, M., and Simon, E., 1968a, Kaltetremor wacher, chronisch spinalisierter Kaninchen im Vergleich zum Kaltezittern intakter Tiere, *Pflug. Arch. 302:*333.

Kosaka, M., and Simon, E., 1968b, Der zentralnervose spinale Mechanismus des Kaltezitterns, *Pflug. Arch. 302:*357.

Kosaka, M., Simon, E., and Thauer, R., 1967, Shivering in intact and spinal rabbits during spinal cord cooling, *Experientia 23:*385.

Kosaka, M., Simon, E., Thauer, R., and Walther, O., 1969, Effect of thermal stimulation of spinal cord on respiratory and cortical activity, *Am. J. Physiol. 217:*858.

Lilienthal, J. L., and Otenasek, F. J., 1937, Decorticate polypneic panting in the cat, *Bull. Johns Hopkins Hosp. 61:*101.

Lipton, J. M., 1968, Effects of preoptic lesions on heat-escape responding and colonic temperature in the rat, *Physiol. Behav., 3:*165.

Lipton, J. M., 1971, Thermal stimulation of the medulla alters behavioral temperature regulation, *Brain Res. 26:*439.

Lipton, J. M., 1973, Thermosensitivity of medulla oblongata in control of body temperature, *Am. J. Physiol. 224:*890.

Lomax, P., 1970, Drugs and body temperature, *Int. Rev. Neurobiol. 12:*1.

Magoun, H. W., Harrison, F., Brobeck, J. R., and Ranson, S. W., 1938, Activation of heat loss mechanisms by local heating of the brain, *J. Neurophysiol. 1:*101.

McCrum, W. R., 1953, A study of diencephalic mechanisms in temperature regulation, *J. Comp. Neurol. 98:*233.

McGinty, D. J., 1969, Somnolence, recovery and hyposomnia following ventromedial diencephalic lesions in the rat, *Electroenceph. Clin. Neurophysiol. 26:*70.

Meurer, K. A., Jessen, C., and Iriki, M., 1967, Kaltezittern wahrend isolierter Kuhlung des Ruckenmarks nach Durchschneidung der Hinterwurzeln, *Pflug. Arch. 293:*236.

Meyer, H. H., 1913, Theorie des Fiebers und seiner Behandlung, *Verhandl. Dtsch. Bes. Inn. Med. 30:*15.

Morishima, M. S., and Gale, C. C., 1972, Relationship of blood pressure and heart rate to body temperature in baboons, *Am. J. Physiol. 223:*387.

Mountcastle, V. B., 1956, The reflex activity of the spinal cord, in *Medical Physiology*, P. Bard, ed., Mosby, St. Louis, pp. 1014–1052.

Murgatroyd, D., and Hardy, J. D., 1970, Central and peripheral temperatures in behavioral thermoregulation of the rat, in *Physiological and Behavioral Temperature Regulation*, J. D. Hardy, A. P. Gagge, and J. A. J. Stolwijk, eds., Thomas, Springfield, Illinois, pp. 874–891.

Myers, R. D., 1969, Temperature regulation: neurochemical systems in the hypothalamus, in *The Hypothalamus*, W. Haymaker, E. Anderson, and W. J. H. Nauta, eds., Thomas, Springfield, Illinois, pp. 506–523.

Myers, R. D., 1970, The role of hypothalamic transmitter factors in the control of body temperature, in *Physiological and Behavioral Temperature Regulation*, J. D. Hardy, A. P. Gagge, and J. A. J. Stolwijk, eds., Thomas, Springfield, Illinois, pp. 648–666.

Myers, R. D., and Veale, W. L., 1970, Body temperature: possible ionic mechanism in the hypothalamus controlling the set point, *Science 170:*95.

Myers, R. D., and Yaksh, T. L., 1971, Thermoregulation around a new 'set-point' established in the monkey by altering the ratio of sodium to calcium ions within the hypothalamus, *J. Physiol.* (London) *218:*609.

Nakayama, T., and Hardy, J. D., 1969, Unit responses in the rabbit's brain stem to changes in brain and cutaneous temperature, *J. Appl. Physiol. 27:*848.

Nakayama, T., Hammel, H. T., Hardy, J. D., and Eisenman, J. S., 1963, Thermal stimulation of electrical activity of single units of the preoptic region, *Am. J. Physiol. 204:*1122.

Ott, I., 1884, The relation of the nervous system to the temperature of the body, *J. Nerv. Men. Dis. 11:*141.

Pinkston, J. O., Bard, P., and Rioch, D. McK., 1934, The responses to changes in environmental temperature after removal of portions of the forebrain, *Am. J. Physiol. 109:*515.

Randall, W. C., 1963, Sweating and its neural control, in *Temperature: Its Measurement and Control in Science and Industry, Vol. 3*, J. D. Hardy, ed., Reinhold, New York, pp. 275–286.

Ranson, S. W., 1940, Regulation of body temperature, *Proc. Soc. Assoc. Res. Nerv. Men. Dis. 20:*342.

Ranson, S. W., and Clark, S. L., 1959, *The Anatomy of the Nervous System*, 10th ed., Saunders, Philadelphia.

Ranson, S. W., and Magoun, H. W., 1939, The hypothalamus, *Ergebn. Physiol. 41:*56.

Richet, C., 1884, La fièvre traumatique nerveuse et l'influence des lésions du cerveau sur la température générale, *Comp. Rend. Soc. Biol. 1:*189.

Roberts, W., 1970, Hypothalamic mechanisms for motivational and species-typical behavior, in *The Neural Control of Behavior*, R. E. Whalen, R. F. Thompson, M. Verzeano, and N. M. Weinberger, eds., Academic Press, New York, pp. 175–206.

Roberts, W. W., and Mooney, R. D., 1974, Brain areas controlling thermoregulatory grooming, prone extension, locomotion and tail vasodilatation in rat, *J. Comp. Physiol. Psychol. 86:*470.

Rosendorff, C., and Mooney, J. J., 1971, Central nervous system sites of action of a purified leucocytic pyrogen, *Am. J. Physiol., 220:*597.

Ruch, T. C., 1960, Central control of the bladder, in *Handbook of Physiology: Neurophysiology,* sect. 1, vol. 2, Am. Physiol. Soc., Washington, D.C., pp. 1207–1223.

Rudiger, W., and Seyer, G., 1965, On the lateralization of cortico-hypothalamic relations as revealed by thermosensitive behavior in the rat, *Physiol. Bohemoslov. 14:*515.

Rudiger, W., and Seyer, G., 1968, Thermosensitive bar-pressing behavior of the rat with unilateral lesion in the hypothalamus and during cortical spreading depression, *Acta Biol. Exptl.* (Warsaw) *28:*375.

Satinoff, E., 1964, Behavioral thermoregulation in response to local cooling of the rat brain, *Am. J. Physiol. 206:*1389.

Satinoff, E., 1967, Aberrations of regulation in ground squirrels following hypothalamic lesions, *Am. J. Physiol. 212:*1215.

Satinoff, E., and Rutstein, J., 1970, Behavioral thermoregulation in rats with anterior hypothalamic lesions, *J. Comp. Physiol. Psychol. 71:*77.

Satinoff, E., and Shan, S. Y. Y., 1971, Loss of behavioral thermoregulation after lateral hypothalamic lesions in rats, *J. Comp. Physiol. Psychol. 77:*302.

Seckendorf, R., and Randall, W. C., 1961, Thermal reflex sweating in normal and paraplegic man, *J. Appl. Physiol. 16:*796.

Sherrington, C. S., 1924, Notes on temperature after spinal transection, with some observations on shivering, *J. Physiol.* (London) *58:*405.

Simon, E., Klussman, F. W., Rautenberg, W., and Kosaka, M., 1966, Kaltezittern bei narkotisierten spinalen Hunden, *Pflug. Arch. 291:*187.

Squires, R. D., and Jacobson, F. H., 1968, Chronic deficits of temperature regulation produced in cats by preoptic lesions, *Am. J. Physiol. 214:*549.

Stein, L., 1964, Reciprocal action of reward and punishment mechanisms, in *The Role of Pleasure in Behavior,* R. G. Heath, ed., Harper and Row, New York, pp. 113–139.

Stuart, D. G., Kawamura, Y., and Hemingway, A., 1961, Activation and suppression of shivering during septal and hypothalamic stimulation, *Exptl. Neurol. 4:*485.

Stuart, D. G., Kawamura, Y., Hemingway, A., and Price, W. M., 1962, Effects of septal and hypothalamic lesions on shivering, *Exptl. Neurol. 5:*335.

Sundsten, J. W., 1967, Effects of steady and cyclic hypothalamic thermal stimulation in unanesthetized cats, *J. Appl. Physiol. 22:*1129.

Tabatabai, M., 1972a, Respiratory and cardiovascular responses resulting from heating the medulla oblongata in cats, *Am. J. Physiol. 222:*1558.

Tabatabai, M., 1972b, Respiratory and cardiovascular responses resulting from cooling the medulla oblongata in cats, *Am. J. Physiol. 223:*8.

Teague, R. S., and Ranson, S. W., 1936, The role of the anterior hypothalamus in temperature regulation, *Am. J. Physiol. 117:*562.

Teitelbaum, P., and Epstein, A. N., 1962, The lateral hypothalamic syndrome: Recovery of feeding and drinking after lateral hypothalamic lesions, *Psychol. Rev. 69:*74.

Thauer, R., 1935, Warmeregulation und Fieberfahigkeit nach operativen Eingriffen am Nervensystem homoiothermer Saugetiere, *Pflug. Arch. 236:*102.

Thauer, R., 1970, Thermosensitivity of the spinal cord, in *Physiological and Behavioral Temperature Regulation,* J. D. Hardy, A. P. Gagge, and J. A. J. Stolwijk, eds., Thomas, Springfield, Illinois, pp. 472–492.

Thompson, G. E., and Stevenson, J. A. F., 1965, The temperature response of the male rat to treadmill exercise, and the effect of anterior hypothalamic lesions, *Canad. J. Physiol. Pharm. 43:*279.

Toth, D., 1973, Temperature regulation and salivation following preoptic lesions in the rat, *J. Comp. Physiol. Psychol. 82:*480.

Villablanca, J., and Myers, R. D., 1965, Fever produced by microinjection of typhoid vaccine into hypothalamus of cats, *Am. J. Physiol. 208:*703.

Wampler, R. S., 1970, Changes in sleep and arousal accompanying the lateral hypothalamic syndrome in rats, Ph.D. thesis, University of Pennsylvania.

Weiss, B., and Laties, V. G., 1961, Behavioral thermoregulation, *Science 133:*1338.

Wit, A., and Wang, S. C., 1968, Temperature-sensitive neurons in preoptic/anterior hypothalamic region: effects of increasing ambient temperature, *Am. J. Physiol. 215:*1151.

Woods, J. W., 1964, Behavior of chronic decerebrate rats, *J. Neurophysiol. 27:*635.

CHAPTER 3

Neural and Hormonal Determinants of Mating Behavior in Adult Male Rats. A Review

Charles W. Malsbury* and Donald W. Pfaff

Rockefeller University
New York, N. Y.

During the last 40 years evidence has accumulated that mating behavior results from interactions of steroid sex hormones with neural tissues. In order to study brain mechanisms of mating responses, one wants to describe carefully the elements of the behavior to be accounted for, to know the chemical nature of the inducing hormones, to know where these hormones act in the brain, and finally to study participation in the control of the behavior by pathways to and from hormone-sensitive neural regions. Analyses of these sorts have been applied to a comprehensive study of the neural control over the lordosis reflex of female rodents, during the past few years in our laboratory (Pfaff *et al.,* 1973; Pfaff *et al.,* 1974).

The present review is restricted to the study of mechanisms underlying male mating behavior, primarily in rats. It includes a brief description of the male's responses to the female rat during mounting (Section 1.); analyses of the chemical nature of the hormones which facilitate male sex behavior (Section 2.1.); and a review of sites of action of testicular androgens in the male rat brain (Sections 2.2. and 2.3.). For a complete physiological analysis of male mating behavior mechanisms, it is not sufficient just to explain the hormone-sensitive links of these phenomena. Rather, it is also necessary to identify the neural pathways participating in the sensory-motor aspects of masculine mating behavior, and then to discover the anatomical and physiological links between these pathways and

---

* Present address: Western Psychiatric Institute and Clinic University of Pittsburgh Medical School, Pittsburgh, Pennsylvania, 15261.

the sites of hormone-sensitive mechanisms. It is presumably in the sensory, motor, and higher-order "internuncial" neural pathways that the integration underlying coordinated adaptive male mating behavior takes place. Thus, Section 3 reviews our knowledge on the participation by different levels of the neuraxis in the control of masculine mating behavior.

1.   Brief Description of Male Rat Mating Behavior

Information has been gathered on male mating behavior patterns by studying movie films (Stone and Ferguson, 1940; Bermant, 1965), by electrically monitoring male–female contact (Peirce and Nuttall, 1961) and by quantifying several measures of frequency and duration of male responses toward the female (Dewsbury, 1967, 1968). Our recent work has added detail by analyzing frame-by-frame, high-speed (54 frames per second) color movie pictures of rat mating encounters, taken both from the side and from below (Pfaff, 1971a; Pfaff et al., 1973). Following is a brief description of a "typical" encounter between a highly motivated, sexually experienced male rat and a behaviorally receptive, estrous female rat, which ends with an intromission. At the end of a darting and hopping sequence, the female halts in a crouching posture. The male approaches from behind, and mounts by grasping her flanks with his forepaws, putting his head and chin against her back or neck, and beginning rapid alternating movements with his forepaws on her skin. While palpating her flanks, he moves his hindquarters forward by "walking up" with his hindlegs until his knees and legs are pressing against the backs of her legs and hips, and his pelvic region is pressing on the dorsal surface of her rump and tailbase. Then, he begins rapid pelvic thrusting movements against the rear end of the female. Before and during the initial pelvic thrusts the female is beginning to raise her rump and tailbase both by rear leg extension and by extension (*dorsiflexion*) of the vertebral column. Initial penile thrusts by the male may not be near the vaginal region, usually being off to one side or too far posterior. If the encounter is to end in an intromission, subsequent thrusts approach the vagina as the female lifts her rear end higher, approaching a lordosis posture. Eventually, with the female in or near a lordosis posture, a penile thrust hits the lip of the vagina and either it or the next thrust will include penile insertion into the vagina (*intromission*). By the time of intromission, the female has raised her rump and tailbase so far, and the male has bent his pelvic region so far underneath, that in movies taken from below the male's hindquarters obscure view of the female's ventral pelvic region. Immediately after withdrawal of the penis, if the intromission is not accompanied by ejaculation, the male dismounts with a backward springing movement. The female remains briefly in the lordosis posture, before returning to a normal standing or running posture.

Analyses of the sensory basis of the lordosis reflex in the female rat show that movements by the female play an active role in permitting the male to apply adequate stimulation for her lordosis and in turn for his intromission (Pfaff *et al.*, 1973). Since the successful mating encounter between male and female rat is characterized by active responses from both partners, it is clear that normal fertilization requires the interaction of reflexes in the male and the female. Thus, the male may be thought of as initiating the encounter by mounting the female, but the female's response to his mount and to early stimuli in her pelvic region—namely, her early elevation of the rump and tailbase—allow the male subsequently to apply perivaginal stimulation necessary to bring the estrous female into a lordosis posture. In turn, the assumption of lordosis posture by the female allows the male to bend his hindquarters underneath hers, achieving a position requisite for penile insertion.

2. Hormonal Basis of Mating Responses in Male Rats

2.1. Systemically Circulating Hormones

2.1.1. Testicular Androgens

It is well known that castration results in the decline or disappearance of masculine mating behavior in many male animals (reviewed by Beach, 1948; Young, 1961; Davidson, 1969). The decline of mating response frequencies after castration may be very prolonged, lasting up to several months in male rats (Davidson, 1966a). At least in male cats, the vigor of mating behavior remaining a given time after castration may be related to degree of sexual experience before castration (Rosenblatt and Aronson, 1958).

Administration of testosterone can restore mating behavior in castrated male animals (Reviewed by Beach, 1948; Young, 1961; Davidson, 1969). Recent studies, following up Beach's early work (Beach and Holz-Tucker, 1949) on the doses required, suggest that 50–75 μg testosterone propionate per day given to a 400-g castrated male rat is sufficient to maintain mating behavior scores at precastration levels (Davidson and Bloch, 1969).

Testosterone has at least two types of functional effects in brain: one related to mating behavior and the other to feedback control over the pituitary. The action of testosterone on mating behavior could be direct, by triggering behavior-controlling neurons, or indirect, by altering neurons controlling the pituitary as an intermediate and then by subsequent pituitary hormone changes actually affecting mating behavior control systems. Studies with hypophysectomized castrated male rats allowed independent manipulation of pituitary hormones and testosterone (Pfaff, 1970a). They showed that testosterone injections can increase the vigor of male sex behavior in hypophysectomized castrated male rats as well as in castrated males with pituitaries intact. These experiments were replicated in adrenalectomized hypophysectomized castrated male rats (Pfaff, 1971b). Thus, testosterone has a direct triggering action in the brain affecting male sex behavior, independent of effects mediated by the pituitary.

Testosterone is not the only steroid hormone capable of influencing mating behavior in male rats. Ball (1937), Beach (1942c), and Davidson and Bloch (1969) all have shown that estradiol injections can facilitate male sex behavior in male rats. Recent quantitative studies (Pfaff, 1970b) show that estradiol benzoate can stimulate simple mounting and mounts with thrusts in castrated male rats almost as effectively as testosterone propionate, even though only 10 μg of estradiol benzoate was given per day, compared to 200 μg testosterone propionate. Estradiol also significantly stimulated intromissions, though not as effectively as testosterone. In the same study (Pfaff, 1970b), responses of individual male and female rats to testosterone and estradiol injections were compared. The same individual rats which responded best to androgenic stimulation of masculine behavior also tended to respond best with masculine behavioral responses to estrogenic stimulation. Thus, the two types of hormonal stimulation may be acting on the same or similar neural substrates.

2.1.2. Metabolism of Testosterone

The simplest hypothesis is that testosterone stimulates male sex behavior acting chemically in the brain as testosterone. However, some recent data have raised the possibility that testosterone acts on male sex behavior via chemical conversion either to dihydrotestosterone-5α or to estrogens.

In peripheral androgenic target tissues, such as the prostate, radioactive dihydrotestosterone can be found concentrated in cell nuclei following administration of labeled testosterone (Bruchovsky and Wilson, 1968; Anderson and Liao, 1968; Wilson and Gloyna, 1970). Such chemical conversion has also been observed in the nervous system. Conversion from labeled testosterone to dihydrotestosterone has been detected in a wide variety of brain regions (reviewed by McEwen et al., 1974), and, in general, the conversion to dihydrotestosterone-5α is higher in the hypothalamus than in cerebral cortex (Sholiton et al., 1966; Jaffe, 1969; Kniewald et al., 1970, 1971; Stern and Eisenfeld, 1971; McEwen et al., 1974).

Feder (1971) studied both male sex behavior responses and anti-gonadotrophic feedback functions in male rats following dihydrotestosterone injections, and uncovered the interesting possibility that the chemical specificity for androgen activation of these two functions is not the same. Dihydrotestosterone was not effective in activating male sex behavior responses of adult castrated male rats, but did appear to have anti-gonadotrophic activity in that it reduced testicular weight when injected into immature intact male rats. Thus, behavioral activation might require testosterone as opposed to dihydrotestosterone, while feedback control over the pituitary can be exerted at least as well by dihydrotestosterone as testosterone. McDonald *et al.* (1970) also found that dihydrotestosterone did not activate sex behavior in the castrated male rat. Androstenedione can stimulate male sex behavior as effectively as testosterone, and under the same experimental conditions dihydrotestosterone is barely more effective than control oil injections (Whalen and Luttge, 1971).

Experiments were also undertaken independently in our own laboratory to compare a variety of androgens in their effects on male sex behavior and testicular weight, including comparisons among dihydrotestosterone, androstenedione, testosterone, and control oil injections. In addition, we used the compound fluoxymesterone, a steroid found by Beach and Westbrook (1968) to be ineffective in activating male sex behavior even though it had peripheral androgenic action. In our experiment sexually inexperienced, intact male rats (Sprague–Dawley, from Charles River or Hormone Assay Laboratories) were castrated on one side and that testis was weighed. The next day one of four subcutaneous injection regimes was begun: control oil injections, or 500 μg/rat/day of dihydrotestosterone-5α or testosterone or androstenedione. Twenty-eight days later the second testis was removed, weighed and compared to the first. Injections were continued daily, as before. At this point another group of castrated, sexually inexperienced male rats was added to the experiment and injected subcutaneously with fluoxymesterone 500 μg/rat/day. Three weeks after castrations were completed, sex behavior tests were begun. These were 5-minute tests conducted with receptive female rats two times per week until eight tests were completed for each rat. Each rat was tested individually. The frequencies of the usual male sex behavior responses were scored: simple mounts, mounts with thrusts, intromissions, and ejaculations.

Testosterone and androstenedione both stimulated high frequencies of masculine sex behavior responses (Table 1). In contrast, dihydrotestosterone-5α stimulated less vigorous masculine sex behavior, and fluoxymesterone did not stimulate performance above the control oil-injected level. One characteristic of male sex behavior in this study was high variability. The experiment was actually run in two squads; half the males in each

TABLE 1.   Effects of Subcutaneous Injections of Different
Androgens on Frequencies of Masculine Sex Behavior
Responses in Castrated Adult Male Rats
(Pfaff, Unpublished Data)

Injection	No. of rats	Mean no. total mounts[a] per rat per set of 8 tests 5 min each	Mean no. intromissions[b] per rat per set of 8 tests 5 min each
Sesame oil (0.1 ml/rat/day)	8	8.2	1.2
Dihydrotestosterone-5α (500 μg/rat/day)	8	21.5	4.9
Testosterone (500 μg/rat/day)	8	48.9	14.4
Androstenedione (500 μg/rat/day)	8	58.5	18.1
Fluoxymesterone (500 μg/rat/day)	8	7.0	0.2

[a] Includes simple mounts, mounts with thrusts, intromissions, and ejaculations.
[b] Includes only intromissions and ejaculations.

treatment group being run in the first squad, and the other half in the second. Mean performance within some of the treatment groups varied between the two squads. Furthermore, many individual males' performance varied considerably from test to test. In groups with low mean performance rates this variability took the form of small "bursts" of responsiveness; after tests in which no masculine sex behavior was scored an individual rat might display several mounts and even some intromissions on the next test. Overall, the averaged results are in good agreement with the comparative androgen study by Whalen and Luttge (1971) and the results with fluoxymesterone reported by Beach and Westbrook (1968), as well as agreeing with other authors that dihydrotestosterone is significantly less effective in stimulating male sex behavior than testosterone.

When the ability of different androgens to inhibit testicular growth was measured (Table 2) a different pattern of results was seen. The degree of testicular compensatory hypertrophy was small. However, dihydrotestosterone seemed to be the most effective androgen in preventing testicular growth (Table 2). This evidence of possible antigonadotrophic effects of dihydrotestosterone even in the absence of significant behavioral effects agrees with Feder's (1971) results as well as with Beyer's results with female rats (Beyer *et al.*, 1971) and Davidson's results with dihydrotestosterone implantation in the medial basal hypothalamus (Johnston and Davidson, 1972; Davidson, 1972).

The data above indicate that conversion of testosterone to dihydrotestosterone is not necessary for the stimulation of male sex behavior. Similar arguments apply regarding the conversion of testosterone to estrogen. Initial impetus for study in this field was provided by Beyer and his colleagues (Beyer *et al.*, 1970a,b; Beyer and Komisaruk, 1971), who showed that several measures of female sex behavior could be stimulated by administration of androgens which could be chemically converted (aromatized) to estrogens, while androgens which could not be so converted were not effective. Moreover, Naftolin and his colleagues (Naftolin *et al.*, 1972) showed that small amounts of androstenedione could indeed be converted by brain tissue into estrogens. However, Whalen *et al.* (1972) found that administration of an antiestrogen was not effective in blocking the effect of testosterone on male sex behavior of male rats, even though the same antiestrogenic compound was effective in blocking effects of testosterone on female behavior in female rats. These results indicate that androgen acts on male sex behavior neither by conversion to an estrogenic

TABLE 2. Effects of Subcutaneous Injections of Different Androgens on "Testicular Compensatory Hypertrophy" in Adult Male Rats (Pfaff, Unpublished Data)

Injection	No. of rats	Mean body weight at sacrifice (g)	Mean testis weights (g)		Mean percent change testis weight
			1st	2nd	
Sesame oil (0.1 ml/rat/day)	8	453	1.62	1.76	9% increase
Dihydrotestosterone-5α (500 μg/rat/day)	9	449	1.64	1.38	16% decrease
Testosterone (500 μg/rat/day)	8	462	1.73	1.63	6% decrease
Androstenedione (500 μg/rat/day)	7	434	1.66	1.68	1% increase

hormone nor by acting through receptor sites specific for estrogens. Along these lines, several authors have reasoned that if testosterone acts to stimulate male mating behavior through two separate actions, centrally, as an estrogen, and, peripherally, by maintaining genital structure, then the following "formula" would substitute effectively for testosterone in maintaining high levels of male sex behavior: injections of estrogen (to act on male sex behavior mechanisms in the brain) plus injections of dihydrotestosterone (to act as a peripheral androgen). Although this formula is effective in stimulating male sex behavior (Baum and Vreeburg, 1973; Feder *et al.*, 1974; Larsson *et al.*, 1973) these results do not prove that in the normal case testosterone conversion to estrogen is a necessary step in the activation of male rat mating behavior (Feder *et al.*, 1974).

2.2. Hormones Implanted in Brain

A useful tool in discovering possible sites of androgenic action facilitating male sex behavior has been the implantation of testosterone crystals directly into particular regions of the brain. Previous work using implants of natural or synthetic estrogens into the preoptic area and hypothalamus of ovariectomized female cats (Michael, 1965; Harris *et al.*, 1958) and rats (Lisk, 1962) had revealed that estrogens in these areas can restore female sex behavior, even when the likelihood of leakage of substantial amounts of hormone into the blood was reduced by control procedures. Davidson (1966b) found that pellets (200 μg in weight) of crystalline testosterone propionate best restored male sex behavior of castrated male rats when implanted in the medial preoptic area. Implantation throughout the extent of the hypothalamus, posterior to the preoptic area, was somewhat less effective. Implantation outside the preoptic area or hypothalamus led only to masculine behavior which was infrequent and of poor quality. After medial preoptic implants, rats intromitted enough to reach ejaculation on 57% of the tests, while implantation outside the preoptic–hypothalamic region led to this result on only 20% of tests. Other experiments by Davidson in which smaller testosterone implants were used yielded no positive tests following extrahypothalamic implantation, while the positive regions within the preoptic area and hypothalamus were similar to those found with the large testosterone implants. An essentially similar localization of positive effects has been reported by Johnston and Davidson (1972). Lisk (1967) also found that testosterone implantation in the anterior hypothalamic–preoptic region can trigger male sex behavior in castrated male rats, but little or no masculine behavior was observed in animals bearing testosterone implants in other regions of the brain.

It appears that experiments in which male sex behavior was stimulated successfully by direct application of testosterone to the brain have used larger implants than the size of estrogen implants needed to stimulate female sex behavior in female rats. This apparent inequality of androgen and estrogen implant size may reflect the substantially higher testosterone blood levels in normal male rats (as compared to estrogen levels in estrous female rats) (Resko *et al.,* 1968; Brown-Grant *et al.,* 1970) and consequently, the higher doses required for successful replacement therapy by injection of testosterone in castrated male rats (compared to estrogen injections required in ovariectomized female rats). Finally, this inequality may reflect quantitative differences in the strength of estrogen and androgen binding in the brain (see Section 2.3.). In view of these possible parallels with normal blood levels and with binding studies it seemed worthwhile to compare quantitatively the stimulation of female behavior in female rats by preoptic–hypothalamic estradiol benzoate implants with the stimulation of male behavior in male rats by preoptic–hypothalamic implantation of testosterone propionate.

All animals, both male and female, in our study (Pfaff, unpublished observations) were Sprague–Dawley rats gonadectomized before brain implantation. Before castration, all of the males had tested positively for the presence of mounting and intromissions, but were not given extensive sexual experience with multiple ejaculations. Some but not all of the female rats had been tested for lordosis during natural estrus. Stainless steel 21-gauge guide tubes were implanted in all the rats under Equithesin anesthesia and were directed to the preoptic area or anterior hypothalamus. Prior to behavioral testing either blank 28-gauge stainless steel implant tubes were inserted, or the insert tubes had their lumens filled with crystalline estradiol benzoate (for the female rats) or testosterone propionate (for the male rats). All implanted rats were tested first in blank-tube control tests until low or zero levels of feminine behavior (for the female rats) and masculine behavior (for the male rats) had been recorded repeatedly. Then, the hormone-bearing insert tubes were prepared by dipping the 28-gauge stainless steel tubing into molten testosterone propionate (for males) or estradiol benzoate (for females). The sides of the tubes were cleaned off with a razor blade and with alcohol during examination under a dissecting microscope, so that only the lumen was filled with steroid hormone. We were able to substitute hormone-bearing tubes for the blank tubes either without anesthesia or with brief ether anesthesia.

Since the most important variable for "equating" procedures in males and females probably is the surface area of testosterone or estradiol, respectively, contacting the brain, we attempted to hold this variable constant for all animals in our study by using the same implant tube sizes and hormone-loading procedure.

Females were tested for female behavior as soon as 2 days after implantation, and were often tested at 2-day intervals following, usually with progesterone supplementation (0.5 mg, subcutaneous, 3–5 hours before the test). Males were tested repetitively for male sex behavior with estrous "lure" female rats. A female rat was designated *positive* in response to estradiol benzoate if her lordosis quotient during testing with the hormone was significantly higher than during blank-tube control tests. Male rats were designated positive in response to testosterone propionate implants if the numbers of intromissions during their hormone tests were significantly higher than during blank-tube control tests.

After testing was completed, animals were sacrificed by cardiac perfusion with formalin, and their brains processed histologically to verify implantation sites. The locations of implants in both males and females were found to be in a range of preoptic and anterior hypothalamic sites, reducing the probability that inequalities between the sexes in elicited behavior were due to implants being very near a female sex "center," for instance, while being far from a male sex "center." In addition, seminal vesicle and prostate weights were measured in the male rats and compared to castrated, unimplanted male rats and to normal intact male rats to test for the possibility of testosterone leakage from the site of implantation. The uteri of female rats were weighed and compared to ovariectomized, unimplanted female rats and estrogen-injected female rats to test for the possibility of estrogen leakage from the brain. With these procedures we found no significant leakage of testosterone from the male rat brain. Regarding the female rats, a few showed evidence of estrogen leakage as measured by uterine weight increases, but these were not primarily the rats that showed significant responses to implantation, and no correlation was seen between uterine weight at autopsy and the level of behavior. In other work not reported here, leakage of estrogen from brain implantation sites frustrated our systematic brain-wide studies attempting to define well-circumscribed positive and negative sites for effects of estrogen on female rat mating behavior. However, in the study reported here, leakage did not appear to interfere with interpretation of the results.

In this study, a significantly higher proportion of female rats responded positively with female behavior responses to preoptic or anterior hypothalamic implantation of estrogen than did male rats, with masculine behavior responses, to preoptic or anterior hypothalamic implantation of testosterone (Table 3). Twenty out of twenty-seven females showed significantly higher lordosis quotients with estradiol benzoate implants than during control blank-tube tests, while only five out of sixteen male rats showed numbers of intromissions significantly higher during testosterone implantation tests than during blank-tube controls. This result occurred

TABLE 3. Effects of Anterior Hypothalamic–Preoptic Implants[a] of Testosterone Propionate in Castrated Male Rats and Estradiol Benzoate in Ovariectomized Female Rats on Homotypical Sex Behavior Responses (Pfaff, Unpublished Observations)

Rats and Tests	No. of rats studied	Behavioral response to brain implant (compared to blank-tube control)	
		Positive	Negative
Ovariectomized females, tested for feminine behavior	27	20	7
Castrated males, tested for masculine behavior	16	5	11
		$p < 0.03$ (x^2 test, 2-tailed)	

[a] 28-gauge stainless steel tubes with only lumen filled with steroid hormone. Unilateral placements only. Locations confirmed histologically.

even though the male rats had been tested and found positive for masculine behavior responses before gonadectomy and brain implantation.

Perhaps the simplest interpretation of these results is that it is easier to restore female behavior to female rats with estrogen from a localized source in the basal forebrain than it is to restore masculine responses of male rats with testosterone. This interpretation may be consistent with differences between the affinities of male and female brains for testosterone and estradiol, respectively, as mentioned below.

2.3. Testosterone in the Male Rat Brain: Concentration by Neurons and Electrophysiological Effects

Following the initial demonstration that radioactivity could be detected in the brain following systemic injection of tritiated testosterone (Resko *et al.*, 1967), efforts were made to describe precisely the distribution of radioactive testosterone to cells in the brain of the male rat. Castrated male rats were injected intravenously with tritiated testosterone, and the distribution of radioactivity throughout their brain and spinal cord studied by autoradiography (Pfaff, 1968a). At short times (30 minutes) after injection, high levels of radioactivity were detected in many regions of the brain and spinal cord. At longer times (3 hours) after injection it could be seen that certain limbic and hypothalamic structures had retained radioactivity longer than other parts of the brain. The overall distribution of radioactive testosterone in the male rat brain is similar to that of radioactive estradiol in the female rat brain in that limbic–hypothalamic structures showed higher, longer lasting uptake than cells in most other regions of the nervous system (Pfaff, 1968b, 1972; Pfaff and Keiner, 1973). However, within the limbic–hypothalamic distribution of sex-steroid-concentrating neurons, there were differences in detail between the highest points of testosterone and estradiol uptake. Highest levels of testosterone uptake were seen in the preoptic area, prepiriform cortex, lateral septum, olfactory tubercle, and bed nucleus of the stria terminalis. While radioactive estradiol was seen concentrated in these structures as well, it was also taken up (more highly than testosterone) in the amygdala and in structures in the midline hypothalamus.

Conclusions from the autoradiographic work were confirmed by scintillation counting of finely dissected regions of neural tissue following injections of radioactive testosterone (McEwen et al., 1970a,b). Limbic, preoptic, and hypothalamic structures tended to have higher levels of radioactivity following systemic injections and tended to show better binding site competition effects than structures elsewhere in the brain. Scintillation counting results demonstrated some similarity, as shown also with autoradiography, between the overall topography of estradiol-concentrating and testosterone-concentrating neural systems (McEwen and Pfaff, 1970). In addition, with the quantitative results available from scintillation counting, it was clear that estradiol was concentrated more highly from the blood than was testosterone, had a somewhat more specific anatomical distribution, and showed larger binding site competition effects. Finally, the high level of nuclear concentration shown for radioactive estradiol (Zigmond and McEwen, 1970) has not been seen with radioactive testosterone. This pattern of comparisons between radioactive testosterone and estradiol uptake in the rat brain—similarity in overall topography, with quantitative differences in strength of uptake—is especially interesting in view of the pattern of comparisons between the behavioral effects of estradiol and testosterone (Pfaff, 1971c).

Somewhat stronger binding of testosterone by brain cells has been seen in birds. Compared to rats, the results gathered from cell-fractionation studies in ring doves (Zigmond et al., 1972) and from autoradiographic studies in castrated male chaffinches (Zigmond et al., 1972) have been quantitatively more impressive for their demonstrations of significantly higher levels of testosterone binding in preoptic and hypothalamic tissue.

Concentration of radioactive testosterone by cells in the preoptic area and anterior hypothalamus can be accompanied by electrophysiological effects on those neurons or nearby neurons. Systemic injections of testosterone, or direct application of testosterone to the preoptic region, can alter spontaneous discharge rates or reactivity of preoptic neurons to peripheral stimuli, in urethane-anesthetized castrated male rats (Pfaff and Pfaffmann, 1969a). In part, attempts to interpret these and other electrophysiological effects in terms of behavioral mechanisms have been based on the pattern of electrophysiological effects of testosterone. Thus, the neural coding of olfactory input to the preoptic area, as studied by the differential responsiveness of individual cells to different odor stimuli, appears not to be androgen-sensitive (Pfaff and Pfaffmann, 1969b; Pfaff and Gregory, 1971a). Neither is the behavioral identification of sex odors affected by androgenic hormones (Carr and Caul, 1962; Carr et al., 1962). Thus it seems possible that the coding of responses to female rat odors by preoptic neurons in male rats,—which is androgen-insensitive,—corresponds to the behavioral detection and discrimination of female rat odors by male rats, which also is not affected by testicular androgens. In contrast, behavioral preferences for female rat odors are androgen-sensitive (Lemagnen, 1952; Carr et al., 1965, 1966; Pfaff and Pfaffmann, 1969b). Candidates for the electrophysiological correlate of the testosterone effect on sex odor preferences and other aspects of sexual arousal in the male rat presently would include testosterone effects on preoptic neuronal resting discharge, absolute magnitude of preoptic neurons' responses to odors, and relation of single unit firing to the cortical EEG (Pfaff and Gregory, 1971b; Pfaff et al., 1973).

2.4. Philosophy of Studying Neuroendocrine Mechanisms Underlying Behavior

A strategic advantage in studying neural mechanisms of mating behavior is its hormone dependency, because the tools of experimental endocrinology can be used analytically. Sources of sex hormones can be removed, replacement injections of hormones achieve quantitative control over blood levels, hormones can be implanted to achieve high local concentrations in selected brain regions, and hormones can be labeled radioactively and their distribution studied, all in the effort to gain more information about behaviorally relevant neural mechanisms which hormones affect. Yet, a related danger in studying mating behavior is the tendency to expect that the impact of hormones on individual neurons in the preoptic area and hypothalamus (see Section 2.3.) will explain the entire neural control of mating behavior. Effects of hormones on behavior cannot be explained merely by studying individual hormone-sensitive neurons. Rather, effects of hormones on behavior must depend upon hormone-sensitive neural circuits, in which hormone-induced changes in individual neurons alter the operations of such circuits, so that the "transfer functions" from relevant sensory inputs to mating behavior outputs through sensory and motor pathways and internuncial nets are changed. Viewed in this light, the study of hormone effects on behavior clearly involves tracing circuits using neurophysiological (in addition to neuroendocrinological) methods. In our laboratory, work on the analysis of the lordosis reflex of female rodents has been performed during the past several years with this point of view in mind (Pfaff *et al.*, 1973; Pfaff *et al.*, 1974).

In the section below we review studies designed to show which regions of neural tissue participate in the control of male mating behavior in animals. If lesion and stimulation studies on the neural control of male sex behavior give a coherent picture of which brain regions are involved, then potential neural circuits underlying male mating behavior can be studied with more detailed neurophysiological methods.

3. Neural Basis of Mating Responses in Male Rats

3.1. Introduction

Neural mechanisms of male copulatory behavior may be *sensitized* by androgens perinatally and are partially dependent on the presence of androgens for *activation* in later life. We have some degree of confidence in the preceding statement because (1) we assume a neural basis for copulatory behavior, and (2) experimental evidence has demonstrated the influence of androgens on this behavior (Section 2). However, comparatively few data relate the presence or absence of androgens directly to detailed measures of neural function. This is why the terms sensitization and activation are placed in italics. At the present time they are useful terms when applied to hormonal effects on behavior, but can be given little weight as explanatory concepts concerning hormonal effects on the presumed neural mechanisms of this behavior (Beach, 1971). What do androgenic sensitization and activation mean at the level of individual neurons or neuronal circuits? Answering this question depends on knowing which neurons and which particular aspects of neural function to examine.

The laboratory rat (*R. norvegicus*) has been the species most widely used in studies of mating behavior in mammals. Mating behavior in the sexually experienced adult male rat consists of a relatively complex series of stereotyped actions which are easily quantified by an experienced observer. Elements involved are: recognition of a suitable mate, approach and investigation, mounting, clasping and palpation of the female's sides, pelvic thrusting, penile intromission, and after repeated mounts with and without intromissions, ejaculation (Section 1). Following ejaculation there is a brief period (4–8 minutes) of sexual inactivity termed the postejaculatory interval or refractory period. Sexual arousal can be defined as the state of the animal necessary for the initiation of mounting and intromission. Thus, the degree of sexual arousal has been measured by the latency to initiate copulation after introduction of the female or after ejaculation has occurred (Beach and Jordan, 1956). Large individual differences occur on measures of copulatory activity, but within an individual, provided that tests are given under constant conditions at regular intervals, the behavior pattern often remains stable over long periods of time. For several reasons—ease of elicitation and measurement, marked hormone sensitivity, the availability of previous data describing the elements of the behavior and relevant environmental variables, and its obvious biological importance—copulatory activity of the male rat seems an appropriate subject for the neural analysis of behavior. The material reviewed below concentrates on evidence relevant to such an analysis in the rat, with the addition of comparative data where they are available.

3.2. Sensory Systems

Information about the environment is essential for the initial aspects of the mating pattern: the approach, investigation, and recognition of a suitable mate. Sensory information must be processed by the nervous system and on this basis a "decision" must be made either to ignore, to continue investigating, or to try to mount the mating partner.

Early studies of the effects of sensory deprivations on male copulatory behavior have been reviewed by Beach (1947). In one study both sexually experienced and virgin male rats were deprived of various senses including vision, olfaction, and cutaneous sensitivity in the head region (Beach, 1942a). No individual sense modality was necessary for the appearance of mating, although each of the three types of deafferentation increased the proportion of virgin males which failed to copulate. A combined removal of any two sense modalities in inexperienced animals blocked the development of copulatory activity, but did not abolish the response in experienced males. No particular combination of sensory deficits seemed critical. Beach concluded that the initial arousal of copulatory behavior depends not on any single class of sensory input such as odor or vision, but upon a multisensory pattern.

The limited data from primates seem to follow the same general rule. Michael and Keverne (1968) found that peripheral anosmia in two sexually experienced male rhesus monkeys did not significantly affect measures of sexual arousal or performance when they were tested with an ovariectomized female treated with subcutaneous estrogen injections (control female). They had previously copulated with this control female while showing little interest in two other ovariectomized untreated females (experimental females) before becoming anosmic. Operant responding to gain access to the females was included as a means of testing sexual arousal while eliminating direct contact between the animals. Previous research had shown that the administration of intravaginal estrogen in ovariectomized females increased male sexual interest and mounting. When the experimental females were given this treatment after the males were rendered anosmic, no increase over the original low level of male sexual interest in these females was seen. Intravaginal estrogen did not produce changes in the invitational behavior of the females or changes in the coloration of the sexual skin. Thus, anosmia caused by nasal plugs prevented lever pressing for access to the experimental females when visual cues of behavioral receptivity were also absent while lever pressing and copulation with the control female continued. With olfaction restored after removal of the plugs, the males did work to gain access to and copulate with the experimental females, still in the absence of visual evidence of behavioral receptivity, indicating that olfactory cues, in this case arising from intravaginal estrogen administration, can contribute to sexual arousal in this species. This experiment also demonstrates that neither visual nor olfactory cues of behavioral receptivity are critical for sexual arousal and performance in experienced male rhesus monkeys, but that their combined absence can result in a lack of interest in the female.

Hård and Larsson (1968) have suggested that although no one sensory modality may be absolutely necessary for the occurrence of mating, specific stimulus modalities still may be contributing to sexual responsiveness, and the extent of this contribution may vary from one modality to another. Of course, the importance of an individual sensory modality may vary greatly from one species to another as well (Beach, 1951; Schein and Hale, 1965). Beach's (1942a) findings with experienced male rats agree with the suggestion by Hård and Larsson, as a marked impairment of copulatory activity followed olfactory bulb lesions while no comparable decrease was found in blinded animals. The relative unimportance of visual information for successful copulation in experienced males has been confirmed (Hård and Larsson, 1968) and is also supported by Larsson's (1964) report of normal mating behavior in rats with large occipital cortex lesions, although some difficulty in locating the female and maintaining bodily contact with her was reported in that study.

3.2.1. Olfaction

Deficits in copulatory activity of male rats after olfactory bulb lesions (Beach, 1942a) have been confirmed in several experiments (Bermant and Taylor, 1969; Heimer and Larsson, 1967; Larsson, 1969). In the male golden hamster and in Swiss–Webster mice bilateral olfactory bulbectomy has been reported to eliminate mating behavior completely (Doty et al., 1971; Murphy and Schneider, 1970; Rowe and Edwards, 1972). The effects on male rats are much less severe. Heimer and Larsson (1967) found that after such lesions experienced males were less likely to initiate mounting, and in any given 30-minute session 25–50% of the males failed to ejaculate. When ejaculation did occur, latencies to ejaculate and postejaculatory intervals were prolonged. The number of mounts and intromissions preceding ejaculation was unchanged. Bermant and Taylor (1969) report similar results and also find that the effects of olfactory bulb lesions depend to some extent on the previous sexual experience of the males. Treatment with gonadal or gonadotrophic hormones fails to restore normal levels of copulatory performance after such lesions, thus ruling out the possibility that the deficits are due to disruption of the pituitary–gonadal system (Larsson, 1969). Kaada et al. (1969) studied the effects of lesions in several forebrain areas in a situation in which rats had to cross an electrified grid to approach a rat of the opposite sex. In general agreement with previous studies, olfactory bulb lesions resulted in some loss of sexual motivation as shown by significantly fewer grid crossings for both sexes postoperatively. Although intercopulatory intervals may be prolonged, no obvious disruption of the actual performance of mounts and intromissions has been seen in animals which do begin mounting in any of the preceding studies.

Electrophysiological and anatomical evidence indicates that olfactory stimulation can influence activity in the lateral preoptic area and lateral hypothalamus (i.e., medial forebrain bundle, MFB) in rats, mice, and hamsters (Scott and Pfaffmann, 1967; Pfaff and Pfaffmann, 1969a,b; Scott and Pfaff, 1970; Scott and Leonard, 1971) and that in the case of the male rat, this influence may be modified by the hormonal state of the animal (Pfaff and Pfaffmann, 1969a). It is likely that olfactory structures participate in the initiation of male mating activity through these connections to the MFB and/or those with the medial preoptic–anterior hypothalamic continuum via the amygdala and stria terminalis (see Section 3.5., Limbic System).

Although neither vision nor olfaction are critical for the initiation of mounting in the male rat, it should be pointed out that the importance of distance receptors probably is reduced by the usual procedure of testing animals in confined spaces. These conditions minimize the discriminatory importance of such stimuli while emphasizing their purely motivational effects. Perhaps under more natural conditions these sensory losses would stop males from copulating, not by a direct effect on mechanisms of sexual arousal or performance, but by making it difficult to locate a receptive female. Competition for females with other males might also increase the importance of sensory losses under natural conditions.

Interpretations of mating behavior deficits after olfactory bulb lesions must be limited by the difficulty of interpreting data from bulbectomized animals in terms of simple anosmia (Bermant and Taylor, 1969; Marks *et al.*, 1971; Phillips, 1970). Widespread changes in central neural functioning aside from simple sensory loss may follow such lesions. Alterations of norepinephrine levels after bulbectomy are seen in several brain areas, including brainstem regions not receiving direct olfactory projections (Pohorecky *et al.*, 1969a,b). However, in male rats destruction of the olfactory epithelium and separation of olfactory bulbs from the rest of the forebrain produced similar deficits in male copulatory behavior (Larsson, 1971). This indicates that in this species loss of olfactory input alone is sufficient to produce the deficits.

Another method of producing a simple loss of olfactory input in rats has been reported by Alberts and Galef (1971). They bathed the olfactory mucosa with a dilute zinc sulfate solution, producing a loss of ability to use olfactory cues in a food-motivated task. The effects produced by this method were partially reversible, and are easier to interpret than those resulting from olfactory bulbectomy. Systematic comparisons of the effects of both treatments would be useful in arriving at a more complete picture of olfactory bulb participation in controlling the copulatory behavior of different species. Such a comparison has been reported in the mouse (Rowe and Smith, 1972). They found that although bilateral bulbectomy eliminates male copulatory behavior, peripheral anosmia using zinc sulfate has little effect, indicating that nonsensory olfactory bulb function plays a role in the initiation of male sexual behavior in that strain and species.

3.2.2. Genital Sensations

The importance of the sensory role of the male genitalia has been demonstrated by several studies. Temporary anesthetization of the penis of the rat by topical application of lidocaine or tetracaine interferes with intromission, but not mounting or thrusting (Adler and Bermant, 1966; Carlsson and Larsson, 1964; Sachs and Barfield, 1970). Erection does not seem to be prevented by this procedure in either the rat (Adler and Bermant, 1966; Carlsson and Larsson, 1964) or the cat (Aronson and Cooper, 1968). Adler and Bermant have concluded that lack of sensation from the penis disrupts the process of locating the vagina, which depends on several very rapid shallow thrusts and is normally followed by a single deep penetration or intromission. A disruption of the intromission response attributed to "loss of genital orientation" has also been reported in the male cat as a result of either chemical or surgical desensitization of the penis (Aronson and Cooper, 1968). Sexual arousal was not immediately affected by either method.

Thus, stimulation of the penis in both the male rat and cat is necessary for the performance of the intromission response but not for the initial arousal of mounting behavior. Eventually, mounting attempts by the male rat do wane if intromission continues to be impossible (Adler and Bermant, 1966; Carlsson and Larsson, 1964). Similarly, surgical desensitization of the glans penis of the cat, in addition to causing immediate disruption of sensory-motor coordination in copulation, will eventually produce decrements in sexual arousal developing over a period of many months (Aronson and Cooper, 1968). An excellent study of immediate and longer-term deficits resulting from surgical desensitization of the penis is now available for the rhesus monkey as well (Herbert, 1973).

Although genital stimulation is important for intromission in rat and cat and is necessary for ejaculation during normal copulation, little information is available concerning the effects of such stimulation on central neural activity. Electrical stimulation along the course of the spinothalamic tract has produced genital scratching and seminal discharge in the male squirrel monkey (MacLean et al., 1963) suggesting that sensory information from the genitals may reach the brain through this pathway. A polyspike EEG pattern has been seen in the posterior hypothalamic–MFB area following mounting, intromission, and ejaculation in the male rat, but it is not clear whether this effect is a result of genital stimulation (Ward and Newton, 1970). Chhina et al. (1968) have observed an increase in high-voltage, low-frequency EEG activity from the supraoptic area and mammillary-body region as a result of penile stimulation in the immature male rhesus monkey. These changes were observed only after repeated testosterone injections and were specific to genital stimulation. Although more data are needed to clarify this point, these results suggest that penile stimulation may influence activity in specific hypothalamic areas known to be important for male copulatory behavior.

Strong somatosensory stimulation unrelated to that produced by the receptive female can facilitate certain measures of male copulatory behavior (Barfield and Sachs, 1968), elicit copulation from persistent noncopulators (Caggiula and Eibergen, 1969; Malsbury, 1972), and hasten the appearance of copulatory responses in developing male rats (Goldfoot and Baum, 1972). The concept of an "optimal level of arousal" for copulation may be important in understanding this phenomenon, but it seems that somatosensory stimulation is particularly effective in directing the male's response toward the female. Other types of "arousing" stimulation have been ineffective (Caggiula and Eibergen, 1969). Further research is needed to understand how this artificial stimulation acts to facilitate mechanisms of sexual arousal in the male.

3.3. The Spinal Level

The neural mechanisms necessary for penile erection and ejaculation are organized in the spinal cord below the midthoracic level and are capable of functioning in isolation from other levels of the nervous system. In 1897, Spina (cited in Bacq, 1931) noted that when a spinal transection was made between the 12th thoracic and 1st lumbar levels in the male guinea pig, erection and ejaculation soon followed. Bacq (1931) repeated these experiments and found that within 1 to 7 minutes after transection, rhythmic movements of the anogenital region began spontaneously and were followed by a full erection and then ejaculation.

Bacq also found that sympathetic denervation of the genital organs prior to spinal transection prevented ejaculation, but not rhythmic movements of the anogenital region or erection. Erection seems to depend on parasympathetic activation. Sympathetic denervation of the genital organs was also carried out in rats which later were tested for copulatory behavior. Although these animals were unable to successfully impregnate females, their copulatory activity was described as "normal." However, no details were given. Recently Larsson and Swedin (1971), using standardized quantitative measures of mating behavior, confirmed and extended Bacq's findings for the rat. It was concluded that sympathetic smooth muscle innervation of the genital organs was not necessary for normal mating behavior, including the behavioral response associated with ejaculation.

In general agreement with earlier workers using the guinea pig, Hart (1968b) has found with the male rat that not only are the basic genital reflexes independent of higher levels of the nervous system, but also that they are released from tonic inhibition by spinal transection. Transections were made between the 6th and 9th thoracic levels and testing, which consisted of retracting the sheath of the penis while the animal was restrained on its back, was begun 20 days postoperatively. Four reflexes were described: erections, quick flips of the penis, long flips, and violent leg kicking. The occurrence of the responses in clusters suggested a spinal timing mechanism that might be involved in the normal rat's postejaculatory refractory period. These genital reflexes occur to a greater degree if testosterone is present neonatally (sensitization) as well as when testing takes place (activation) (Hart, 1967b, 1968a). It is unlikely that the androgenic activational effect is a result of changes in penile sensitivity, since facilitation has also been demonstrated with androgen pellets implanted in the spinal cord (Hart and Haugen, 1968). The relatively complex penile responses were seen more frequently in spinal animals than in normal males (Hart, 1968b), supporting the contention that, for vertebrates in general, spinal mechanisms mediating copulatory reflexes are under tonic inhibitory control by more anterior levels of the nervous system (Beach, 1967).

Unlike Hart's (1967a) finding using the spinal dog, ejaculation in response to penile stimulation was never observed in the rat. However, evidence of spontaneous ejaculation was seen. Thus the necessary sympathetic mechanism was left intact. Hart speculated that transections at midthoracic levels prevented afferent stimulation from reaching a higher level of the cord where ejaculation normally may be triggered during copulation.

3.4. Midbrain and Hypothalamic Control

3.4.1. Inhibitory Mechanism

Although the presence of a supraspinal inhibitory influence on copulatory reflexes has been demonstrated for the rat and may be a rather general phenomenon (Beach, 1967), little is known concerning the location and functioning of any particular inhibitory mechanism. Large lesions of the medial brainstem at the level of the diencephalic–mesencephalic junction have produced an enhancement of copulatory performance in male rats (Heimer and Larsson, 1964a). In about 50% of the lesioned males, ejaculation occurred after fewer intromissions and with shorter latency postoperatively. The postejaculatory refractory period was drastically shortened from the normal 5–6 minutes, to 1–3 minutes. Thus, not only was the spinal reflex for ejaculation facilitated, but sexual arousal, part of the appetitive phase of the mating pattern, was enhanced as well. As a result, many more ejaculations were observed in a standard 30-minute test session. The lesions included the posterior, medial part of the hypothalamus, the posterior parts of the medial thalamic nuclei, and the rostral portion of the mesencephalic central grey.

One of the structures destroyed by these very large lesions was the posterior mammillary region, which has been the subject of investigations giving conflicting results. Soulairac (1963), for example, found gonadal atrophy and disruption of copulatory behavior after lesions which included the mammillary bodies. Testosterone injections did not succeed in restoring copulatory activity. In contrast, other workers have found little or no change in this behavior after lesions confined to the mammillary region (Giantonio et al., 1970; Heimer and Larsson, 1964b).

The studies of Lisk (1966a,b, 1969) provide the strongest evidence that an inhibitory mechanism includes basal midline structures at the level of the posterior mammillary region and interpeduncular nucleus. However, most of Lisk's data are not based on direct observations of copulatory behavior. An indirect measure of frequency of ejaculation was taken based on daily counts of the number of copulation plugs found below the cages in which single males had free access to continuously receptive females [see Beach (1966) for a discussion of this method]. Using this technique, Lisk found that small lesions in the mammillary region resulted in an increase in the number of copulation plugs formed and in the percentage of days on which plugs were found (Lisk, 1966a,b). In a later experiment (Lisk, 1969), lesioned males were observed directly in repeated 10-minute tests with receptive females. More ejaculations occurred per test following lesioning, due mainly to a decrease in latency to ejaculate. In contrast to the results of Heimer and Larsson (1964a) who had made much larger lesions, no decrease was seen in the duration of the postejaculatory refractory period or in the number of intromissions preceding ejaculation. Mammillary-body lesions were also capable of increasing the number of copulation plugs found per day for previously sexually inactive males.

3.4.2. Facilitation

3.4.2.1. Medial Forebrain Bundle (MFB). Whereas the inhibition of the mating pattern may involve medial structures at the level of the posterior hypothalamus, much research on the activation of the pattern has focused on more anterior hypothalamic levels. The relative contributions of the lateral and medial preoptic regions to this excitatory mechanism have been studied extensively. Fisher (1956) first reported eliciting male mating behavior in an exaggerated form by injecting minute amounts of a testosterone solution into the brains of male rats. No quantitative measures of the effects produced were given in this pioneering report. Components of maternal behavior or copulatory behavior were seen depending on the site of the cannula. Fisher suggested that the medial preoptic area (MPO) was the effective locus for activation of maternal behavior and the lateral preoptic (LPO) for male copulatory behavior. However, from photographs of representative brain sections, it appears that the effective cannulae for eliciting copulation were actually on the lateral edge of the MPO (Fisher, 1966). The same exaggerated form of male behavior was seen in a few animals using electrical stimulation of an area described as the "anterior dorsolateral hypothalamus" (Vaughan and Fisher, 1962). However, no histological verification or diagrammatic representation of the electrode loci was provided. Madlafousek *et al.* (1970) have demonstrated rather weak facilitatory effects by electrical stimulation of the medial portion of the LPO. Caggiula and Hoebel (1966) and Caggiula (1970), also using electrical stimulation, have shown that facilitation of male copulatory performance can be produced by stimulation of the posterior lateral hypothalamus at points ranging from the level of the ventromedial nucleus to the mammillary bodies. Recently facilitatory effects have been found continuing posteriorly into the ventral, caudal extension of the MFB all the way to the ventral tegmental area of Tsai (Eibergen and Caggiula, 1973).

In summary, the changes attributed to electrical stimulation of the lateral hypothalamic and preoptic medial forebrain bundle (MFB) region have included: stimulation-bound mounting behavior (Caggiula, 1970; Caggiula and Hoebel, 1966; Madlafousek *et al.*, 1970; Vaughan and Fisher, 1962), reduction of the postejaculatory interval (Caggiula, 1970; Caggiula and Hoebel, 1966; Vaughan and Fisher, 1962), and reduction in the number of intromissions preceding ejaculation (Vaughan and Fisher, 1962; Caggiula and Szechtman, 1972). Conversely, bilateral lesions of the middle and posterior MFB can seriously reduce copulatory behavior in male rats without producing gonadal atrophy (Caggiula *et al.*, 1973; Hitt *et al.*, 1970). These studies indicate that portions of the lateral preoptic–hypothalamic continuum, from the most anterior to the most posterior extent of the MFB, are involved in the excitatory aspect of copulatory behavior in male rats.

3.4.2.2. Medial Preoptic Area (MPO). Other studies suggest that the MPO plays a crucial role in the mediation of the male copulatory pattern. Although the LPO–MFB and MPO regions are intimately related anatomically (Matano *et al.*, 1969; Millhouse, 1969), functional differences have been demonstrated. Bilateral MPO lesions can abolish male rat mating behavior without producing gonadal atrophy (Giantonio *et al.*, 1970; Heimer and Larsson, 1966/1967; Larsson and Heimer, 1964; Lisk, 1968;. Soulairac, 1963; but see Lott, 1966). Bilateral lesions of the LPO–anterior hypothalamic MFB are relatively ineffective (Giantonio *et al.*, 1970; Heimer and Larsson, 1966/1967; Larsson and Heimer, 1964) (see

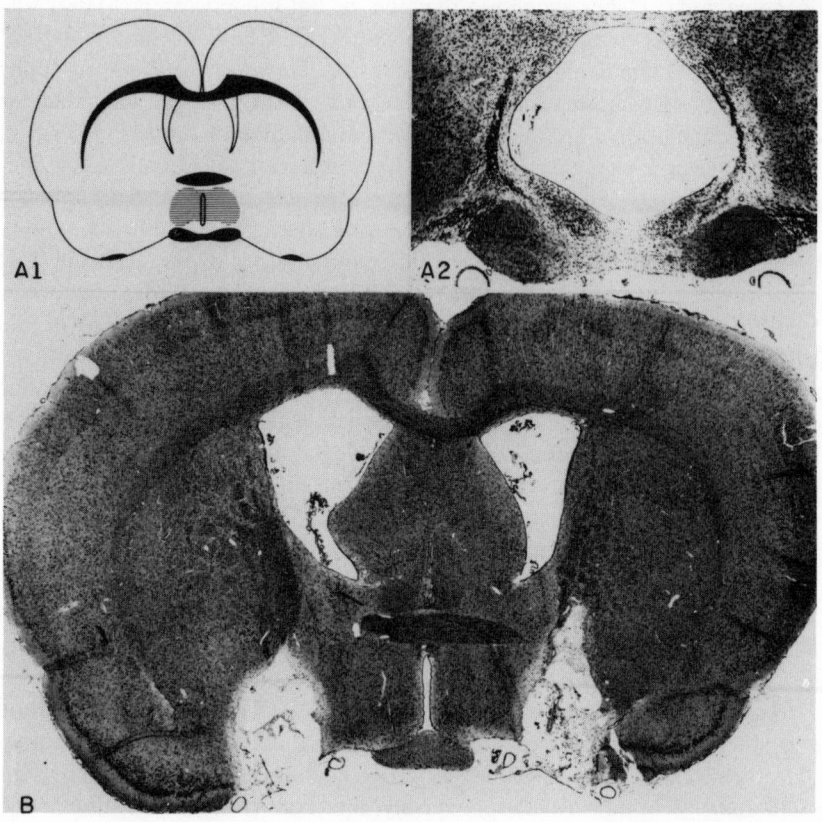

FIG. 1. Coronal sections of rat brains at the preoptic level. A1: Schematic drawing of a bilateral lesion in the medial preoptic area which eliminated male mating behavior. A2: Photograph of the stained section demonstrating how the scar tissue has transformed the normally slit-shaped third ventricle into a round cavity. The intact supraoptic and suprachiasmatic nuclei are seen lateral and medial to the optic tract, respectively. B: Extensive bilateral destruction of the lateral preoptic area which did not cause any change in mating behavior. The medial forebrain bundle is completely destroyed at this level. (From Heimer and Larsson, 1966/1967).

Fig. 1). In the two reports using electrical stimulation to explore both areas, MPO, but not LPO, stimulation was found to facilitate various aspects of male copulatory behavior (Malsbury, 1971a; Roberts *et al.*, 1967).

Roberts *et al.* (1967) explored both the LPO and MPO in the opossum using a very large number of loci (see Fig. 2). They were able to elicit separate elements of male sexual behavior such as teeth clicking, or

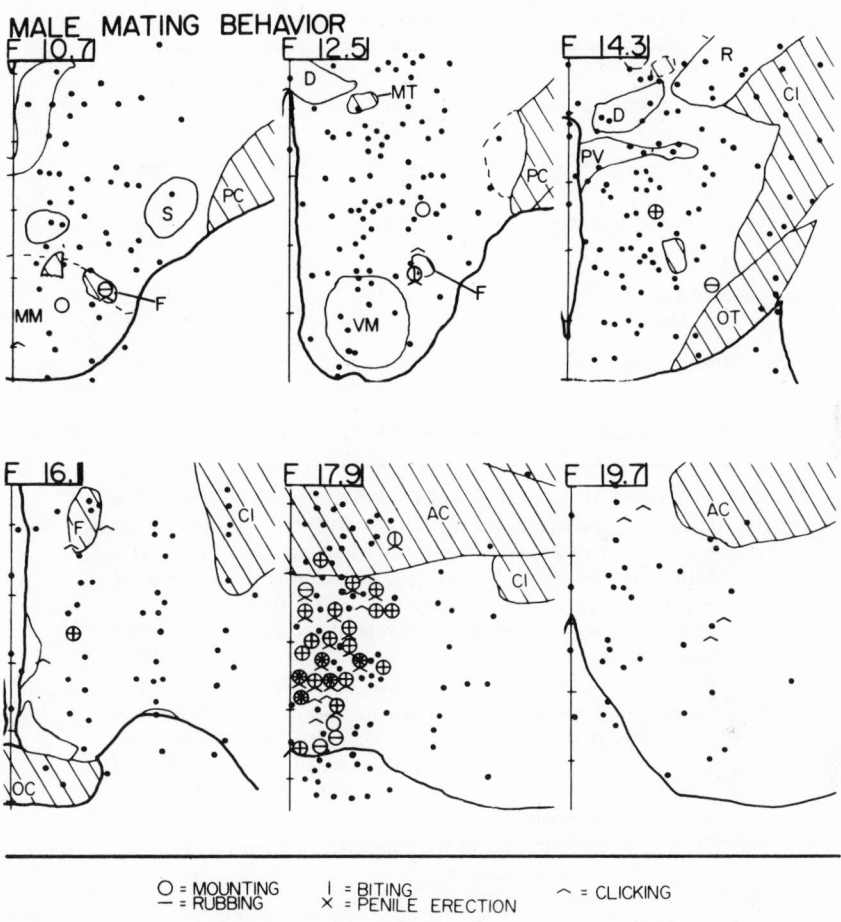

O = MOUNTING   I = BITING   ⌒ = CLICKING
— = RUBBING   X = PENILE ERECTION

FIG. 2. Locations of positive and negative points for elicitation of components of male mating behavior in the opossum plotted on coronal plane diagrams through the hypothalamus and preoptic
area 10.7 to 19.7 mm anterior to the interaural axis. Negative points are indicated by small solid
circles (From Roberts et al., 1967). AC: commissura anterior, AM: nucleus anterior medialis
thalami, AV: nucleus anterior ventralis thalami, C: nucleus centralis, CD: nucleus caudatus, CI:
capsula interna, D: nucleus dorsalis hypothalami; F; columna fornicus; H; hippocampus; HA: nucleus habenularis, HC: commissura hippocampi, HP: tractus habenulopeduncularis, LH: nucleus
lateralis hypothalami, MM: corpus mamillare, MT: tractus mamillothalamicus, OC: chiasm opticum,
OT: tractus opticus, PC: pedunculus cerebri, PV: nucleus filiformis pars paraventricularis, R: nucleus
reticularis, S: nucleus subthalamicus, SE: area septalis, SM: stria medullaris, TH: thalamus, VM:
nucleus ventromedialis hypothalami.

TABLE 4.   Facilitation of Male Rat Copulatory Behavior by Electrical Stimulation of the Medial Preoptic Area[a]

	Control		Stimulation	
	Mean	SEM	Mean	SEM
Duration of ejaculatory series[b]	11.1	1.8	1.2[d]	0.5
Refractory periods[b]	5.4	0.1	0.7[d]	0.1
Incomplete mounts	6.2	1.8	2.2[c]	0.8
Intromissions	18.8	2.0	6.8[d]	0.6

[a] Means (SEM) are calculated from four test days under each condition for a single animal (No. 38). Testing was conducted at two-day intervals and was continued to the first mount with thrusts following the first ejaculation in order to measure the duration of the postejaculatory refractory period. The duration of the ejaculatory series represents the time from the first mount with thrusts following introduction of the female to ejaculation. Stimulation consisted of a 30-sec-on–30-sec-off pattern of $100\text{-}\mu\text{A}$ square-wave stimulation. Stimulation test days alternated with control days. Decreases in measures under the stimulation condition indicate a facilitation of male rat copulatory activity. See Malsbury (1971a) for exact electrode location and details.

[b] Times are given to nearest 0.1 minute.

[c] $p < 0.05$. One-tailed T-tests.

[d] $p < 0.01$. One-tailed T-tests.

mounting, as well as the complete integrated behavior pattern from the MPO, but not the LPO–MFB region in both males and females. Recently, electrical stimulation of the MPO has been shown to produce a dramatic increase of copulatory activity in rats as well. All the facilitatory effects attributed to lateral hypothalamic–MFB stimulation (section 3.4.2.1.) have also been seen with MPO stimulation (Malsbury, 1971a; van Dis and Larsson, 1971). See Table 4 for a comparison of control and MPO-stimulation scores in the case of a single animal showing facilitation on all measures of copulatory behavior. In addition, after castration, at a time when interest in the female had completely disappeared, MPO stimulation in one male continued to produce approach, mounting, and even a few intromissions, but no ejaculation (van Dis and Larsson, 1971).

In testosterone-injected female rats (Doerner *et al.*, 1969; Singer, 1968) male, but not female, mating behavior has been selectively eliminated by MPO lesions. Further substantiation for the importance of the medial area is provided by testosterone-implantation studies. Doerner *et al.* (1968) found male mounting behavior could be produced in ovariectomized females by implants in the MPO–anterior hypothalamus. The most effective sites for reactivation of male copulatory behavior after castration are also in the hypothalamic–preoptic region, with the most consistent reactivation resulting from MPO implants (Davidson, 1966b; Johnston and Davidson, 1972; Lisk, 1967).

The MPO–anterior hypothalamic region also is involved in patterns of male courtship and copulatory behavior in several nonmammalian forms. Lesions here have disrupted copulatory behavior in frogs (Aronson and Noble, 1945; Schmidt, 1968) and chicks (Meyer and Salzen, 1970); electrical stimulation has produced elements of courtship behavior in frogs (Schmidt, 1968), fish (Demski and Knigge, 1971), and birds (Akerman, 1966), and testosterone implants have activated courtship and copulatory behavior in several species of birds (Barfield, 1969, 1971; Gardner and Fisher, 1968; Hutchison, 1970, 1971).

A convergence of evidence from studies using several different techniques has given more information about the function of the MPO–anterior hypothalamic continuum than any other neural area in male copulatory behavior. However more detailed study could possibly be of great value in understanding the way in which testosterone interacts with the nervous system to influence this behavior.

Activation of the MPO is probably greatly influenced by the presence of testosterone. The preoptic region, along with other hypothalamic and limbic areas, preferentially takes up radioactively labeled testosterone into its cell bodies (Pfaff, 1968a; Sar and Stumpf, 1971, 1972). Testosterone-implant studies point to a selective effect of testosterone on MPO neurons as far as facilitation of copulatory behavior is concerned. Although little is known about specific physiological inputs to this area, perhaps MPO neurons are activated by stimuli resulting from the presence of a receptive female and/or genital stimuli, the level of such activation being influenced by testosterone. Thus the MPO may be an integrating area where peripheral stimuli and hormonal levels interact to control certain aspects of the male copulatory pattern.

3.4.3. Intrahypothalamic and Midbrain Connections

Paxinos and Bindra (1971) have presented evidence that connections between medial and lateral hypothalamic areas, but not connections within the medial hypothalamus, are important for male rat copulatory behavior.

Long bilateral parasaggital knife cuts were used to sever the medio–lateral connections of the hypothalamus, resulting in abolition or impairment of this behavior. In most of these rats, cuts were long enough to separate all medio–lateral connections from the level of the preoptic area to that of the mammillary bodies. In contrast, coronal cuts restricted to the width between the fornices at levels either anterior or posterior to the ventro-medial hypothalamic nuclei did not affect the behavior. The lack of deficits in the anterior coronal-cut group confirms earlier work of Clark (1942) and Rodgers (1969). In further experiments Paxinos and Bindra (1973) used smaller bilateral saggital cuts at three separate anterior–posterior levels and concluded that cuts lateral to the MPO–anterior hypothalamic con-tinuum were sufficient to disrupt copulation in male rats.

Although bilateral LPO–MFB lesions have had relatively little effect in comparsion with MPO lesions (Giantonio et al., 1970; Heimer and Larsson, 1966/1967), more posterior MFB lesions have been shown to sig-nificantly reduce male rat mating behavior (Caggiula et al., 1973; Hitt et al., 1970). Results using small knife cuts confirm this picture, as bilateral cuts in the coronal plane are ineffective if placed in the LPO–MFB but sig-nificantly impair male rat copulatory behavior if placed in the ventral pos-terior MFB (Paxinos and Bindra, 1973). The perifornical, medial MFB is the area where Caggiula (1970) most consistently obtained positive stimulation effects. Mating responses elicited by MPO stimulation in the male opossum can be abolished or attenuated by ipsilateral posterior MFB lesions demonstrating a descending output for MPO stimulation effects (Bergquist, 1970). As yet there is no information on how MPO activity may be influenced by afferent fibers ascending in the MFB.

Recently it has been reported that small bilateral lesions just caudal to the LPO in the rostral MFB can disrupt male copulatory behavior in male and testosterone-injected female rats (Hitt et al., 1973; Modianos et al., 1973). These data along with the results of Paxinos and Bindra (1973) indi-cate that the medio–lateral hypothalamic connections important for this behavior are made at the level of the anterior hypothalamic nuclei.

In summary, the preceding studies suggest that much of the LPO–MFB does not contain fibers as crucial for male rat mating behavior as the more posterior MFB, which is part of a necessary circuit, possibly excited by MPO stimulation via medio–lateral intrahypothalamic connec-tions at the level of the anterior hypothalamus. Activation of these descending pathways in the MFB probably results in facilitation of brainstem and spinal cord systems where mounting, intromission, and ejaculation are organized.

The MFB receives input via reticular formation (Wolf and DiCara, 1971) and projects back to the mesencephalic reticular formation (Nauta and Haymaker, 1969). Although the posterior MFB is involved in the facilitation of copulatory responses, only a few studies have explored the possibility that the reticular formation might also be a part of the neural substrate of male copulatory behavior. A slight decrease in sexual arousal (an increase in the latency to the first mount) was the only change in the male rat mating pattern noted after small bilateral reticular formation lesions (Goodman *et al.*, 1971). Large bilateral knife cuts in the coronal plane of the reticular formation at the level of the posterior tip of red nucleus resulted in a reduction in the number of ejaculations in a standard 40-minute session for a group of four male rats (Paxinos and Bindra, 1973). It was later found that invasion of the ventral reticular formation was probably responsible for the deficits (Paxinos, 1973).

Evidence has been presented that various hypothalamic and midbrain areas are involved in the control of male rat copulatory behavior. Basal midline structures at the level of the posterior mammillary region seem to be involved in the inhibition of this behavior, while the MPO–anterior hypothalamic continuum and posterior lateral hypothalamic–MFB region are involved in its activation. How these systems normally interact with each other or with other brain areas is unknown.

3.5. Limbic System

3.5.1. Hippocampus

MacLean and Ploog (1962) have noted EEG afterdischarge activity in the dorsal hippocampus accompanying "throbbing" erection after stimulation of the septum and rostral diencephalon in the male squirrel monkey. These and other behavioral–EEG observations on cats and rats (MacLean, 1957b) have led to investigations of possible hippocampal involvement in some aspect of male copulatory behavior (Kim, 1960; Kimble *et al.*, 1967). Inferences about a specific role for the hippocampus based on this type of evidence are somewhat suspect considering that hippocampal afterdischarge can easily propagate throughout the limbic system (MacLean, 1957a; Creutzfeldt and Meyer-Mickeleit, 1953). Only one group has used more direct methods to study hippocampal influences on male copulatory behavior for species other than the rat. Gol *et al.*, (1963) reported that sexual activity was never observed following bilateral ablations restricted to the hippocampus in cats, monkeys, and baboons, but no preoperative observations of copulatory behavior were mentioned.

Studies using ablation of various areas of the hippocampus in the male rat have failed to find dramatic changes in copulatory behavior postoperatively. Kim (1960) made suction removals of the dorsal hippocampus in sexually active male rats. Such ablations increased the frequency of "mounting acts," including mounts with and without intromission, in standard 15-minute sessions. Ablation of the overlying neocortex alone decreased the frequency of mounting acts. Kim concluded that the hippocampus tends to suppress the sexual mechanism in rats. However, these findings are of limited value as no other measures of the copulatory pattern are given. Kimble *et al.* (1967) also made bilateral suction ablations of the dorsal hippocampus and compared the copulatory behavior of sexually naive hippocampectomized and unoperated male rats. Mounts, intromissions, and ejaculations were scored separately, and no differences were found between the groups.

In two subsequent studies (Bermant *et al.*, 1968; Dewsbury *et al.*, 1968) the effects of both dorsal and ventral hippocampal lesions were examined using more complete descriptions of copulatory behavior. Only sexually active males were used in both studies. Bermant *et al.* (1968) suggested that the locus of damage within the hippocampus is an important variable in determining the effect on copulatory activity. Electrolytic lesions involving the ventral hippocampus or both dorsal and ventral hippocampus produced no significant changes in copulatory behavior as compared to sham-operated males. However, dorsal hippocampal lesions alone did result in significant changes. Intercopulatory and postejaculatory intervals progressively decreased during the second and third postoperative tests, reaching levels which were significantly less than preoperative values. When these data were transformed into a measure of frequency of mounting acts they confirmed the results of Kim (1960). Thus the changes produced by dorsal hippocampal damage may be characterized as decreases in the intervals between copulatory events. No changes were seen in the number of mounts or intromissions preceding ejaculation or in the ability to execute copulatory responses. Dewsbury *et al.* (1968) made suction ablations of dorsal hippocampus, dorsal and ventral hippocampus, and neocortex. The only significant effects of total hippocampal ablation were increases in mount latency and intromission latency. Dorsal hippocampal and neocortical lesions failed to produce significant changes in any measure taken. However, there was a consistent trend for dorsally lesioned males to show reduced intercopulatory and postejaculatory intervals in the direction seen by Bermant *et al.* (1968). Dewsbury *et al.* concluded that differences between their data and those of Bermant *et al.* may have been of degree rather than kind.

Considering all of the data collected using lesion techniques, the hippocampal formation does not appear to play a crucial role in the mediation of male rat copulatory behavior, but the dorsal hippocampus may be involved in the timing of copulatory events through an inhibitory influence.

3.5.2. Septum

The septal area is another region of the limbic system which has been implicated in the neural control of male mating behavior. MacLean and Ploog (1962) have called the medial septo–preoptic region one of the "nodal points" in a circuit involved in producing penile erection in the squirrel monkey. The medial preoptic region has since been found to be crucial for male rat copulatory activity. However, large lesions of the septal area have little effect on the behavior of sexually active male rats (Goodman *et al.*, 1969; Heimer and Larsson, 1966/1967). Species differences may be involved, since feelings of pleasure and increased heterosexual interest have been induced in one epileptic male patient by electrical stimulation in the septal region (Moan and Heath, 1972).

3.5.3. Amygdala

The amygdala has also been studied with regard to a possible controlling function in male mating behavior, since "hypersexuality" was seen as part of the syndrome following temporal lobe resection in monkeys (Klüver and Bucy, 1939). Male monkeys increased their frequency of copulation and masturbation after complete bilateral lobectomies which included parts of the ventral hippocampus, amygdala, and temporal neocortex. The observations of increased sexual activity in monkeys have since been confirmed and the critical region localized to the amygdala (Kling, 1968; Schreiner and Kling, 1956).

Amygdaloid lesions have also been shown to produce changes in the mating behavior of male cats. Wood (1958) found increased copulatory activity in two of five male cats with bilateral electrolytic lesions restricted to the lateral amygdaloid nucleus and ventral claustrum. Suction ablations confined to the amygdala and piriform cortex have produced mounting of other species and inanimate objects as well as "tandem" copulation with other males (Schreiner and Kling, 1953). However, similar "abnormal" behaviors have been observed in normal male cats after repeated copulatory experience in a particular testing room and treatment with exogenous hormones (Green *et al.*, 1957). Green *et al.* (1957) observed changes in copulatory behavior which might be called "hypersexual" only in a rather qualified sense. After lesions in the region of the amygdala, male cats were observed copulating with a variety of partners, including other males, kittens, other species, anesthetized animals, and inanimate objects in an unfamiliar testing room. Untreated males displayed no sexual responses under such circumstances. These authors also found that small bilateral lesions of the piriform cortex were just as effective as combined lesions of the amygdala and piriform cortex in producing this effect. These studies indicate that the amygdala and piriform cortex may be involved in inhibiting the initiation of mating behavior, since the removal of this influence through bilateral lesions results in an increase in mating in situations where it would not normally be seen. No evidence has been reported to indicate that the basic copulatory pattern seen in lesioned males is different from that seen in normal active males.

Electrical stimulation of the amygdala in a single male cat has produced erection, copulatory movements, and ejaculation (Shealy and Peele, 1957), but it is difficult to interpret these data in terms of a specific role for the amygdala, as this structure is prone to afterdischarge activity which can spread through the limbic system. The electrophysiological state of the amygdala itself was not monitored in this study. More recently, Schwartz and Whalen (1965) recorded the electroencephalograpic activity from two male cats during mating behavior and found a decrease in 40 Hz spindling from electrodes in the basolateral amygdala during intromission and an increase in this activity upon withdrawal. No change that could be correlated with mating behavior was seen in activity recorded from suprasylvian cortex, anterior and posterior hypothalamus, or reticular formation.

Unlike monkeys and cats, male rats do not seem to show any increase in copulatory behavior after amygdala lesions. In fact, damage to the amygdala usually results in some decrement in this behavior. Schwartz and Kling (1964) have reported that bilateral amygdala lesions in prepuberal rats resulted in aphagia and adipsia in the majority of the operated animals. The surviving (force-fed) aphagic males did not mate, but this failure was attributed to the debilitation produced by the aphagia. Operated nonaphagic males showed normal copulatory activity. Bermant *et al.* (1968) found that bilateral amygdala lesions produced a large but transient decrease in the rate of copulatory responding, while no changes were noted in number of mounts or intromissions preceding ejaculation. In this study sexually active males were given three postoperative tests begun 13–15 days after surgery and spaced seven days apart. Large increases in intercopulatory and postejaculatory intervals were seen during the first postoperative test, but these changes disappeared by test three. Giantonio *et al.* (1970) also found decrements in copulatory activity in sexually active male rats postoperatively. Their data suggest that specific areas within the amygdala are responsible for this effect. No changes occurred following bilateral lesions of lateral basolateral amygdala, anterior amygdala, or piriform cortex, while lesions of the stria terminalis, and to a lesser extent, basomedial–corticomedial amygdala, produced an increase in latency to ejaculate and a slight decrease in number of ejaculations to exhaustion. These changes did not disappear over the three postoperative tests given at 2-week intervals. In agreement with studies using direct measures of copulatory behavior, Kaada *et al.* (1969) found that bilateral amygdala lesions resulted in a decrease in sexual motivation as measured with their obstruction box method. Interestingly, they also reported that small lesions of the overlying piriform cortex resulted in an increase in the number of grid crossings to reach an animal of the opposite sex. Although Green et al. (1957) have proposed this for the cat, this is the only report suggesting that the piriform cortex may be involved in the inhibition of sexual responsiveness in the rat.

Bilateral destruction of portions of the amygdala in the sexually active male rat results in decrements less severe, but similar to, those following olfactory bulbectomy. This is not too surprising considering that well-established anatomical connections link the olfactory bulbs with the amygdala (Heimer, 1968; Powell et al., 1965; White, 1965) and link the amygdala with the MPO–anterior hypothalamic continuum (Heimer and Nauta, 1969; Leonard and Scott, 1971). The demonstration that amygdala neurons in the male rat respond to natural olfactory stimuli provides further evidence for a close physiological link between olfactory bulbs and amygdala (Cain and Bindra, 1972). Lesions of the amygdala, like bulbectomy, may produce increases in intercopulatory and postejaculatory intervals resulting in longer latencies to ejaculate and decreases in the number of ejaculations to exhaustion. Olfactory bulbectomy sometimes produces more severe deficits in that some lesioned males initiate mounting only irregularly during postoperative testing (Bermant and Taylor, 1969; Heimer and Larsson, 1967; Larsson, 1969). It is possible that the use of a variety of testing conditions might reveal additional olfactory-related control functions of the amygdala in male rat copulatory behavior. In the cat, the amygdala and/or piriform cortex acts to inhibit male mating behavior in unfamiliar situations (Green et al., 1957). It is not known whether this inhibition normally depends on olfactory cues.

In summary, the olfactory bulbs and certain amygdaloid nuclei participate in the excitatory aspect of male rat copulatory behavior, possibly by influencing the activity of the MPO–anterior hypothalamic continuum. In contrast, lesions of the dorsal hippocampus sometimes produce a decrease in intercopulatory and postejaculatory intervals, suggesting that this structure may be involved in a hypothetical inhibitory system. The hippocampus does have strong connections through the fornix to the mammillary bodies, an area suggested by Lisk's work (1966a,b, 1969) to be part of an inhibitory mechanism. None of these extrahypothalamic structures seems to have any influence on the number of mounts or intromissions preceding ejaculation or on the performance of the consummatory responses of mounting and intromission. The influence they do exert on the copulatory pattern is quite weak as compared to that demonstrated for hypothalamic areas. This reinforces the idea that their influence is normally exerted via modulation of activity in the crucial hypothalamic mechanisms.

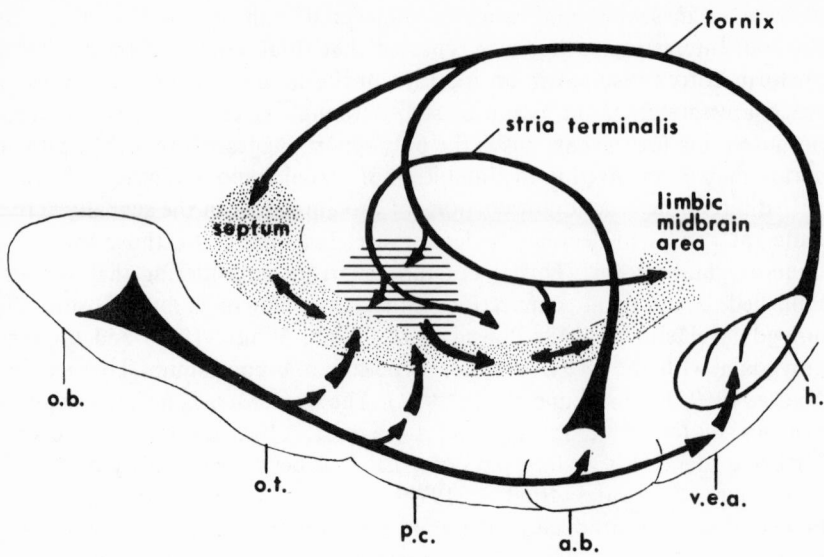

FIG. 3.   A schematic representation of some of the limbic and hypothalamic connections involved in the control of male copulatory behavior. Medial preoptic–anterior hypothalamic continuum is represented by the hatched area, medial forebrain bundle by the stippled area. The connection leaving the MPO and descending in the MFB is based more on physiological grounds than on obvious anatomical evidence. Diagram modified from Heimer and Larsson (1966/1967). o.b.: olfactory bulb, o.t.: olfactory tubercle, p.c.: prepiriform cortex, a.b.: amygdaloid body, v.e.a.: ventral entorhinal area, h.: hippocampus.

Seen in this way, the hypothalamus could be a region of convergence for olfactory and limbic influences on male copulatory behavior (Fig. 3).

3.6.   Neocortex

Complete removal of the neocortex abolishes male mating behavior in rats (Beach, 1940) and cats (Beach *et al.*, 1956) but does not disrupt this behavior in rabbits (Brooks, 1937). Temporary functional decortication after the application of a 25% KCl solution to the neocortex also stops male rat mating behavior for approximately two hours (Larsson, 1962a).

In an effort to understand the influence of the neocortex upon male rat mating behavior in more detail, smaller lesions have also been made (Beach, 1940). Lesions of less than 20% of the cortical surface did not affect the behavior, while lesions including 60% or more effectively eliminated it. Testosterone injections did not restore the behavior, and no gonadal abnormalities were seen, indicating that the deficits were not secondary to disruption of the pituitary–gonadal system. No particular area was determined to be crucial for these effects. The size, not the locus of the lesions seemed to be the important factor. Beach concluded that the cerebral cortex of the rat was involved in sexual arousal, maintaining the excitability of subcortical areas.

In subsequent studies certain cortical areas were found to be more important than others. Larsson (1962b) found that using relatively small lesions of approximately 12% of the cortical surface, lateral lesions were more effective in eliminating male rat mating behavior than medial cortical lesions. The bilateral lateral lesions involved the parieto–temporal area while the medial lesions destroyed the medial parts of the frontal, parietal, and occipital areas. The behavior of the 4 out of 20 lateral-lesioned animals that stopped copulating could not be restored with testosterone injections, and no gonadal abnormalities were seen. In a later study it was found that lesions of the frontal area caused even greater deficits (Larsson, 1964). Eight out of twenty frontally lesioned males stopped copulating postoperatively, while lesions in the posterior cortical areas were ineffective. Kaada et al. (1969) found similar localization of cortical lesion effects using their obstruction-box technique. Taken together, these studies suggest that the sensorimotor cortex, especially the "precentral" frontal area, is important for the initiation of male rat copulatory activity. Kaada et al. (1969) have suggested that an even smaller region, the lumbosacral (genital) division of the sensorimotor cortex, is crucial for these effects.

The apparent contradiction between more recent studies and Beach's conclusion that the locus of neocortical lesions is unimportant can be partially resolved by inspection of diagrams of the individual lesions. Very few animals received extensive bilateral destruction of the important frontal areas, and most lesions were not confined to localized regions in the earlier study (Beach, 1940). Under these conditions it was possible to conclude that the size, not the locus of the lesions was the important factor.

Somewhat different effects have been found with regard to the participation of cortical areas in male cat mating behavior (Beach et al., 1955, 1956; Zitrin et al., 1956). Although copulatory behavior was also most affected by frontal cortex lesions, these deficits seemed, in cats, to be due to motor impairment rather than a lack of sexual motivation (Beach et al., 1955). In contrast, rats which continue to copulate postoperatively display little or no change in the basic motor patterns of mounting and intromission after neocortical lesions. This is true regardless of the size or location of the lesions (Beach, 1940; Kaada et al., 1969; Larsson, 1964). The cortex of the rat seems to be involved more in the arousal of interest in the female and the initiation of mounting attempts rather than in the organization and execution of the responses themselves. Beach (1942b) has suggested that the neocortex may be a locus of intersensory summation and facilitation, its output participating in activating subcortical mechanisms.

It is not known whether the relevant neocortical areas influence hypothalamic mechanisms of this behavior. Evidence for direct anatomical projections of neocortex to hypothalamus is sparse (Nauta and Haymaker, 1969). Indirect anatomical connections could allow the cortex to influence the hypothalamus. However, it is also possible that the neocortex acts on mating behavior via connections to brainstem systems further caudal than the hypothalamus.

3.7. Discussion

3.7.1. Functional Differences Among Medial Preoptic Area, Medial Forebrain Bundle, and Peripheral Stimulation

Beach and Jordan (1956) proposed that two at least partially independent neurophysiological mechanisms are involved in male rat sexual behavior: an arousal mechanism (AM) which mediates the increase of sexual excitement leading to copulation, and a copulatory–ejaculatory mechanism (CEM) which mediates the behavioral components of mounting, intromitting, and ejaculation. The state of the arousal mechanism was held to be indicated by the latency to the first intromission after the female is introduced, and by the refractory period after ejaculation. The state of the copulatory mechanism was held to be indicated by the number of intromissions necessary to achieve ejaculation and by the duration of the ejaculatory series. This theoretical framework has since been elaborated and modified by Beach and his co-workers (Beach, 1956; Beach and Whalen, 1959). Other authors have pointed out its weaknesses and suggested their own revisions of the same theme (Cherney and Bermant, 1970; McGill, 1965).

The two mechanisms were originally postulated as a result of careful and detailed behavioral observation and analysis. Recently some of the strongest support for the proposal that separate mechanisms mediate various components of male behavior comes from studies using direct manipulation of the neural elements involved.

MacLean and Ploog (1962) have called the medial septo–preoptic region one of the "nodal points" in a brain circuit involved in producing penile erection in the squirrel monkey (*S. sciureus*). As erection is also seen in noncopulatory social situations in this species (Ploog and MacLean, 1963), this demonstration alone does not show conclusively that the area is involved in the mediation of erection during copulatory activity. The medial preoptic area (MPO) is the only area from which a normal-looking projectile ejaculation preceded by erection has been elicited in the monkey (*M. mulatta*), although erection without ejaculation has been elicited by stimulation of many other loci in this species (Robinson and Mishkin, 1966, 1968). This does support the idea of a specific involvement of the MPO in genital responses during copulation in the monkey. Seminal emission preceding erection has also been produced from certain other loci in the monkey brain (MacLean et al., 1963). Since these studies all have been carried out in restrained animals, the possible relation of the stimulation effects to other measures of copulatory behavior is unknown. The importance of testing for stimulation effects in freely moving animals is emphasized by the results of Perachio et al. (1969). Although electrical stimulation of points in both the putamen and anterior hypothalamus produced penile erection in the restrained rhesus monkey, only putamen stimulation facilitated mounting of a receptive female in the unrestrained condition.

In summary, electrical stimulation of many points in the monkey brain will produce erection without emission while other points will produce emission preceding penile erection, thus demonstrating a *fractionation* of the control of genital responses in the brain. The MPO is distinguished by being an area from which erection can consistently be elicited in both *S. sciureus* and *M. mulatta* and also the only area from which a normal-looking projectile ejaculation following erection has been elicited.

Roberts et al. (1967) found that the MPO was the only one of a great number of hypothalamic regions tested in which electrical stimulation produced penile erection in the opossum (see Fig. 2). MPO stimulation in the male rat has been found to greatly reduce the number of intromissions to ejaculation and in some cases, in the absence of a female, produced partial penile erections and dribbling from the penis (Malsbury, 1971a,b; van Dis and Larsson, 1971). The release of genital fluid containing sperm not accompanied by erection has been associated with electrical stimulation of the MPO as well as many other areas of the brain in restrained male rats (van Dis and Larsson, 1970). However, the relation of seminal-fluid release seen in a restrained male rat to the mating behavior of the animal is somewhat obscure, as sperm have also been found in fluid released by the male rat during the "marking" of inanimate objects (Pottier and Baran, 1971). The use of chronically implanted electrodes in the freely moving animal was necessary to demonstrate the facilitation of the ejaculatory response during actual copulatory behavior. In summary, it seems that in several species MPO activation facilitates the genital responses of erection and ejaculation, measures of the CEM of Beach and Jordan (1956). These data suggest that neurons in the region of the MPO–anterior hypothalamic continuum form part of the neural basis of the CEM.

Measures of sexual arousal may also be facilitated by stimulation of the MPO and posterior MFB (Caggiula and Hoebel, 1966; Caggiula, 1970; Malsbury, 1971a; Roberts *et al.*, 1967; van Dis and Larsson, 1971). Although activation of the AM seems relatively common with MFB stimulation, this effect is rarely seen with MPO stimulation. Malsbury (1971a) has reported that MPO stimulation in two animals produced short-latency approach and mounting, greatly reduced refractory periods, and dramatically reduced the number of intromissions to ejaculation. However, there were several MPO animals in this study that showed a significant facilitation of ejaculation without showing signs of increased sexual arousal during stimulation. Thus, in some cases MPO stimulation is able to facilitate ejaculation independent of measures of sexual arousal. Activation of components of the CEM independent of the AM has also been reported in the telestimulation experiments of Perachio *et al.* (1969) with the male rhesus monkey. Penile erections induced by anterior hypothalamic stimulation were sometimes accompanied by *withdrawal* from sexually presenting estrus females.

At this time a true facilitation of measures of sexual arousal (AM) without facilitation of ejaculation (CEM) has not conclusively been demonstrated using brain stimulation, but in studies of posterior MFB stimulation the possibility of a functional separation of the two systems has not always been rigorously tested (Caggiula, 1970; Caggiula and Hoebel, 1966; but see Stephan *et al.*, 1971). A comparison of control and stimulation scores within the same subjects as well as tests for post-stimulation inhibition to check for a "true" facilitation of the AM are necessary for this demonstration [see experiment 2, Malsbury (1971)]. In a recent study of MFB stimulation in five rats comparisons of control and stimulation scores revealed that facilitation of sexual arousal was always accompanied by facilitation of ejaculation (Caggiula and Szechtman, 1972).

However, facilitation of measures of sexual arousal without facilitation of ejaculation has been demonstrated using strong somatosensory stimulation in the form of electric shock through safety pins inserted in the skin of the back (Sachs and Barfield, 1974). In the shock condition, males intromitted at more frequent intervals and resumed mounting and intromission sooner after ejaculation (measures of sexual arousal), but the number of intromissions preceding ejaculation (CEM) was unaffected. The neural areas which mediate these effects of peripheral shock are presently unknown.

Data from a study of persistently sexually inactive male rats also supports the assumption of separate arousal and copulatory–ejaculatory neural mechanisms (Malsbury, 1971b, 1972). Fourteen sexually inactive, adult male hooded rats were selected out of a group of 100 animals on the basis of either 15 sessions, 15-minutes each (9 out of 40 animals) or 20 half-hour sessions (5 out of 60 animals) in which they were the only males exhibiting no mounting responses toward receptive females. Repeated tests with electrical stimulation in the region of the MPO (15 of 19 electrode placements) was found to be ineffective in eliciting copulatory responses. Thirteen of these animals were then tested using strong somatosensory stimulation. Back shock was delivered according to the technique of Barfield and Sachs (1968). If no mounts had occurred by 15 minutes into a session, peripheral stimulation was begun. A single shock or tail pinch was delivered every 60 seconds until the first intromission occurred or until a total of 10 stimulations. If 15 minutes elapsed without a second intromission, testing was terminated. If no intromissions had occurred by 10 stimulations using back shock, five closely spaced shocks were given in a last effort to elicit copulation in that session.

Although sexual responses were not elicited from the 14 persistent noncopulators during the brain stimulation tests, the subsequent peripheral stimulation tests were effective in eliciting copulation from 8 of 13 animals tested. (See Table 5 for results.) During sessions in which peripheral stimulation was used to elicit the first intromission, subjects would continue copulating to ejaculation without further stimulation. This occurred in 15 out of 18 instances. It was concluded that the primary deficit in these noncopulators lay in the mechanism which produces the initial intromission response, the sexual arousal mechanism, and not in the copulatory–ejaculatory performance mechanism. This conclusion is also supported by the fact that several males became quite vigorous copulators, ejaculating rapidly during sessions without peripheral stimulation, once this behavior was established (see animals No. 7 and 9, Table 5).

In this experiment MPO stimulation did not elicit copulation from persistent noncopulators. However, in one animal, once copulation had been established using peripheral stimulation, facilitation of mounting behavior by MPO stimulation was seen. During repeated MPO stimulation sessions this animal displayed a mean of 77% of its mounts during *stimulation-on* periods. No evidence of post-stimulation inhibition was seen in this animal when tested in the manner described by Malsbury (1971a).

In an earlier study the most common change produced by MPO stimulation in sexually active males was a reduction of both the number of mounts and intromissions preceding ejaculation. Facilitation of measures of sexual arousal was relatively rare although dramatic when it did occur (Malsbury, 1971a). These data and those from other investigators already mentioned suggests that the MPO is primarily concerned with genital responses. In the rare instances where it occurs, facilitation of sexual arousal by MPO stimulation may depend on prior conditioning whereby genital sensations become associated with the appetitive responses of pursuit and mounting during the development of copulatory behavior in the normal male. Once this conditioning process has occurred, a sudden increase in genital sensations as a result of electrical stimulation of the MPO might initiate approach and mounting. Viewed in this way the sensations produced by MPO stimulation in persistent noncopulators would be meaningless until the full copulatory pattern can be established.

See Table 6 for a schematic summary of the differential effects demonstrated for hypothalamic and peripheral somatosensory stimulation on proposed neural mechanisms of male rat copulatory behavior.

TABLE 5. Development of Copulatory Behavior in Sexually Inactive Males During Peripheral Stimulation Tests. Latency to Ejaculate Is Given to the Nearest Second for Each Rat (Malsbury, 1972)

Rat No.	Tail pinch session[a]				
	1	2	3	4	5
1	X*	34:07*	33:36*	17:13	16:41
2	62:06*	42:49*	42:17	30:14	29:04
3	X*	31:04*	I*	8:05	43:05
4	X*	X*	X*	X*	X*
5	X*	X*	X*	X*	X*
	Back shock session[a]				
6	I*	30:45*	23:25*	23:25*	23:45*
7	32:15*	3:35	5:45	7:45	3:35
8	X*	X*	X*	X*	X*
9	23:45*	7:35	5:15	4:28	5:15
10	X*	X*	X*	X*	32:10*
11	X*	I*	28:10*	27:50*	25:38*
12	X*	X*	X*	X*	X*
14	X*	X*	X*	X*	X*

[a] Tail pinch sessions conducted every other day, back shock sessions given daily.

* Indicates that peripheral stimulation was used. I: Intromission, but no ejaculation; X: No intromission.

TABLE 6.   Differential Effects of Hypothalamic and
Peripheral Somatic Stimulation on Male Rat
Copulatory Activity [a]

Stimulation		Arousal mechanism	Ejaculatory mechanism
Medial preoptic	Common	—	↑
	Rare	↑	↑
Medial forebrain bundle		↑	↑
Peripheral somatic		↑	—

[a] ↑ : facilitation; — : no effect

The importance of olfactory, cortical, and limbic forebrain areas in mediating the initial appetitive aspects of the pattern has already been mentioned. Several studies show that some degree of sexual arousal is still present even after MPO lesions have completely eliminated intromissions and ejaculation. Perhaps the important extrahypothalamic areas are able to maintain arousal by exciting the posterior MFB in the absence of the MPO. Giantonio *et al.* (1970) report that postoperatively, males showed sniffing and pursuit behavior and even palpation of the female's sides, but never any pelvic thrusting. They state that the animals were aroused, but incapable of consummatory responding. Heimer and Larsson (1966/1967) describe almost identical behavior for their lesioned males. Soulairac (1963) reported that in the first postoperative test, intromissions became rarer and were replaced by mounts and thrusts without penile intromission. Over 10 to 15 days all interest in the female disappeared. This successive disappearance of arousal may have been based on learning that successful copulatory responses were no longer possible. These reports indicate that with loss of MPO function experienced males can still be behaviorally aroused by the introduction of the female, but this arousal no longer results in successful copulatory attempts.

3.7.2.   Centers vs. Systems

Bard (1940) and Sawyer (1960) have discussed the concept of a center or centers for mating behavior in the central nervous system. Although other properties are ascribed to the hypothetical center, one of these is that it is a "... locus of integration of the component activities of a total pattern" (Sawyer, 1960), or that "... an outstanding feature of the center is its capacity to weld together individual responses to form a complex reaction pattern" (Bard, 1940). Destruction of the MPO–anterior hypothalamic continuum can eliminate copulatory behavior in the male rat, and electrical stimulation of the region can trigger the entire well-organized mating pattern. This area also seems to be a neural locus for hormonal influences on this behavior as shown by testosterone implant and autoradiographic evidence.

However, it is unlikely that neurons in one particular anatomical region (e.g., the MPO) *weld* together all individual response elements into the complex pattern of male rat copulatory behavior. The review of the evidence in this chapter seems to show that certain neural structures are more concerned with one particular subset of responses than they are with another. The complicated sequence of responses that make up the male behavior pattern can more fruitfully be considered to be the result of the interactions of several relevant neural subsystems, in a temporal pattern partially determined by the behavior of the female (Pfaff *et al.*, 1973). The individual response elements are not integrated entirely by one particular neural area, but by interactions among all relevant neural systems, coordinated by changing sensory input.

The evidence in this section suggests that it is possible to functionally dissect the nervous system with regard to separate components of male copulatory behavior, and that this effort can be guided by a theoretical approach to the data coming from purely behavioral studies. Perhaps *mechanisms* of mating behavior first proposed as hypothetical constructs as a result of behavioral analysis (Beach and Jordan, 1956) may actually be studied directly in certain areas of the nervous system.

ACKNOWLEDGMENTS

Preparation of this chapter was supported by a grant from The Rockefeller Foundation to the Rockefeller University, and NIH grant HD05751 awarded to Dr. Pfaff. Dr. Malsbury was supported by NIH Training Grant GM 01789 as a postdoctoral fellow. Research on testosterone metabolites and on brain implants was supported by The Rockefeller Foundation grant. Research on sexually inactive male rats was supported by National Research Council of Canada Grant No. A.P.A. 66 awarded to Dr. P. M. Milner and a Bursary from the National Research Council of Canada awarded to Dr. Malsbury while at McGill University. The authors would like to thank Drs. Peter Milner, James Campbell, George Paxinos, and Michael Corcoran for critically reading early versions of Section 3. Invaluable bibliographic assistance for this review chapter was given by the UCLA Brain Information Service.

4. References

Adler, N., and Bermant, G., 1966, Sexual behavior of male rats: Effects of reduced sensory feedback, *J. Comp. Physiol. Psychol. 61:*240–243.

Akerman, B., 1966, Behavioural effects of electrical stimulation in the forebrain of the pigeon. I. Reproductive behaviour, *Behav. 26:*323–338.

Alberts, J. R., and Galef, B. G., 1971, Acute anosmia in the rat: A behavioral test of a peripherally-induced olfactory deficit, *Physiol. Behav. 6:*619–621.

Anderson, K. M., and Liao, S., 1968, Selective retention of dihydrotestosterone by prostatic nuclei, *Nature 219:*277–279.

Aronson, L. R., and Cooper, M. L., 1968, Desensitization of the glans penis and sexual behavior in cats, in M. Diamond ed., *Perspectives in Reproduction and Sexual Behavior,* Indiana University Press, Bloomington, pp. 51–82.

Aronson, L. R., and Noble, G. K., 1945, The sexual behavior of anura. 2. Neural mechanisms controlling mating in the male leopard frog *Rana pipiens, Bull. Am. Museum Natl. Hist. 86:*83–139.

Bacq, Z. M., 1931, Impotence of the male rodent after sympathetic denervation of the genital organs, *Am. J. Physiol. 96:*321–330.

Ball, J., 1937, Sex activity of castrated male rats increased by estrin administration, *J. Comp. Psychol. 24:*135–144.

Bard, P., 1940, The hypothalamus and sexual behavior. *Res. Publ. Assoc. Res. Nerv. Men. Dis. 20:*551–579.

Barfield, R. J., 1969, Activation of copulatory behavior by androgen implanted into the preoptic area of the male fowl, *Horm. Behav. 1:*37–52.

Barfield, R. J., 1971, Activation of sexual and aggressive behavior by androgen implanted into the male ring dove brain, *Endocrinol. 89:*1470–1476.

Barfield, R. J., and Sachs, B. D., 1968, Sexual behavior: Stimulation by painful electric shock to the skin in male rats, *Science 161:*392–394.

Baum, M. J., and Vreeburg, J. T. M., 1973, Copulation in castrated male rats following combined treatment with estradiol and dihydrotestosterone, *Science 182:*283–285.

Beach, F. A., 1940, Effects of cortical lesions upon copulatory behavior of male rats, *J. Comp. Psychol. 29:*193–244.

Beach, F. A., 1942a, An analysis of the stimuli adequate to elicit mating behavior in the sexually inexperienced male rat, *J. Comp. Psychol. 33:*163–207.

Beach, F. A., 1942b, Central nervous mechanisms involved in the reproductive behavior of vertebrates, *Psychol. Bull. 39:*200–226.

Beach, F. A., 1942c, Copulatory behavior in prepuberally castrated male rats and its modification by estrogen administration, *Endocrinol. 31:*679–683.

Beach, F. A., 1947, A review of physiological and psychological studies of sexual behavior in mammals, *Physiol. Rev. 27:*240–307.

Beach, F. A., 1948, *Hormones and Behavior,* Cooper Square Publishers, Inc., New York.

Beach, F. A., 1951, Instinctive behavior: Reproductive activities, in *Handbook of Experimental Psychology,* S. S. Stevens, ed., Wiley, New York. pp. 387–434.

Beach, F. A., 1956, Characteristics of masculine "sex-drive," in *The Nebraska Symposium on Motivation,* M. R. Jones, ed., University of Nebraska Press, Lincoln. pp. 1–32.

Beach, F. A., 1966, Sexual behavior in the male rat, *Science 153:*769–770.

Beach, F. A., 1967, Cerebral and hormonal control of reflexive mechanisms involved in copulatory behavior, *Physiol. Rev. 47:*289–316.

Beach, F. A., 1971, Hormonal factors controlling the differentiation, development, and display of copulatory behavior in the ramstergig and related species, in *The Biopsychology of Development,* E. Tobach, L. R. Aronson, and E. Shaw, eds., Academic Press, New York, pp. 249–296.

Beach, F. A., and Holz-Tucker, A. M., 1949, Effects of different concentrations of androgen upon sexual behavior in castrated male rats, *J. Comp. Physiol. Psychol. 42:*433–453.

Beach, F. A., and Jordan, L., 1956, Sexual exhaustion and recovery in the male rat. *Quart. J. Expl. Psychol. 8:*121–133.

Beach, F. A., and Westbrook, W. H., 1968, Dissociation of androgenic effects on sexual morphology and behavior in male rats, *Endocrinol. 83:*395–398.

Beach, F. A., and Whalen, R. E., 1959, Effects of ejaculation on sexual behavior in the male rat, *J. Comp. Physiol. Psychol. 52:*249–254.

Beach, F. A., Zitrin, A., and Jaynes, J., 1955, Neural mediation of mating in male cats: II. Contribution of the frontal cortex, *J. Expl. Zool. 130:*381–401.

Beach, F. A., Zitrin, A., and Jaynes, J., 1956, Neural mediation of mating in male cats: I. Effects of unilateral and bilateral removal of the neocortex, *J. Comp. Physiol. Psychol. 49:*321–327.

Bergquist, E. G., 1970, Output pathways of hypothalamic mechanisms for sexual, aggressive, and other motivated behaviors in opossum, *J. Comp. Physiol. Psychol. 70:*389–398.

Bermant, G., 1965, Rat sexual behavior: Photographic analysis of the intromission response, *Psychon. Sci. 2:*65–66.

Bermant, G., and Taylor, L., 1969, Interactive effects of experience and olfactory bulb lesions in male rat copulation, *Physiol. Behav. 4:*13–17.

Bermant, G., Glickman, S. E., and Davidson, J. M., 1968, Effects of limbic lesions on copulatory behavior of male rats, *J. Comp. Physiol. Psychol. 65:*118–125.

Beyer, C., and Komisaruk, B., 1971, Effects of diverse androgens on estrous behavior, lordosis reflex, and genital tract morphology in the rat, *Horm. Behav. 2:*217–225.

Beyer, C., McDonald, P., and Vidal, N., 1970a, Failure of 5-α-dihydrotestosterone to elicit estrous behavior in the ovariectomized rabbit, *Endocrinol. 86:*939–941.

Beyer, C., Vidal, N., and Mijares, A., 1970b, Probable role of aromatization in the induction of estrous behaviour by androgens in the ovariectomized rabbit, *Endocrinol. 87:*1386–1389.

Beyer, C., Morali, G., and Cruz, M., 1971, Effect of 5-α-dihydrotestosterone on gonadotropin secretion and estrous behavior in the female Wistar rat, *Endocrinol. 89:*1158–1161.

Brooks, C. M., 1937, The role of the cerebral cortex and of various sense organs in the excitation and execution of mating activity in the rabbit, *Am. J. Physiol. 120:*544–553.

Brown-Grant, K., Exley, D., and Naftolin, F., 1970, Peripheral plasma oestradiol and luteinizing hormone concentrations during the oestrus cycle of the rat, *J. Endocrinol. 48:*295–296.

Bruchovsky, N., and Wilson, J. D., 1968, The conversion of testosterone to 5α-androstan-17B-ol-3-one by rat prostate *in vivo* and *in vitro, J. Biol. Chem. 243:*2012–2021.

Caggiula, A. R., 1970, Analysis of the copulation-reward properties of posterior hypothalamic stimulation in male rats, *J. Comp. Physiol. Psychol. 70:*399–412.

Caggiula, A. R., and Eibergen, R., 1969, Copulation of virgin male rats evoked by painful peripheral stimulation, *J. Comp. Physiol. Psychol. 69:*414–419.

Caggiula, A. R., and Hoebel, B. G., 1966, "Copulation-Reward Site" in the posterior hypothalamus, *Science 153:*1284–1285.

Caggiula, A. R., and Szechtman, H., 1972, Hypothalamic stimulation: A biphasic influence on copulation of the male rat, *Behav. Biol. 7:*591–598.

Caggiula, A. R., Antelman, S. M., and Zigmond, M. J., 1973, Disruption of copulation in male rats after hypothalamic lesions: A behavioral, anatomical and neurochemical analysis, *Brain Res. 59:*273–287.

Cain, D. P., and Bindra, D., 1972, Response of amygdala single units to odors in the rat, *Expl. Neurol. 35:*98–110.

Carlsson, S. G., and Larsson, K., 1964, Mating in male rats after local anesthetization of the glans penis, *Z. Tierpsychol. 21:*854–856.

Carr, W. J., and Caul, W. F., 1962, The effect of castration in the rat upon the discrimination of sex odors, *Anim. Behav. 10:*20–27.

Carr, W. J., Loeb, L. S., and Dissinger, M. L., 1965, Responses of rats to sex odors, *J. Comp. Physiol. Psychol. 59:*370–377.

Carr, W. J., Loeb, L. S., and Wylie, N. R., 1966, Responses to feminine odors in normal and castrated male rats, *J. Comp. Physiol. Psychol. 62:*336–338.

Carr, W. J., Solberg, B., and Pfaffmann, C., 1962, The olfactory threshold for estrous female urine in normal and castrated male rats, *J. Comp. Physiol. Psychol. 55:*415–417.

Cherney, E. F., and Bermant, G., 1970, The role of stimulus female novelty in the rearousal of copulation in male laboratory rats (*Rattus norvegicus*), *Anim. Behav. 18:*567–574.

Chhina, G. S., Chakrabarty, A. S., Kaur, K., and Anand, B. K., 1968, Electroencephalographic responses produced by genital stimulation and hormone administration in sexually immature rhesus monkeys, *Physiol. Behav. 3:*579–584.

Clark, G., 1942, Depressed sexual activity by lesion in medial part of anterior hypothalamus, *Am. J. Physiol. 137:*746.

Creutzfeldt, O. D., and Meyer-Mickeleit, R. W., 1953, Patterns of convulsive discharges of the hippocampus and their propagation, *Electroenceph. Clin. Neurophysiol.* (Suppl. 3), 43.

Davidson, J. M., 1966a, Characteristics of sex behavior in male rats following castration, *Anim. Behav. 14:*266–272.

Davidson, J. M., 1966b, Activation of the male rat's sexual behavior by intracerebral implantation of androgen, *Endocrinol. 79:*783–794.

Davidson, J. M., 1969, Hormonal control of sexual behavior in adult rats, in: *Advances in the Biosciences, Vol. 1.* Schering Symposium on Endocrinology, G. Raspe, ed., Pergamon, Oxford, pp. 119–141.

Davidson, J. M., 1973, Feedback of steroid hormones in relation to reproduction, *Progress in Endocrinology, Proceedings of the IV International Congress of Endocrinology,* (C. Gual, ed.) Excerpt Medica Internat. Congress Series.

Davidson, J. M., and Bloch, G. J., 1969, Neuroendocrine aspects of male reproduction. *Biol. Reproduction 1:*67–92.

Demski, L. S., and Knigge, K. M., 1971, The telencephalon and hypothalamus of the bluegill (*Lepomis macrochirus*): Evoked feeding, aggressive and reproductive behavior with representative frontal sections, *J. Comp. Neurol. 143:*1–16.

Dewsbury, D. A., 1967, A quantitative description of the behavior of rats during copulation, *Behav. 24:*154–178.

Dewsbury, D. A., 1968, Copulatory behavior in rats: Changes as satiety is approached. *Psychol. Rep. 22:*937–943.

Dewsbury, D. A., Goodman, E. D., Salis, P. J., and Bunnell, B. N., 1968, Effects of hippocampal lesions on the copulatory behavior of male rats, *Physiol. Behav. 3:*651–656.

Doerner, G., Doecke, F., and Hinz, G., 1969, Homo- and hypersexuality in rats with hypothalamic lesions, *Neuroendocrinol. 4:*20–24.

Doerner, G., Doecke, F., and Moustafa, S., 1968, Homosexuality in female rats following testosterone implantation in the anterior hypothalamus, *J. Reproduction Fertility 17:*173–175.

Doty, R. L., Carter, C. S., and Clemens, L. G., 1971, Olfactory control of sexual behavior in the male and early-androgenized female hamster, *Horm. Behav. 2:*325–335.

Eibergen, R. D., and Caggiula, A. R., 1973, Ventral midbrain involvement in copulatory behavior of the male rat, *Physiol. Behav. 10:*435–442.

Feder, H. H., 1971, The comparative actions of testosterone propionate and 5α-androstan-17B-ol-3-one propionate on the reproductive behaviour, physiology and morphology of male rats, *J. Endocrinol. 51:*241–252.

Feder, H. H., Naftolin, F., and Ryan, K. J., 1974, Male and female sexual responses in male rats given estradiol benzoate and 5α-androstan-17β-ol-3-one propionate, *Endocrinol. 94:*136–141.

Fisher, A. E., 1956, Maternal and sexual behavior induced by intracranial chemical stimulation, *Science 124:*228–229.

Fisher, A. E., 1966, Chemical and electrical stimulation of the brain in the male rat, in *Brain and Behavior, III, The Brain and Gonadal Function,* R. A. Gorski, and R. E. Whalen, eds., University of California Press, Berkeley, pp. 117–130.

Gardner, J. E., and Fisher, A. E., 1968, Induction of mating in male chicks following preoptic implantation of androgen, *Physiol. Behav. 3:*709–712.

Giantonio, G. W., Lund, N. L., and Gerall, A. A., 1970, Effect of diencephalic and rhinencephalic lesions on the male rat's sexual behavior, *J. Comp. Physiol. Psychol. 73:*38–46.

Gol, A., Kellaway, P., Shapiro, M., and Hurst, C. M., 1963, Studies of hippocampectomy in the monkey, baboon and cat, *Neurol. 13:*1031–1041.

Goldfoot, D. A., and Baum, M. J., 1972, Initiation of mating behavior in developing male rats following peripheral electric shock, *Physiol. Behav. 8:*857–864.

Goodman, E. D., Bunnell, B. N., Dewsbury, D. A., and Boland, B., 1969, Septal lesions and male rat copulatory behavior, *Psychon. Sci. 16:*123–124.

Goodman, E. D., Jansen, P. E., and Dewsbury, D. A., 1971, Midbrain reticular formation lesions: Habituation to stimulation and copulatory behavior in male rats, *Physiol. Behav. 6:*151–156.

Green, J. D., Clemente, C. D., and De Groot, J., 1957, Rhinencephalic lesions and behavior in cats, *J. Comp. Neurol. 108:*505–545.

Hård, E., and Larsson, K., 1968, Visual stimulation and mating behavior in male rats, *J. Comp. Physiol. Psychol. 66:*805–807.

Harris, G. W., Michael, R. P., and Scott, P. P., 1958, Neurological site of action of stilboestrol in eliciting sexual behavior, in *Ciba Foundation Symposium on the Neurological Basis of Behavior,* G. E. W. Wolstenholme, and C. M. O'Connor, eds., Little, Brown & Co., Boston.

Hart, B. L., 1967a, Sexual reflexes and mating behavior in the male dog, *J. Comp. Physiol. Psychol. 64:*388–399.

Hart, B. L., 1967b, Testosterone regulation of sexual reflexes in spinal male rats, *Science 155:*1283–1284.

Hart, B. L., 1968a, Neonatal castration: Influence on neural organization of sexual reflexes in male rats, *Science 160:*1135–1136.

Hart, B. L., 1968b, Sexual reflexes and mating behavior in the male rat, *J. Comp. Physiol. Psychol. 65:*453–460.

Hart, B. L., and Haugen, C. M., 1968, Activation of sexual reflexes in male rats by spinal implantation of testosterone, *Physiol. Behav. 3:*735–738.

Heimer, L., 1968, Synaptic distribution of centripetal and centrifugal nerve fibers in the olfactory system of the rat. An experimental anatomical study, *J. Anat. 103:*413–432.

Heimer, L., and Larsson, K., 1964a, Drastic changes in the mating behaviour of male rats following lesions in the junction of diencephalon and mesencephalon, *Experientia 20:*460–461.

Heimer, L., and Larsson, K., 1964b, Mating behavior in male rats after destruction of the mammillary bodies, *Acta Neurol. Scand. 40:*353–360.

Heimer, L., and Larsson, K., 1966/67, Impairment of mating behavior in male rats following lesions in the preoptic-anterior hypothalamic continuum, *Brain Res. 3:*248–263.

Heimer, L., and Larsson, K., 1967, Mating behavior of male rats after olfactory bulb lesions, *Physiol. Behav. 2:*207–209.

Heimer, L., and Nauta, W. J. H., 1969, The hypothalamic distribution of the stria terminalis in the rat, *Brain Res. 13:*284–297.

Herbert, J., 1973, The role of the dorsal nerves of the penis in the sexual behaviour of the male rhesus monkey, *Physiol. Behav. 10:*293–300.

Hitt, J. C., Hendricks, S. E., Ginsberg, S. I., and Lewis, J. H., 1970, Disruption of male, but not female, sexual behavior in rats by medial forebrain bundle lesions, *J. Comp. Physiol. Psychol. 73:*377–384.

Hitt, J. C., Bryon, D. M., and Modianos, D. T., 1973, Effects of rostral medial forebrain bundle and olfactory tubercle lesions upon the sexual behavior of male rats, *J. Comp. Physiol. Psychol. 82:*30–36.

Hutchison, J. B., 1970, Influence of gonadal hormones on the hypothalamic integration of courtship behaviour in the Barbary dove, *J. Reproduction Fertility, 11* (Suppl.):15–41.

Hutchison, J. B., 1971, Effects of hypothalamic implants of gonadal steroids on courtship behavior in Barbary doves (Streptopelia risoria), *J. Endocrinol. 50:*97–113.

Jaffe, R. B., 1969, Testosterone metabolism in target tissues: Hypothalamic and pituitary tissues of the adult rat and human fetus, and the immature rat epiphysis, *Steroids 14:*483–489.

Johnston, P., and Davidson, J. M., 1972, Intracerebral androgens and sexual behavior in the male rat, *Horm. and Behav. 3:*345–357.

Kaada, B. R., Rasmussen, E. W., and Bruland, H., 1969, Approach behavior towards a sex incentive following forebrain lesions in rats, *Int. J. Neurol. 6:*306–323.

Kim, C., 1960, Sexual activity of male rats following ablation of hippocampus, *J. Comp. Physiol. Psychol. 53:*553–557.

Kimble, D. P., Rogers, L., and Hendrickson, C. W., 1967, Hippocampal lesions disrupt maternal, not sexual, behavior in the albino rat, *J. Comp. Physiol. Psychol. 63:*401–407.

Kling, A., 1968, Effects of amygdalectomy and testosterone on sexual behavior of male juvenile macaques, *J. Comp. Physiol. Psychol. 65:*466–471.

Klüver, H., and Bucy, P. C., 1939, Preliminary analysis of functions of the temporal lobes in monkeys, *Arch. Neurol. Psychiat. 42:*979–1000.

Kniewald, Z., Massa, R., and Martini, L., 1970, The transformation of testosterone into dihydrotestosterone by the anterior pituitary and the hypothalamus, in *Abstracts Book, Third International Congress on Hormonal Steroids,* International Congress Series, Excerpta Medica, Amsterdam, p. 210.

Kniewald, Z., Massa, R., Motta, M., and Martini, L., 1971, Feedback mechanisms and the control of the hypothalamohypophysial complex, in *Steroid Hormones and Brain Function,* C. H. Sawyer, and R. A. Gorski, eds., UCLA Forum Med. Sci. No. 15, University of California Press, Los Angeles, pp. 289–300.

Larsson, K., 1962a, Spreading cortical depression and the mating behaviour in male and female rats, *Z. Tierpsychol. 19:*321–331.

Larsson, K., 1962b, Mating behavior in male rats after cerebral cortex ablations: I. Effects of lesions in the dorsolateral and the median cortex, *J. Expl. Zool. 151:*167–176.

Larsson, K., 1964, Mating behavior in male rats after cerebral cortex ablation: II. Effects of lesions in the frontal lobes compared to lesions in the posterior half of the hemispheres, *J. Expl. Zool. 155:*203–214.

Larsson, K., 1969, Failure of gonadal and gonadotrophic hormones to compensate for an impaired sexual function in anosmic male rats, *Physiol. Behav. 4:*733–738.

Larsson, K., 1971, Impaired mating performances in male rats after anosmia induced peripherally or centrally, *Brain, Behav. Evol. 4:*463–471.

Larsson, K., and Heimer, L., 1964, Mating behaviour of male rats after lesions in the preoptic area, *Nature 202:*413–414.

Larsson, K., and Swedin, G., 1971, The sexual behavior of male rats after bilateral section of the hypogastric nerve and removal of the accessory genital glands, *Physiol. Behav. 6:*251–253.

Larsson, K., Sodersten, P., and Beyer, C., 1973, Induction of male sexual behaviour by oestradiol benzoate in combination with dihydrotestosterone, *J. Endocrinol. 57:*563–564.

Le Magnen, J., 1952, Les phenomenes olfacto-sexuels chez le rat blanc, *Arch. Sci. Physiol. 6:*295–331.

Leonard, C. M., and Scott, J. W., 1971, Origin and distribution of the amygdalofugal pathways in the rat: An experimental neuroanatomical study, *J. Comp. Neurol. 141:*313–330.

Lisk, R. D., 1962, Diencephalic placement of estradiol and sexual receptivity in the female rat. *Am. J. Physiol. 203:*493–496.

Lisk, R. D., 1966a, Increased sexual behavior in the male rat following lesions in the mammillary region, *J. Exptl. Zool. 161:*129.

Lisk, R. D., 1966b, Inhibitory centers in sexual behavior in the male rat, *Science 152:*669–670.

Lisk, R. D., 1967, Neural localization for androgen activation of copulatory behavior in the male rat, *Endocrinol. 80:*754–761.

Lisk, R. D., 1968, Copulatory activity of the male rat following placement of preoptic-anterior hypothalamic lesions *Exptl. Brain Res. 5:*306–313.

Lisk, R. D., 1969, Reproductive potential of the male rat: Enhancement of copulatory levels following lesions of the mammillary body in sexually non-active and active animals. *J. Reproduction Fertility 19:*353–356.

Lott, D. F., 1966, Effect of preoptic lesions on the sexual behavior of male rats, *J. Comp. Physiol. Psychol. 61:*284–288.

MacLean, P. D., 1957a, Chemical and electrical stimulation of hippocampus in unrestrained animals. Part I. Methods and electroencephalographic findings, *Am. Med. Assoc. Arch. Neurol. Psychiat. 78:*113–127.

MacLean, P. D., 1957b, Chemical and electrical stimulation of hippocampus in unrestrained animals. Part II. Behavioral findings, *Am. Med. Assoc. Arch. Neurol. Psychiat. 78:*128–142.

MacLean, P. D., and Ploog, D. W., 1962, Cerebral representation of penile erection, *J. Neurophysiol. 25:*29–55.

MacLean, P. D., Dua, S., and Denniston, R. H., 1963, Cerebral localization for scratching and seminal discharge, *Arch. Neurol. 9:*485–497.

Madlafousek, J., Freund, K., and Grofova, I., 1970, Variables determining the effect of electrostimulation in the lateral preoptic area on the sexual behavior of male rats, *J. Comp. Physiol. Psychol. 72:*28–44.

Malsbury, C. W., 1971a, Facilitation of male rat copulatory behavior by electrical stimulation of the medial preoptic area, *Physiol. Behav. 7:*797–805.

Malsbury, C. W., 1971b, The effects of electrical stimulation of the preoptic area of the hypothalamus on male rat copulatory behavior, Ph.D. Thesis, McGill University.

Malsbury, C. W., 1972, Effects of preoptic area and peripheral stimulation in sexually inactive male rats. Paper presented at the meeting of the Eastern Psychological Association, Boston, Massachusetts, April.

Marks, H. E., Remley, N. R., Seago, J. D., and Hastings, D. W., 1971, Effects of bilateral lesions of the olfactory bulbs of rats on measures of learning and motivation, *Physiol. Behav. 7:*1–6.

Matano, S., Sakai, A., and Ban, T., 1969, Dendritic arborization of the hypothalamus in mouse, *Med. J. Osaka Univ. 20:*1–6.

McDonald, P., Beyer, C., Newton, F., Brien, B., Baker, R., Tan, H. S., Sampson, C., Kitching, P., Greenhill, R., and Pritchard, D., 1970, Failure of 5α-dihydrotestosterone to initiate sexual behavior in the castrated male rat, *Nature 227:*964–965.

McEwen, B. S., and Pfaff, D. W., 1970, Factors influencing sex hormone uptake by rat brain regions. I. Effects of neonatal treatment, hypophysectomy and competing steroids on estradiol uptake, *Brain Res. 21:*1–16.

McEwen, B. S., Pfaff, D. W., and Zigmond, R. E., 1970a, Factors influencing sex hormone uptake by rat brain regions. II. Effects of neonatal treatment and hypophysectomy on testosterone uptake, *Brain Res. 21:*17–28.

McEwen, B. S., Pfaff, D. W., and Zigmond, R. E., 1970b, Factors influencing sex hormone uptake by rat brain regions. III. Effects of competing steroids on testosterone uptake, *Brain Res. 21:*29–38.

McEwen, B. S., Denef, C. J., Gerlach, J. L., and Plapinger, L., 1974, Chemical studies of the brain as a steroid hormone target tissue, in *The Neurosciences, Vol. III,* F. O. Schmitt *et al.,* eds., Massachusetts Institute of Technology Press, Boston, pp. 599–620.

McGill, T. E., 1965, Studies of the sexual behavior of male laboratory mice: Effects of genotype, recovery of sex drive, and theory, in *Sex and Behavior,* F. A. Beach, ed., Wiley, New York, pp. 76–88.

Meyer, C. C., and Salzen, E. A., 1970, Hypothalamic lesions and sexual behavior in the domestic chick, *J. Comp. Physiol. Psychol. 73:*365–376.

Michael, R. P., 1965, Oestrogens in the central nervous system, *Brit. Med. Bull. 21:*87–90.

Michael, R. P., and Keverne, E. B., 1968, Pheromones in the communication of sexual status in primates, *Nature 218:*746–749.

Millhouse, O. E., 1969, A Golgi study of the descending medial forebrain bundle, *Brain Res. 15:*341–363.

Moan, C. E., and Heath, R. G., 1972, Septal stimulation for the initiation of heterosexual behavior in a homosexual male, *J. Behav. Ther. Exptl. Psychiat. 3:*23–30.

Modianos, D. T., Flexman, J. E., and Hitt, J. C., 1973, Rostral medial forebrain bundle lesions produce decrements in masculine, but not feminine, sexual behavior in spayed female rats, *Behav. Biol. 8:*629–636.

Murphy, M. R., and Schneider, G. E., 1970, Olfactory bulb removal eliminates mating behavior in the male golden hamster, *Science 167:*302–304.

Naftolin, F., Ryan, K. J., and Petro, Z., 1972, Aromatization of androstenedione by the anterior hypothalamus of adult male and female rats, *Endocrinol. 90:*295–298.

Nauta, W. J. H., and Haymaker, W., 1969, Hypothalamic nuclei and fiber connections, in *The Hypothalamus,* W. Haymaker, E. Anderson, and W. J. H. Nauta, eds., Charles C. Thomas, Springfield, pp. 136–209.

Paxinos, G., 1973, Midbrain and motivated behavior, *J. Comp. Physiol. Psychol. 85:*64–69.

Paxinos, G., and Bindra, D., 1971, Hypothalamic knife cuts: Effects on eating, drinking, irritability, aggression and copulation in the male rat, *J. Comp. Physiol. Psychol. 79:*219–229.

Paxinos, G., and Bindra, D., 1973, Hypothalamic and midbrain neural pathways involved in eating, drinking, irritability, aggression and copulation in rats, *J. Comp. Physiol. Psychol. 82:*1–14.

Peirce, J. T., and Nuttall, R. L., 1961, Duration of sexual contacts in the rat, *J. Comp. Physiol. Psychol. 54:*585–587.

Perachio, A. A., Alexander, M., and Robinson, B. W., 1969, Sexual behavior evoked by telestimulation, in *Proceedings of the Second International Congress on Primatology, Vol. 3.* Karger, Basel/New York, pp. 68–74.

Pfaff, D. W., 1968a, Autoradiographic localization of radioactivity in rat brain after injection of tritiated sex hormones, *Science 161:*1355-1356.

Pfaff, D. W., 1968b, Uptake of estradiol-17B-H^3 in the female rat brain. An autoradiographic study. *Endocrinol. 82:*1149-1155.

Pfaff, D. W., 1970a, Mating behavior of hypophysectomized rats, *J. Comp. Physiol. Psychol. 72:*45-50.

Pfaff, D. W., 1970b, Nature of sex hormone effects on rat sex behavior: Specificity of effects and individual patterns of response, *J. Comp. Physiol. Psychol. 73:*349-358.

Pfaff, D. W., 1971a, Movie analysis of female rat mating behavior. Presented to Eastern Psychological Association, New York, April.

Pfaff, D. W., 1971b, Mating behavior of adrenalectomized rats, *Am. Zool. 11:*Abstract No. 2.

Pfaff, D. W., 1971c, Steroid sex hormones in the rat brain: Specificity of uptake and physiological effects, in *Steroid Hormones and Brain Function,* C. H. Sawyer, and R. A. Gorski, eds., UCLA Forum Med. Sci. No. 15. University of California Press, Los Angeles, pp. 103-112.

Pfaff, D. W., 1972, Interactions of steroid sex hormones with brain tissue: Studies of uptake and physiological effects, in *The Regulation of Mammalian Reproduction,* S. Segal, ed., Thomas, Springfield, Illinois, pp. 5-22.

Pfaff, D. W., and Gregory E., 1971a, Olfactory coding in olfactory bulb and medial forebrain bundle of normal and castrated male rats, *J. Neurophysiol. 34:*208-216.

Pfaff, D. W., and Gregory, E., 1971b, Correlation between preoptic area unit activity and the cortical EEG: Difference between normal and castrated male rats, *Electroenceph. Clin. Neurophysiol. 31:*223-230.

Pfaff, D., and Keiner, M., 1973, Atlas of estradiol-concentrating cells in the central nervous system of the female rat, *J. Comp. Neurol. 151:*121-158.

Pfaff, D. W., and Pfaffmann, C., 1969a, Olfactory and hormonal influences on the basal forebrain of the male rat, *Brain Res. 15:*137-156.

Pfaff, D. W., and Pfaffmann, C., 1969b, Behavioral and electrophysiological responses of male rats to female rat urine odors, in *Olfaction and Taste,* III, C. Pfaffmann, ed., Rockefeller University Press, New York, pp. 258-267.

Pfaff, D., Lewis, C., Diakow, C., and Keiner, M., 1973, Neurophysiological analysis of mating behavior responses as hormone-sensitive reflexes, in *Progress in Physiological Psychology, Vol. 5,* E. Stellar, and J. Sprague, eds., Academic Press, New York, pp. 253-297.

Pfaff, D. W., Diakow, C., Zigmond, R. E., and Kow, L.-M., 1974, Neural and hormonal determinants of female mating behavior in rats, in *The Neurosciences, Vol. III,* F. O. Schmitt *et al.,* ed., Massachusetts Institute of Technology Press, Boston, pp. 621-646.

Phillips, D. S., 1970, Effects of olfactory bulb ablation on visual discrimination, *Physiol. Behav. 5:*13-15.

Ploog, D. W., and MacLean, P. D., 1963, Display of penile erection in squirrel monkey (Saimiri sciureus), *Anim. Behav. 11:*32-39.

Pohorecky, L. A., Larin, F., and Wurtman, R. J., 1969a, Mechanism of changes in brain norepinephrine levels following olfactory bulb lesions, *Life Sci. 8:*1309-1317.

Pohorecky, L. A., Zigmond, M. J., Heimer, L., and Wurtman, R. J., 1969b, Olfactory bulb removal: Effects on brain norepinephrine, *Proc. Natl. Acad. Sci. U.S. 62:*1052-1055.

Pottier, J. J., and Baran, D., 1971, Persistent failure to mate in the male laboratory rat: Behavioural observations. Paper presented at the meeting of the Eastern Psychological Association, New York City, April.

Powell, T. P. S., Cowan, W. M., and Raisman, G., 1965, The central olfactory connections. *J. Anat. 99:*791-813.

Resko, J. A., Goy, R. W., and Phoenix, C. H., 1967, Uptake and distribution of exogenous testosterone-1, 2-^{3}H in neural and genital tissues of the castrate guinea pig, *Endocrinol. 80:*490–498.

Resko, J. A., Feder, H. H., and Goy, R. W., 1968, Androgen concentrations in plasma and testis of developing rats, *J. Endocrinol. 40:*485–491.

Roberts, W. W., Steinberg, M. L., and Means, L. W., 1967, Hypothalamic mechanisms for sexual, aggressive, and other motivational behaviors in the opossum, *Didelphis Virginiana, J. Comp. Physiol. Psychol. 64:*1–15.

Robinson, B. W., and Mishkin, M., 1966, Ejaculation evoked by stimulation of the preoptic area in monkey, *Physiol. Behav. 1:*269–272.

Robinson, B. W., and Mishkin, M., 1968, Penile erection evoked from forebrain structures in Macaca mulatta, *Arch. Neurol. 19:*184–198.

Rodgers, C. H., 1969, Total and partial surgical isolation of the male rat hypothalamus: Effects on reproductive behavior and physiology, *Physiol. Behav. 4:*465–470.

Rosenblatt, J. S., and Aronson, L. R., 1958, The decline of sexual behavior in male cats after castration with special reference to the role of prior sexual experience, *Behav. 12:*285–338.

Rowe, F. A., and Edwards, D. A., 1972, Olfactory bulb removal: Influences on the mating behavior of male mice, *Physiol. Behav. 8:*37–41.

Rowe, F. A., and Smith, W. E., 1972, Effects of peripherally induced anosmia on mating behavior of male mice, *Psychon. Sci. 27:*33–34.

Sachs, B. D., and Barfield, R. J., 1970, Temporal patterning of sexual behavior in the male rat, *J. Comp. Physiol. Psychol. 73:*359–364.

Sachs, B. D., and Barfield, R. J., 1974, Copulatory behavior of male rats given intermittent electric shocks: Theoretical implications, *J. Comp. Physiol. Psychol., 86:*607–615.

Sar, M., and Stumpf, W. E., 1971, Androgen localization in the brain and pituitary. *Fed. Proc. 30:*363.

Sar, M., and Stumpf, W. E., 1972, Cellular localization of androgen in the brain and pituitary after the injection of tritiated testosterone, *Experientia 28:*1364–1366.

Sawyer, C. H., 1960, Reproductive behavior, in *Handbook of Physiology, Section I, Vol. II. Neurophysiology,* H. W. Magoun, J. Field, and V. E. Hall, eds., Williams & Wilkins, Baltimore, pp. 1225–1240.

Schein, M. W., and Hale, E. B., 1965, Stimuli eliciting sexual behavior, in *Sex and Behavior,* F. A. Beach, ed., Wiley, New York, pp. 440–482.

Schmidt, R. S., 1968, Preoptic activation of frog mating behavior, *Behav. 30:*239–257.

Schreiner, L., and Kling, A., 1953, Behavioral changes following rhinencephalic injury in cat, *J. Neurophysiol. 16:*643–659.

Schreiner, L., and Kling, A., 1956, Rhinencephalon and behavior, *Am. J. Physiol. 184:*486–490.

Schwartz, A. S., and Whalen, R. E., 1965, Amygdala activity during sexual behavior in the male cat, *Life Sci. 4:*1359–1366.

Schwartz, N. B., and Kling, A., 1964, The effect of amygdaloid lesions on feeding, grooming and reproduction in rats, *Acta Neurovegetat. 26:*12–34.

Scott, J. W., and Leonard, C. M., 1971, The olfactory connections of the lateral hypothalamus in the rat, mouse and hamster, *J. Comp. Neurol. 141:*331–344.

Scott, J. W., and Pfaff, D. W., 1970, Behavioral and electrophysiological responses of female mice to male urine odors, *Physiol. Behav. 5:*407–411.

Scott, J. W., and Pfaffmann, C., 1967, Olfactory input to the hypothalamus: Electrophysiological evidence, *Science 158:*1592–1594.

Shealy, C. N., and Peele, T. L., 1957, Studies on amygdaloid nucleus of cat, *J. Neurophysiol.* *20:*125–139.

Sholiton, L. J., Marnell, R. T., and Werk, E. E., 1966, Metabolism of testosterone-4-C[14] by rat brain homogenates and subcellular fractions, *Steroids 8:*265–275.

Singer, J. J., 1968, Hypothalamic control of male and female sexual behavior in female rats, *J. Comp. Physiol. Psychol. 66:*738–742.

Soulairac, M. L., 1963, Étude expérimentale des régulations hormono-nerveuses du comportement sexuel du rat mâle, *Ann. Endocrinol. 24*(Suppl.):1–98.

Stephan, F. K., Valenstein, E. S., and Zucker, I., 1971, Copulation and eating during electrical stimulation of the rat hypothalamus, *Physiol. Behav. 1:*587–594.

Stern, J. M., and Eisenfeld, A. J., 1971, Distribution and metabolism of ^{3}H-testosterone in castrated male rats: Effects of cyproterone, progesterone and unlabelled testosterone. *Endocrinol. 88:*1117–1125.

Stone, C. P., and Ferguson, L. W., 1940, Temporal relationships in the copulatory acts of adult male rats, *J. Comp. Psychol. 30:*419–433.

van Dis, H., and Larsson, K., 1970, Seminal discharge following intracranial electrical stimulation, *Brain Res. 23:*381–386.

van Dis, H., and Larsson, K., 1971, Induction of sexual arousal in the castrated male rat by intracranial stimulation, *Physiol. Behav. 6:*85–86.

Vaughan, E., and Fisher, A. E., 1962, Male sexual behavior induced by intracranial electrical stimulation, *Science 137:*758–759.

Ward, O. B. Jr., and Newton, F. A., 1970, Subcortical brain activity during copulation in the male rat, *Proceedings of the 78th Annual Convention of the American Psychological Association,* 239–240.

Whalen, R. E., and Luttge, W. G., 1971, Testosterone, androstenedione and dihydrotestosterone: Effects on mating behavior of male rats, *Horm. Behav. 2:*117–125.

Whalen, R. E., Battie, C., and Luttge, W. G., 1972, Anti-estrogen inhibition of androgen-induced sexual receptivity in rats, *Behav. Biol. 7:*311–320.

White, L. E., 1965, Olfactory bulb projection of the rat, *Anat. Rec. 152:*465–480.

Wilson, J. D., and Gloyna, R. E., 1970, Intranuclear metabolism of testosterone in the accessory organs of reproduction, in *Recent Progress in Hormone Research, Vol. 26,* E. B. Astwood, ed., Academic Press, New York.

Wolf, G., and DiCara, L. V., 1971, A third ascending hypothalamopetal pathway, *Exptl. Neurol. 33:*69–77.

Wood, C. D., 1958, Behavioral changes following discrete lesions of temporal lobe structures, *Neurol. 8:*215–220.

Young, W. C., 1961, The hormones and mating behavior, in *Sex and Internal Secretions,* W. C. Young, ed., Williams & Wilkins, Baltimore, pp. 1173–1239.

Zigmond, R. E., and McEwen, B. S., 1970, Selective retention of estradiol by cell nuclei in specific brain regions of the ovariectomized rat, *J. Neurochem. 17:*889–899.

Zigmond, R. E., Stern, J. M., and McEwen, B. S., 1972, Retention of radioactivity in cell nuclei in the hypothalamus of the ring dove after injection of ^{3}H-testosterone, *Gen. Comp. Endocrinol. 18:*450–453.

Zigmond, R. E., Nottebohm, F., and Pfaff, D. W., 1973, Distribution of androgen-concentrating cells in the brain of the chaffinch, *Progress in Endocrinology, Proceedings of the IV International Congress on Endocrinology,* Internat. Congress Series, Excerpta Medica, Amsterdam.

Zitrin, A., Jaynes, J., and Beach, F. A., 1956, Neural mediation of mating in male cats: III. Contribution of the occipital, parietal and temporal cortex, *J. Comp. Neurol. 105:*111–125.

CHAPTER 4

A Model of Agonistic Behavior: Endocrine and Autonomic Correlates

Douglas K. Candland and Alan I. Leshner

Department of Psychology
Bucknell University
Lewisburg, Pennsylvania

1. Introduction

Attempts to relate agonistic behavior to fluctuations in a specific physiological system, especially the autonomic nervous system, have been more instructive than conclusive in establishing the relationship between physiological functioning and aggression. Clearly, the variety of behaviors we label *agonistic* or *aggressive* are not the product of the functioning of a single, known system. If we were to select promising candidates, we might be well served to choose autonomic and endocrine functioning. Seeking physiological correlates of aggression in the endocrine system presents technical problems. Endocrine responses are not discrete, and the factors which control the nature and quantity of endocrine secretions are not completely understood. The endocrine system is composed of complex feedback subsystems, a characteristic which presents problems in deciding how and when to interrupt the sequences for measurement and investigation. These problems encourage unwanted disparity among studies and present difficulties in interpretation.

Study of the relation of the endocrine system to aggression has proceeded in two methodologically distinct ways, thus providing two different but harmonious views of the relationship between the endocrine system and aggression. These two aspects of aggression differ in terms of the types of questions they suggest and, it would follow, in terms of the methods used to answer the questions. First, the endocrine glands are related to the type, level, and degree of aggressiveness. Second, the endocrine system is a part of the general physiological response mechanism that is activated during and again following agonistic contact.

The typical techniques employed to study the role of the endocrine system in the determination of aggression are: (1) glandular extirpation and replacement therapy with exogenous hormones, and (2) neonatal treatment with exogenous hormones. In the special case of analyzing the endocrine response to agonistic encounters, measurements of glandular weights and of circulating hormone levels in the plasma are the more common techniques. In the study of these questions, studies have emphasized different glandular changes: Some have concentrated on the pituitary–gonadal axis; others on the pituitary–adrenocortical axis.

The testes have been thought to exert primary control over whether aggressiveness will occur and, if it does, its intensity. This belief emerged from the incorporation of several chains of evidence derived primarily from studies of rodents. It is known that (1) castration reduces aggressiveness, and replacement therapy with androgens restores the level of aggressiveness of castrates to the level of intact animals (Bevan et al. 1957, 1958; Levy and King, 1953; Scott and Fredericson, 1951; Tollman and King, 1956); (2) early postnatal androgenization of females leads to the manifestation of "malelike" levels of aggressiveness following testosterone treatment in adulthood (Bronson and Desjardins, 1970; Edwards, 1968, 1969, 1970); and (3) early treatment of males with testosterone accelerates the development of aggressiveness in juveniles (Levy and King, 1953).

The pituitary–adrenocortical axis has received attention primarily as a system which responds to agonistic encounters and to the stresses of position in a newly formed dominance-hierarchy. Bronson and Eleftheriou (1963, 1965a,b) have published a series of experiments showing that participation in an agonistic encounter leads to increased plasma corticosterone levels and, moreover, that these changes are most marked in a defeated animal. The pituitary–adrenocortical axis is so sensitive to agonistic situations that mere exposure to an experienced fighter leads to increases in adrenocortical secretion in an animal recently defeated.

The relationship between dominance position and adrenocortical function varies according to the species studied. Dominant rodents have lower levels of adrenocortical secretion than subordinates. Among nonhuman primates, the relationship is less clear. Sassenrath (1970), who studied Macaca mulatta, found subordinate animals to be more responsive to ACTH than dominant animals, while Hayama (1966), studying Macaca irus, found dominant monkeys to have heavier adrenals than subordinates. In addition to its role in response to agonistic encounters, the pituitary–adrenal axis now appears to be related to the control of aggression. Sigg and his co-workers (Sigg *et al.*, 1966; Yen *et al.*, 1962) found that adrenalectomy delayed the onset of the aggressiveness which normally follows social isolation. Evidently, longer periods of isolation are needed to induce aggressiveness in adrenalectomized mice than in intact mice. Brain *et al.*, (1971) found adrenalectomy (*cf.* Harding and Leshner, 1972) and ACTH to decrease aggression, and dexamethasone treatment (which blocks ACTH) to increase the aggressiveness of intact mice.

The concept of *dominance* is central to the thesis of this paper and the studies reported. It is a deceptively simple concept bearing many methodological difficulties. Dominance implies only that one animal gains preference (for a mate, food, territory, for example) and that the order of preference is reliable. Many observers of animal behavior (and some of human behavior) believe that dominance orders based on preference transcend the restriction to one class of objects; that is, they suggest that there is a trait which may be called *dominance*. An animal dominant on one order would be dominant, or at least of high rank, on other orders.

For our purposes in this chapter, it is noteworthy that the establishment and maintenance of dominance orders are related to aggression. Indeed, in many species the order is determined by obvious, overt, and injurious aggression. But in other species, of which the squirrel monkey is an ideal example, a species-specific display is substituted for physical aggression. The fact that aggression takes this form does not imply that there are no physiological correlates of aggression. For these reasons, we classify the establishment of dominance orders as one model of aggressiveness, realizing that among the products of natural selection are cases in which species have developed mechanisms other than direct aggression to serve the same apparent purpose as direct aggression.

Our work attempts to elaborate the function of the adrenals in the outcome of aggressive competition and the hormonal responses to agonistic situations. We have concentrated on two orders: Rodentia, a model for species using injurious forms of aggression; and Primates, a model for species using primarily noninjurious forms of competitive aggression. This series of studies suggests a dual role for the adrenal cortex in competitiveness. First, the adrenals are clearly involved in the determination of aggressiveness. The adrenals are necessary for the full expression of aggressiveness, and animals with high baseline levels of adrenocortical activity appear more aggressive than those with low baseline levels. Second, the adrenals are also part of the mechanism by which organisms adapt to the stresses of competition, particularly defeat. Which role will take precedence appears to depend on when, following competition, evaluation is carried out of the relationship between agonistic behavior and adrenocortical function.

2. A Model of Injurious Aggression

In the first experiment on the role of the adrenals in the control of intermale aggression in rodents, we examined the dose–response relationship between corticosterone and aggressiveness in *Mus musculus* CFW. Corticosterone was selected for study because it, rather than cortisol, is the primary glucocorticoid secreted by the mouse adrenal cortex. Sixty-four adult male mice of the CFW strain were assigned randomly to eight groups of a two-way (2 × 4) factorial design. We used two operation conditions (adrenalectomized and sham-operated) and four dosages of injected corticosterone (a placebo, 100 µg/day, 200 µg/day, and 300 µg/day in 0.10-cc steroid suspending vehicle).

We used two aggression tests in this experiment. First, the animals were tested once against a "standard-type" fighting opponent. These opponents had been housed six per cage for five weeks before the tests. Brain and Nowell (1970) have shown that these "standard" animals are relatively nonaggressive while eliciting high degrees of aggressiveness from isolated, intact animals. No opponent was used more than once. The encounter was held in a neutral arena and lasted five minutes. During this period, the latency to attack and the number of attacks, bites, sniffs, and tail-rattles were recorded.

The results of this first test are shown in Table 1. Compared to intact animals, adrenalectomized animals fought in fewer encounters, took longer to attack, and inflicted fewer attacks and bites in the one fight which did occur. The low (100 µg/day) dosage of corticosterone did not affect the ag-

TABLE 1.   Results of Fights Against Fighting Partners

Group	Encounters	Fights	$\bar{X}$ latency to attack (sec)	$\bar{X}$ attacks + bites per fight
Adrenalectomized				
Placebo	8	1	297.8	3
Low	8	0	—	—
Medium	8	4	120.9	22
High	8	4	193.0	12
Sham				
Placebo	8	5	115.1	21
Low	8	3	141.4	9
Medium	8	4	94.4	8
High	8	4	103.5	26

TABLE 2. Results of Round-Robin Encounters

A vs. B		Encounters	Fights	$\bar{X}$ latency to attack (sec)		$\bar{X}$ attacks + bites per fight		% of fights won	
				A	B	A	B	A	B
A–P	A–L[a]	10	4	97.1	49.6	7	12	75	0
A–P	A–M	16	3	60.0	35.5	6	29	33	67
A–P	A–H	12	2	220.7	37.5	15	24	50	50
A–P	S–P	17	6	124.3	83.1	13	26	33	67
A–P	S–L	15	8	102.5	27.0	22	23	38	62
A–P	S–M	17	8	113.8	50.6	12	17	25	75
A–P	S–H	15	3	137.9	195.6	15	5	67	33
A–L	A–M	11	4	270.6	45.8	8	22	25	75
A–L	A–H	7	2	54.5	64.2	5	8	50	50
A–L	S–P	10	4	7.4	16.6	22	19	25	75
A–L	S–L	9	4	87.6	69.6	8	16	0	25
A–L	S–M	11	9	80.2	79.8	10	23	22	78
A–L	S–H	11	5	22.6	93.9	40	12	40	60
A–M	A–H	13	5	51.7	82.1	19	21	40	60
A–M	S–P	16	11	103.4	42.2	13	29	46	54
A–M	S–L	15	8	64.2	40.0	23	26	38	50
A–M	S–M	16	8	67.3	72.4	14	19	38	50
A–M	S–H	17	4	27.5	190.4	22	32	75	25
A–H	S–P	13	6	8.0	52.3	3	25	0	100
A–H	S–L	12	5	118.3	28.3	15	34	40	60
A–H	S–M	11	4	221.8	93.0	14	10	25	50
A–H	S–H	13	4	109.8	160.8	33	14	75	25
S–P	S–L	16	8	96.3	46.0	24	20	63	25
S–P	S–M	14	10	62.4	60.4	15	16	40	40
S–P	S–H	16	7	22.3	—	32	—	100	0
S–L	S–M	17	11	37.7	24.2	22	25	36	64
S–L	S–H	16	4	11.5	166.6	19	9	13	6
S–M	S–H	15	7	115.9	—	12	—	100	0

[a] A: adrenalectomized, S: sham, P: placebo, L: low (100 μg/day), M: medium (200 μg/day), H: high (300 μg/day).

gressiveness of the adrenalectomized mice, but the medium (200 μg/day) and high (300 μg/day) dosages appeared to restore aggressiveness. Since few intact animals fought, we considered the results inconclusive. We decided to test one-half the animals in a round-robin situation. Four animals from each group were used in this second test. Each animal encountered each of the other animals once. The results may be seen in Table 2.

Intact mice, regardless of their injection condition, typically were more aggressive than adrenalectomized mice of the placebo and low-dosage conditions. As measured by the latency to attack, by the number of attacks and bites, and by who won, animals in the adrenalectomized-medium-dosage condition were approximately equivalent in aggressiveness to intact animals. They won an equal proportion of the encounters and attacked as often and as quickly as the intact animals. The high dosage of corticosterone decreased aggressiveness in both intact and adrenalectomized mice.

Summary and Conclusions. This pilot experiment examined the dose–response relationship between corticosterone levels and aggressiveness in isolated CFW mice using two different types of aggression testing. The results showed that (1) 200 μg/day corticosterone is an appropriate replacement dosage to return the level of aggressiveness of adrenalectomized mice to the level of intact animals, and (2) high dosages of corticosterone appear to decrease aggressiveness.

That the lowest dosage of corticosterone used (100 μg/day) did not affect the aggressiveness of adrenalectomized mice suggests that there is not a gradual increment in aggressiveness as corticosterone levels rise. Rather, there appears to be a threshold dosage of corticosterone for the full expression of aggression. Below the threshold, aggressiveness is minimal; above it, aggression occurs.

Whether corticosterone affects aggression directly or through its effects on other endocrine glands remains to be determined. One explanation of the effects of adrenalectomy on aggression is that adrenalectomy exerts its effect through the increase in ACTH which follows this operation (Cox *et al.*, 1958). Since Brain *et al.* (1971) demonstrated that exogenous ACTH decreases the aggressiveness of intact animals, adrenalectomy may reduce aggression by increasing ACTH levels. Since exogenous corticosterone should reduce ACTH through the feedback system which controls ACTH secretion, corticosterone may have restored the aggressiveness of adrenalectomized mice by counteracting the effects of adrenalectomy on ACTH levels. If manipulations of adrenocortical function affect aggression by changing ACTH levels, does ACTH affect aggression directly, or indirectly through its effects on testicular function? Since increases in ACTH lead to decreases in testicular hormone production (Bullock and New, 1971) and this decrease leads to reduced aggressiveness, it may be that adrenalectomy reduces aggression through a concomitant decrease in testicular secretion. We examined this possibility by treating adrenalectomized mice with testosterone in an attempt to raise the circulating androgen levels of these animals. If this treatment increases the aggressiveness of adrenalectomized animals, the hypothesis that adrenalectomy leads to reduced aggression through concomitant lessening of testicular function would receive support.

In an attempt to improve the validity of the measure of aggressiveness, the test and criterion for aggression were revised. In the revised test, an experimental animal encountered a standard opponent once on each of three successive days. In each test, the same behaviors were recorded as when the single test was used. The revised test contributes more precise data than the single test and provides for reliability checks not possible with a single test.

In order to incorporate the behavior which we were able to evaluate and which we believe reflects some aspect of aggressiveness, we devised a *composite aggression score*. This score is weighted by behaviors in proportion to their apparent contribution to the aggressiveness of the animal. The number of attacks and bites is weighted 2; the number of tail-rattlings, 1; the number of sniffs of the opponent, 0.5. For analysis, an animal's mean score over the three tests is used. Our pilot work indicates that the composite score provides a reliable measure of individual and group differences in aggressiveness. It is also more sensitive to the effects of various treatments than are measurements of single behaviors or determinations of whether or not an animal attacked.

For the second experiment, 258 CFW mice were separated into 32 groups according to a four-way ($2 \times 2 \times 2 \times 4$) factorial design. The design of this experiment and the number of subjects in each group is shown in Table 3. There were two adrenalectomy conditions [bilaterally

TABLE 3. Proportion of Animals Attacking in 2/3 Encounters

Drug treatment[a]	Operation condition			
	Sham–sham	Adx[b]–sham	Sham–castrated	Adx–castrated
Plac–Plac	8/8	1/8[e]	1/8[e]	1/7[d]
Cort–Plac	7/8	6/8	2/7[c]	2/8[d]
Plac–LTP	8/9	4/10[d]	7/8	3/10[d]
Cort–LTP	6/8	3/9[d]	6/8	4/8[c]
Plac–MTP	5/8	2/8[d]	3/8[c]	1/6[c]
Cort–MTP	7/9	3/9[d]	3/8[c]	3/8[c]
Plac–HTP	5/8	2/7[d]	7/8	3/7[c]
Cort–HTP	4/8[c]	4/8[c]	8/8	8/8

[a] Plac: placebo, Cort: corticosterone (200 μg/day), LTP: testosterone propionate (50 μg/day), MTP: testosterone propionate (150 μg/day), HTP: testosterone propionate (500 μg/day).
[b] Adx: adrenalectomized.
[c] $p < 0.05$.
[d] $p < 0.01$.
[e] $p < 0.005$.

adrenalectomized (Adx) and sham operated (Sham)], two castration conditions [bilaterally castrated and sham operated], two corticosterone conditions [200 μg/day corticosterone or a steroid suspending vehicle placebo (Plac)], and four testosterone propionate conditions [50 μg/day (LTP), 150 μg/day (MTP), 500 μg/day (HTP), or a peanut oil placebo]. The testosterone propionate dosages represent the range of dosages used in other studies as replacement therapy for the effects of castration on aggression. The extremely high 500 μg/day dosage was necessary (in combination with corticosterone) to provide replacement for the adrenalectomized–castrated mice in this study. To summarize the design of this study, the mice were adrenalectomized, castrated, neither, or both, and were treated with either corticosterone alone, one of three dosages of testosterone alone, or with neither or both. This experimental design provides a means of examining both the effects of testosterone on the aggressiveness of adrenalectomized and adrenalectomized–castrated mice and the effects of corticosterone on the aggressiveness of castrated and adrenalectomized–castrated mice. The possibility of determining the exact treatment necessary to restore the aggressiveness of adrenalectomized–castrated mice is of special importance, for if the adrenals and testes affect aggressiveness separately, treatment with both corticosterone and testosterone should be needed to restore the aggressiveness of these animals.

Figure 1 shows the mean composite aggression score as a function of the drug treatments for the animals of each of the four operation conditions. Table 3 shows, for each group, the proportion of the animals that attacked at least once in at least two of the three encounters. Differences among the groups on the composite aggression score were tested by analyses of variance and on the proportion of animals attacking in at least two of the three encounters by the Fisher exact probability test. The combined results of these two analyses showed that: (1) adrenalectomy, castration, and the combination of adrenalectomy and castration reduced aggressiveness; (2) corticosterone alone restored the aggressiveness of adrenalectomized, but not castrated or adrenalectomized–castrated mice; (3) testosterone alone restored the aggressiveness of castrated, but not adrenalectomized or adrenalectomized–castrated mice; and (4) the combination of corticosterone and the highest (500 μg/day) dosage of testosterone raised the aggressiveness of adrenalectomized–castrated mice to a level even higher than that of intact mice. The composite aggression score of the adrenalectomized–castrated mice indicates that the highest dosage of testosterone restored the aggressiveness of these animals; but only three of seven animals attacked in more than one encounter. We do not consider this to be a definitive restoration of aggressiveness for these animals. The

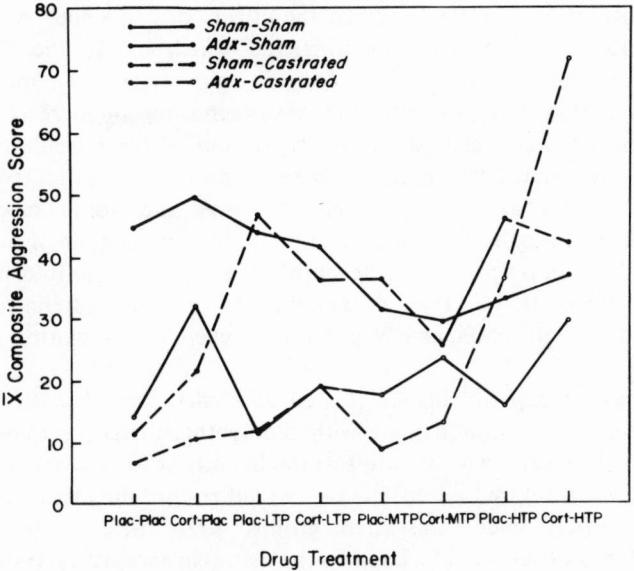

FIG. 1.   Mean composite aggression score as a function of drug treatment
for each operation condition.

finding that the highest dosage of testosterone did not restore the aggressiveness of adrenalectomized mice lends support to our position.

Summary and Conclusions.   The hypothesis that adrenalectomy
decreases aggressiveness through a concomitant decrease in androgen
secretion was tested by treating adrenalectomized and adrenalectomized–castrated mice with exogenous testosterone propionate. The
results of this study showed that: (1) corticosterone, but not testosterone,
restores the aggressiveness of adrenalectomized mice; (2) testosterone, but
not corticosterone, restores the aggressiveness of castrated mice; and (3)
both corticosterone and testosterone are necessary to restore the aggressiveness of adrenalectomized–castrated mice. Because these results
show that the effects of manipulations of the pituitary–adrenocortical axis
on aggression are not due to concomitant effects on testicular functioning,
we suggest that the adrenals and testes may be regarded as two distinct
systems in the determination of aggressiveness.

Since there appears to be an independent role for the pituitary–adrenocortical axis in the control of aggression, an obvious question is, are the effects of manipulations of this axis due to the actions of ACTH directly or
to those of corticosterone? There are several possible ways to examine this

question. Brain *et al.* (1971) studied the effects of exogenous ACTH and dexamethasone, a synthetic glucocorticoid which blocks the release of ACTH from the anterior pituitary, on the aggressiveness of intact mice. They found ACTH to decrease, but dexamethasone to increase, the aggressiveness of these mice. Their interpretation of their results was that ACTH, rather than corticosterone, is the aspect of the pituitary adrenocortical axis that affects aggression. Although their data support this position, their animals were intact and therefore still capable of mobilizing glucocorticoids in response to exogenous ACTH. It is more informative to study the effects of ACTH or dexamethasone on either adrenalectomized mice or those with exogenously controlled levels of circulating corticosterone.

In the next experiment, we treated adrenalectomized, castrated, and adrenalectomized–castrated mice with the synthetic glucocorticoid, dexamethasone. This drug was used to test the hypothesis that blocking the rise in ACTH which follows adrenalectomy would restore the aggressiveness of adrenalectomized mice. Castrated groups were included to measure possible effects of ACTH blockage on the aggressiveness of castrated mice.

Sixty-four CFW mice were separated into eight groups formed according to a three-way ($2 \times 2 \times 2$) factorial design. The operation conditions were the same as in the preceding study, and there were two drug treatment conditions, dexamethasone-injected or placebo-injected. Animals

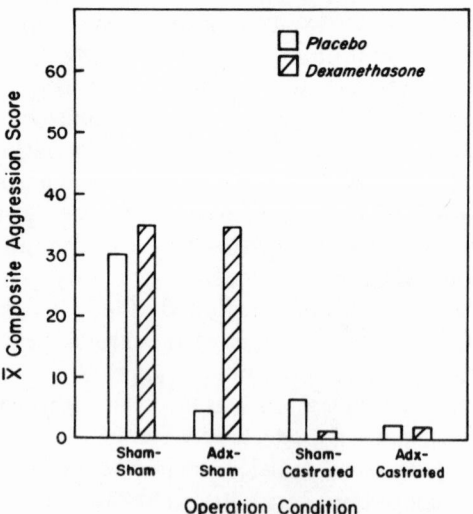

FIG. 2.   Mean composite aggression score as a function of operation condition for mice treated with either dexamethasone or a placebo.

TABLE 4.   Proportion of Animals Attacking in 2/3 Encounters

| | Operation condition | | | |
Drug treatment	Sham–sham	Adx[a]–sham	Sham–castrated	Adx–castrated
Placebo	8/8	2/8[c]	1/8[c]	0/7[c]
Dexamethasone	6/8	6/8	0/8[c]	0/8[c]

[a] Adx: adrenalectomized.
[b] $p < 0.05$.
[c] $p < 0.005$.

receiving dexamethasone were given 0.2 mg dexamethasone in 0.10 cc 10% acacia solution immediately following surgery and 12 hours later, on day 6, and on day 12. Testing was conducted on days 13, 14, and 15.

Figure 2 and Table 4 show the results of this study. Figure 2 shows the mean composite aggression score for each of the operation conditions. Table 4 shows for each group the proportion of the animals which attacked at least once in at least two of the three encounters. Differences among the groups on the composite aggression score were analyzed by analysis of variance, and the differences among the groups on the proportional score were tested by the Fisher exact probability test. Combining the results of these analyses shows that: (1) adrenalectomy, castration, and the combination of adrenalectomy and castration all reduce aggressiveness; and (2) dexamethasone treatment restores the aggressiveness of adrenalectomized mice, but not of castrated or adrenalectomized–castrated mice.

Summary and Conclusions.   The effects of dexamethasone on the aggressiveness of adrenalectomized mice were studied to determine whether ACTH or corticosterone is responsible for the effects of manipulations of the pituitary–adrenocortical axis on aggression. Dexamethasone restored the aggressiveness of adrenalectomized mice. This finding provides strong support for the idea that the effects of adrenalectomy on aggression are due to the increases in ACTH which follow this operation. That dexamethasone can serve as a potent glucocorticoid, however, detracts from the strength of these findings for the ACTH hypothesis.

2.1.   Summary of Series on Injurious Aggression

Three experiments are described which show that: (1) corticosterone restores the aggressiveness of adrenalectomized mice; (2) high doses of corticosterone decrease aggressiveness; (3) the effects of pituitary–adreno-cortical manipulations on aggression are not due to concomitant effects on testicular functioning; and (4) it is probable that the effects of adrena-lectomy on aggressiveness are due to the resulting rise in ACTH. That dexamethasone is a synthetic glucocorticoid may qualify the fourth sug-gestion. The finding of a clear and independent role of the adrenals in the control of injurious aggression is of particular importance to the thesis of this chapter. Future studies in this series will examine the effects of ACTH with controlled levels of circulating corticosterone on the aggressiveness of mice.

3. A Model of Noninjurious Aggression

The primary purpose of this series of studies was to see if we could generalize our findings on the role of the adrenals in aggression in rodents to a species using noninjurious forms of aggression. Does the relationship of adrenocortical activity to aggressiveness apply to different modes of expressing aggression? We decided to study noninjurious aggression by using dominance rank as an index of relative aggressiveness. For this series of studies we selected the squirrel monkey (*Saimiri sciureus*, source: Iquitos).

The male squirrel monkey (the most common new world nonhuman primate) uses the penile display in forming its dominance orders. Penile displays are seen both in laboratory-housed and free-ranging squirrel monkeys. It has been observed in males as young as 28 days of age (Ploog, 1966). The name of the display is an adequate description, although its im-mediacy and intensity are difficult to convey in a paper of this nature. In its extreme form, when two males see one another each extends one leg and lifts an erect penis toward the face of the other. The animals remain in this position for up to 3 minutes. The display is ended by one animal lowering his head, wrapping his tail around himself, and placing his head sub-missively between the legs of the other animal. The animal who is able to avoid submission thereafter enjoys independence of movement. He can chase away a submissive animal and take his tree limb or perch. He is deferred to in the gathering of food and can take food from animals who have submitted. Whether the dominant male also has first choice of a mate is uncertain. Field workers have suggested that he is sometimes too busy displaying to copulate, which leads to reproduction of the mediocre; however, in the laboratory environment it is almost certain that the dominant male has sexual privilege. The dominance order based on the penile display remains highly consistent for years, although occasional attempts at upward mobility take place. Squirrel monkeys in a colonized group rarely challenge each other, although the introduction of an unfamiliar male elicits displays from most males in the colony.

It is difficult to detect highly reliable dominance orders in field conditions, for not all males are seen in proximity, no doubt because their dominance relationships have been established. In order to ascertain whether a reliable order exists in our laboratory situation, we used a round-robin pair comparison procedure. Each combination of two animals was placed in a large chamber with three compartments. An opaque screen behind each animal prevented his seeing his competitor (he may, of course, sense his presence in many other ways). After a period to encourage adaptation to the chamber, the opaque screens were lifted permitting the animals to see, but not to touch one another. Eventually the remaining screens were lifted to permit both animals free access to the chamber. The chamber contained a floor of raised grids to encourage the animals to follow their arboreal habits. Dominance was evaluated by two factors: Independence of movement (i.e., whether one animal consistently displaced another) and submission to penile displays. The development and reliability of this technique is described elsewhere (Candland *et al.*, 1970).

A second function of this series was to test the phylogenetic spread of another set of results from rodent studies. In most rodent studies which examine the relationship of dominance position to adrenocortical function, the subordinates show higher levels of adrenocortical activity than the dominant animals (Barnett, 1955; Christian and Davis, 1956; Louch and Higginbotham, 1967). In the first of our experiments in this series on squirrel monkeys (Leshner and Candland, 1972), we found the opposite relationship. After living together for 4 years, the dominant squirrel monkeys showed higher levels of adrenocortical activity than the subordinates when tested as described below. The second function of this series was to investigate why this relationship is apparently different for rodents and squirrel monkeys.

The third function of this series was to clarify the hormonal mechanisms which mediate the relationship which had been observed in both squirrel monkeys and chickens between autonomic activity, as indexed by heartrate, and dominance rank (Candland *et al.*, 1969; Candland *et al.*, 1970). In this relationship, both the dominant and the subordinate animals show higher eventual heartrates than midranking animals. Figure 3 shows the relationship between baseline heartrate, measured in a novel environment, and eventual dominance rank for squirrel monkeys. Since heartrate is a valid indicator of autonomic activity, and since the catecholamines both function similarly to the autonomic nervous system and dramatically affect heartrate, Candland (1970) suggested that differences in

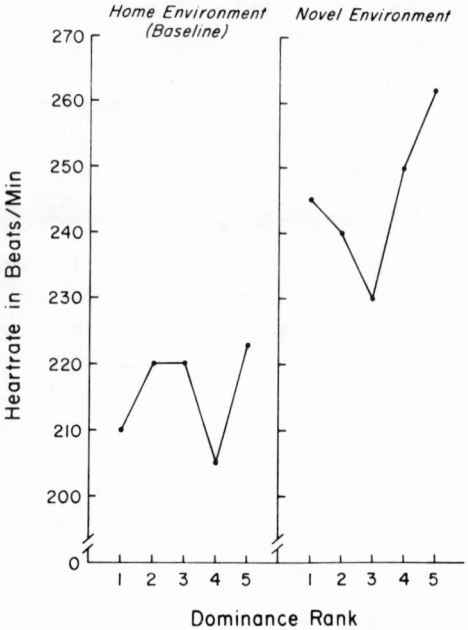

FIG. 3.   The relationship of dominance rank to heart-
rate in squirrel monkeys.

catecholamine secretion levels may account for the relationship of heartrate
to dominance rank. To test this idea we have included a measure of catecholamine secretion levels in the experiments in this series.

  We collected urine samples from the squirrel monkeys and analyzed
the samples for a series of endocrine metabolites. Urine samples were
selected rather than plasma samples since we were unwilling to risk stress
on animals who occupied stable positions in colonized groups. Urine was
collected in specially constructed metabolism cages. The urine flowed
through a double screen filter, a plastic funnel, and another screen and
glasswool filter into a flask immersed in ice. The urine was then collected
and frozen. Prior to analysis, the samples were thawed, pooled over the
four days of collection for each animal, and HCl added at a concentration
of 2 ml/100 ml urine. The samples were then analyzed by the Upjohn Co.,
King of Prussia, Pa., for 17-hydroxycorticosteroid (17-OHCS), total catecholamine, and 17-ketosteroid (17-KS) levels. For this study, Upjohn used
a modification of the Porter–Silber reaction for the 17-OHCS determination, a variant of the trihydroxyindole fluorimetric quantitation method
for the catecholamine determination, and a modification of the Zim-

merman reaction for the 17-KS determination. Levels of 17 OHCS were then used as an index of adrenocortical activity, total catecholamines as an index of adrenal medullary activity; and 17-KS levels as a very general measure of androgenicity.*

We first compared the urinary hormone level of two "groups" of squirrel monkeys (Leshner and Candland, 1972). Both groups were composed of 4 to 5-year-old male squirrel monkeys. One group had been living in visual isolation from one another for 3 years. The second group had been living for 4 years in an environment which encouraged natural behavior, such as arboreal locomotion, seasonal mating, and births and maternal care. The colony was composed of five males, four females, and two juveniles; only the males were used in this study. The social organization was established and had been as stable as those observed in nature for at least 3 years.

Table 5 presents the means of the measurements. There were no differences between the groups in body weight, water intake, daily urine output, or urinary total catecholamine levels. Animals living in the stable colony showed increased 17-OHCS levels and a suggestive but nonsignificant trend toward decreased urinary 17-KS levels compared to the noncolonized animals. We then examined the relationship between dominance rank and urinary hormone levels in the colonized animals. Figure 4

* Since the 17-KS are but a general measure of androgenicity at best, we used this measure only once and then excluded it from future studies.

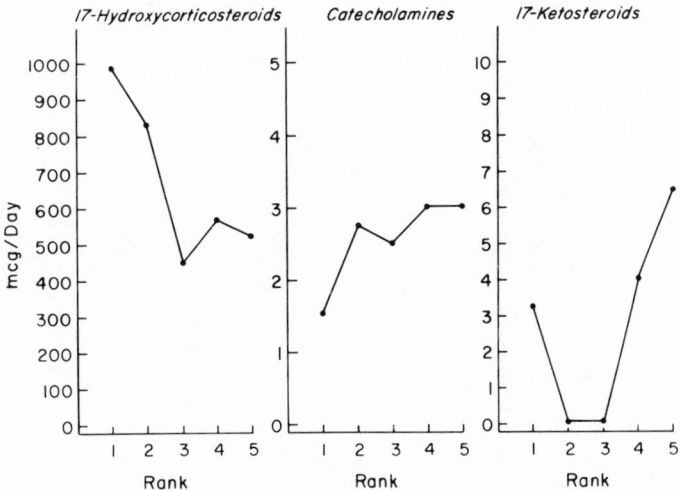

FIG. 4.   The relationship of dominance rank to some hormonal metabolites.

TABLE 5. Means and Standard Deviations of Measurements Taken for Isolated and Colonized Animals

Group	Body weight (g)	Water intake (ml/day)	Urine volume (ml/day)	17-Hydroxy-corticosteroids (µg/day)	Total catecholamines (µg/day)	17-Ketosteroids (µg/day)
Ioslated	927 (204)	71.6 (11.8)	14.7 (5.8)	196.26 (141.18)	4.16 (3.08)	6.14 (2.84)
Group-housed	946 (123)	54.2 (12.6)	18.3 (7.4)	675.80 (228.72)[a]	2.56 (0.59)	2.76 (2.70)[b]

[a] $p < 0.01$.
[b] $p < 0.10$.

TABLE 6. Relation of Dominance Rank to Body Weight, Water Intake and Urine Volume Taken for Colonized Animals

Dominance rank	Body weight (g)	Water intake (ml/day)	Urine volume (ml/day)
1	1130	52.0	31.4
2	856	52.5	17.1
3	999	34.8	14.4
4	824	67.5	13.3
5	923	63.8	15.5

presents the relationships of dominance rank to urinary 17-OHCS, total catecholamines, and 17-KS levels. Table 6 presents the relationship of dominance rank to body weight, water intake, and urine volume.

The findings presented in Fig. 4 and Tables 5 and 6 show that in the novel environment of the metabolism cages dominant animals excreted more 17-OHCS than subordinates, while subordinates excreted more catecholamine. The latter finding may be a result of subordinates being more reactive to a novel environment (metabolism cage) (*cf.* Welch and Welch, 1969). In addition, dominance and weight are correlated positively and 17-KS levels are related to dominance rank according to a J-shaped function with the midranking animals producing no measurable output.

Summary and Conclusions. The relationship between 17-OHCS levels and dominance rank in the squirrel monkey was found to be the reverse of the relationship typically observed between adrenocortical function and dominance rank in rodents. Most studies on rodents have found that subordinate animals show higher levels of adrenocortical activity than dominant animals; our study found that subordinate monkeys showed lower levels. We offer two possible reasons for this difference between rodents and squirrel monkeys. First, rodents typically use injurious forms of aggression in establishing dominance, while squirrel monkeys use a noninjurious, ritualized behavioral display. The relationship between aggression and endocrine function may depend on the type of aggression in which a species engages.

Less engagingly, the difference between rodents and squirrel monkeys may reflect merely when the measurements were taken. In most studies on rodents, the measures of adrenocortical function were taken after relatively short (4–6 weeks) periods of group-housing, when there still may be aggressive encounters. In this case, the subordinates' showing of increased adrenocortical activity relative to the dominant animals would be a reflection of the stress resulting from a recent defeat (Bronson and Eleftheriou, 1963, 1965a,b). The squirrel monkeys of this study were sampled after four years of colonization when there was little, if any, aggression or displaying. The expectation that this absence of competition would be reflected by findings of minimal stress to subordinates was confirmed by the measurements.

To clarify this explanation, we designed a study in which we sampled urine from isolated animals, made an evaluation of the dominance order among the group, and took a second sample. We hoped to accomplish two things. First, we wanted to determine if imposed stresses of intense competition would alter the relationship of endocrine function and dominance rank in squirrel monkeys and, second, we hoped to determine whether an animal's baseline level of adrenal activity is related to his eventual dominance rank or to his relative degree of aggressiveness. The results of this experiment are presented in Figs. 5 and 6. Figure 5 presents the relationship between 17-OHCS levels and dominance rank measured both before and after dominance evaluation. To control for differences in body weight that might affect both dominance rank and endocrine output, we present these values in both absolute levels and in the levels relative to body weight. Figure 6 presents our findings for total catecholamine levels in the urine.

The results of the 17-OHCS determinations show that eventual dominance rank is related to baseline levels of adrenocortical activity. Especially for the high-ranking males, the higher the baseline level of adrenocortical activity, the higher the eventual dominance position. The hormonal measurements taken immediately after the dominance order had been es-

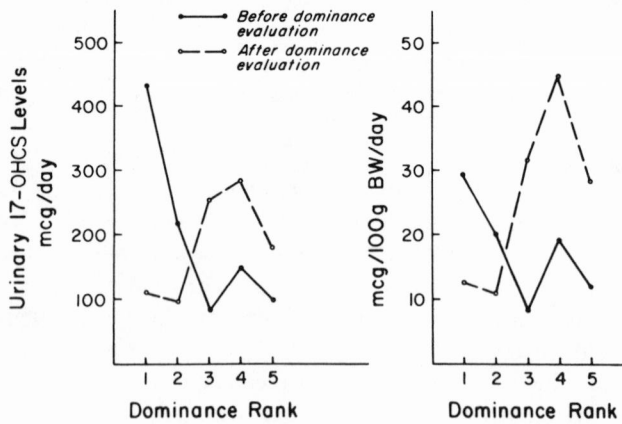

FIG. 5.   The relationship of dominance rank to urinary 17-hydroxycorticosteroid levels.

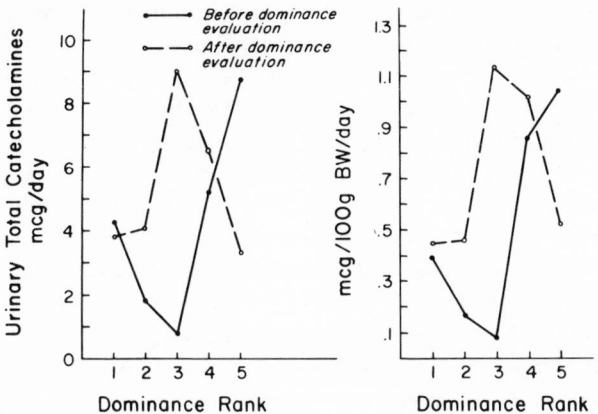

FIG. 6.   The relationship of dominance rank to urinary total catecholamine levels.

tablished showed that subordinate monkeys respond to competition with higher adrenocortical activity than dominant animals.

The total catecholamine determinations made before the dominance-order evaluation showed eventual dominance rank to be related to baseline catecholamine levels according to a J-shaped function: Both dominant and subordinate animals had higher levels than midranking animals. The measurements taken immediately after the establishment of the dominance order reversed the relationship: The dominant and subordinate animals both had lower catecholamine levels than the midranking animals. Relative to their levels prior to the dominance-order evaluation, dominant animals had unchanged catecholamine levels after the dominance order evaluation, the midranking animals had higher levels, and the subordinate animals had lower levels.

Summary and Conclusions.   We measured urinary 17-OHCS and total catecholamine levels of previously isolated squirrel monkeys both before and immediately after they formed a dominance order. Before dominance-order evaluation, the eventually dominant monkeys had higher 17-OHCS levels than the eventually subordinate animals. Immediately after the formation of the order the relationship was reversed: Subordinate monkeys had higher levels than dominant animals. These results suggest that the difference between rodents and squirrel monkeys in the observed relationship of adrenocortical activity and dominance rank is a result of when the determinations are made. If determinations are made either before competition or following stabilization of the dominance order, dominant animals have higher levels of adrenocortical output than subordinates (Leshner and Candland, 1972). If determinations are made shortly following agonistic encounters, subordinates show higher levels.

In a novel environment (the metabolic cage), both baseline catecholamine levels and heartrate corresponded with eventual dominance rank in the J-shaped function (Candland, et al., 1970). This finding supports Candland's (1970) suggestion that the relationship between heartrate and eventual dominance rank is mediated by differences in baseline levels of catecholamine secretion. Since differences in catecholamine levels should affect heartrate, it is probable that these differences in catecholamine secretion mediate the relationship of heartrate to dominance rank.

The relationships between catecholamine levels and dominance rank observed in this experiment differ from those observed by Welch and Welch (1969, 1971) for rodents and by Leshner and Candland (1972) for squirrel monkeys. In these earlier studies, which were conducted after the dominance order was formed and had stabilized, catecholamine levels were lowest for dominant animals and increased as their dominance rank decreased. Welch and Welch (1971) suggest that the relationship of catecholamine levels to competitiveness fluctuates with the intensity of the stresses imposed by a particular situation. They suggest that moderate stress leads to increased catecholamine levels, while severe stress leads to decreased levels. The results of the present study and the differences between these findings and those of Welch and Welch (1971) and our earlier study both suggest that the degree of stress inherent in a particular dominance position depends on whether there have just been numerous encounters or the dominance order has been stable.

The finding that dominant animals had the same catecholamine levels before and after competition while, after competition, the midranking animals had increased levels and the subordinate had decreased levels suggests that the stress of competition is greatest for subordinates, while being only moderate for midranking animals and negligible for dominant animals.

Returning to the issue of the difference in the relationship of adrenocortical function and dominance rank between rodents and squirrel monkeys, we note that the studies presented suggest that when the hormonal measurements are taken is crucial. In order to clarify when the relationship changes from one in which subordinates show higher levels of adrenocortical activity to one in which dominant animals show higher levels, we have been sampling a group of squirrel monkeys at various intervals after placing them in a communal environment. For urine sampling, the animals are removed for two days from the seminaturalistic environment in which they have been living and are placed in the metabolism cages. It should be noted that being moved from one environment to another could impose a stress which would alter the findings, but no alternative technique exists because blood sampling would also be stressful.

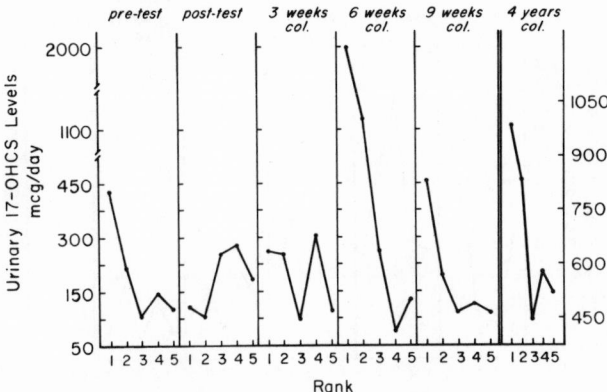

FIG. 7. The relationship of dominance rank to urinary 17-hydroxycorticosteroid levels as a function of duration of group-living.

Results are available on the first few collections from animals put into the communal seminaturalistic environment. Figure 7, urinary 17-OHCS levels, and Fig. 8, urinary total catecholamine levels, show the results of these analyses, (1) as a function of dominance rank and (2) before dominance-order evaluation, immediately after, 3 weeks, 6 weeks, and 9 weeks after dominance-order evaluation. Information on the colony maintained for 4 years is included. These results show that the relationship between dominance rank and urinary 17-OHCS levels changes with time and colonization. After a 6-week colonization period, the relationship is basically similar in form to that observed between baseline 17-OHCS levels and eventual dominance rank and also to the relationship after 4 years of colonization (Leshner and Candland, 1972). After 9 weeks of colonization, the relationship appears to stabilize at the pretest levels, and the amounts excreted are now similar.*

Levels of catecholamine secretion drop following the initiation of group-living and a new function is formed, one which is stable through at least the 9 weeks. At this time, animals ranked 2 and 4 show higher levels of catecholamine excretion than the other animals. Further sampling will show when these levels will return to those of isolates or of long-term colonized animals.

Summary and Conclusions. The variation in the relationships of urinary 17-OHCS to dominance rank was studied before dominance evaluation, immediately after dominance order evaluation, and 3 weeks, 6 weeks, and 9 weeks after evaluation. The 17-OHCS determinations showed that at

* The unusually large 17-OHCS output of alpha and beta males at 6 weeks post-test may be related to the intense aggression between these animals which occurred at this time. The aggression was appreciably less by 9 weeks. Alpha retained his position.

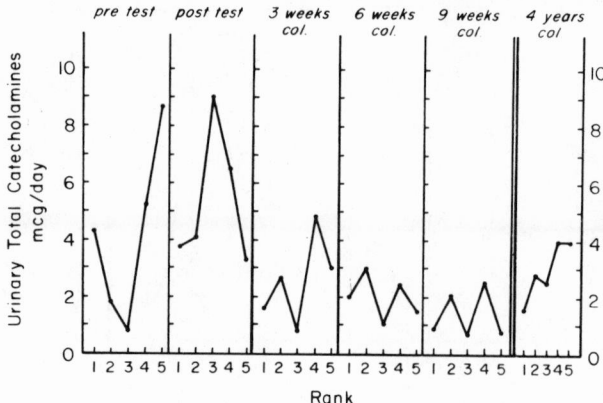

FIG. 8.   The relationship of dominance rank to urinary total catecholamines
as a function of duration of group-living.

6 weeks of group-living the relationship between 17-OHCS and dominance
rank is similar to that observed before the animals are introduced. After introduction and until 6 weeks the relationship is unclear. Catecholamine
level is related to rank in a J-shape function before introduction and dominance evaluation. The J is inverted immediately following evaluation. The
relationship dissipates thereafter. Use of this paradigm has shown that
after 9 weeks of colonization urinary 17-OHCS levels have not risen above
the level of isolates, as was suggested by our earlier study of animals
colonized for 4 years. Perhaps after the animals have been colonized
longer, their 17-OHCS levels will rise. These findings, however, support the
position that *when* the hormonal determinations are taken is crucial to the
determination of the form of the relationship between 17-OHCS levels and
dominance rank.

3.1.   Summary of Series on Noninjurious Aggression

Three experiments were conducted to study the relationship between
adrenal activity and dominance rank in squirrel monkeys. Urine samples
were collected from groups of squirrel monkeys before dominance-order
evaluation (baselines), immediately after competition, and following 3
weeks, 6 weeks, 9 weeks, and 4 years of group-living (colonization), and the
samplings were analyzed for urinary 17-OHCS and total catecholamine
levels. We found that (1) 4-year colonized squirrel monkeys have higher
levels of adrenocortical activity than isolates, (2) eventual dominance rank

is predictable from baseline levels of adrenocortical activity, (3) the form of the relationship between dominance rank and adrenocortical activity changes in time, (4) baseline levels of catecholamine excretion are related to eventual dominance rank by the same form of function which relates heartrate and dominance rank, and (5) the relationship of catecholamine excretion and dominance rank changes over time.

These findings suggest a dual role in noninjurious competition for the hormones of the adrenal cortex. Either before competition or following stabilization of the dominance order, adrenocortical hormones probably contribute to aggressiveness, because dominance rank is predictable from baseline levels, and because the function returns to one of a similar form following stabilization of the order. Immediately following competition, however, adrenocortical hormones are probably involved primarily in the response to the stresses of an agonistic encounter, especially defeat, because the relationship between adrenocortical activity and dominance rank changes to a function similar to that observed in rodent studies in which subordinates have higher levels of adrenocortical activity than dominant animals. The results of the catecholamine determinations support this later suggestion. The nature of the changes in catecholamine levels before and after competition suggest that the subordinate animals undergo more stress in competition than the dominant animals.

4. Conclusions

The results of these studies on mice and squirrel monkeys suggest that the adrenal cortex serves a dual role in agonistic behavior. One role is as a part of the mechanism which formulates aggression and determines its degree. The other role is as a part of the response mechanism by which an animal adapts to the stresses of competition, especially defeat.

The studies of both injurious and noninjurious aggression support the position that the adrenals play a role in the determination of aggressiveness. The series on injurious aggression showed that the adrenals are necessary for aggressive expression, while the findings on noninjurious aggression demonstrate that relative aggressiveness (as measured by dominance) is predictable from baseline levels of adrenocortical activity. The additional finding that after 6 weeks of group-living, when aggressive encounters are few, the relationship between dominance position and adrenocortical activity is similar in form to that observed between baseline adrenocortical activity and eventual dominance rank supports this position by suggesting that when the dominance order is relatively stable, the adrenals function to maintain the dominance position.

The finding that immediately after intense competition, subordinate squirrel monkeys show higher levels of adrenocortical activity combined with the findings of other investigators (e.g., Bronson and Eleftheriou, 1963, 1965a,b) that show similar responses to competition in rodents argues for the second role of the adrenals in agonistic situations; that is, that the adrenals are a part of the mechanism by which an organism responds to the stresses of competition. These findings also support the position that the stresses imposed on defeated animals are greater than those imposed on the victors. The results of the catecholamine determination made immediately after competition lend further support to the idea that as dominance rank decreases the stress of competition increases. Dominant squirrel monkeys showed unchanged catecholamine levels following competition, while midranking animals showed increased and subordinates showed decreased levels. According to Welch and Welch's (1971) formulation, unchanged catecholamine levels reflect negligible stress, while increased levels reflect moderate stress, and decreased levels reflect severe stress.

The findings of these studies also imply that the endocrine mechanisms controlling injurious and noninjurious aggression are similar in at least one respect. Both series of studies showed that the adrenals influence relative aggressiveness. In the rodent series, adrenalectomy reduced aggressiveness independently of the effects of adrenalectomy on testicular function. In the squirrel monkey series, eventual dominance rank was predictable from baseline 17-OHCS levels, which also suggests that the adrenals influence relative aggressiveness. It is yet to be determined whether the other hormonal mechanisms which affect the aggressiveness of rodents, such as the pituitary–gonadal axis, will be found to affect the aggressiveness of those species using noninjurious forms of aggression.

An important implication of these studies is that the observed relationship between aggressiveness and adrenocortical function depends on when the measurements of each are taken. That is, the role of the adrenal cortex in agonistic behavior depends upon how recently intensive competition has occurred. Before competition or when competition is minimal it appears that potentially dominant animals have higher levels of adrenocortical activity than potential subordinates. Immediately after competition, however, the relationship is reversed. Subordinates have higher levels of adrenocortical activity than dominant animals.

Why are the adrenals involved in the control of aggressiveness? A number of explanations are feasible. It may be that the adrenals affect aggressiveness through their role in energy mobilization and utilization. High levels of adrenocortical activity typically reflect high levels of energy mobilization and utilization (Leshner, 1971). Since it is probable that large amounts of energy would be needed to sustain aggressive behaviors, it may be that animals with high levels of adrenocortical activity are better able to mobilize the needed energy than are those with low levels of adrenocortical activity.

Alternatively, the pituitary–adrenocortical hormones may affect directly the neural substrates which control aggression, as has been suggested in the case of the pituitary–gonadal hormones (Bronson and Desjardins, 1970; Edwards, 1968). In this case an area would have to exist within the central nervous system which is both sensitive to circulating corticosterone or ACTH levels and also involved in the neural control of aggression. Direct tests of this possibility need to be performed.

Another explanations is that the pituitary–adrenocortical axis may affect behaviors which control relative aggressiveness. Another line of research from our laboratories (Svare and Lesher, 1973) has suggested that more aggressive animals are more reactive in novel environments and show lower levels of fearfulness than less aggressive animals. Since the pituitary–adrenocortical hormones affect the degree of both reactivity (e.g., Leshner, 1971; Richter, 1927) and fearfulness (reviews of this literature may be found in DeWied and Weijnen, 1970), it may be that this axis affects aggression through its effects on these related behaviors.

This series of studies suggests that (1) the adrenals are necessary for the full expression of aggressiveness; (2) the adrenals affect aggressiveness independently of their effects on testicular functioning; (3) animals with high baseline levels of adrenocortical activity will be more aggressive than those with low levels; (4) the stresses imposed on defeated animals, as measured by both adrenocortical and adrenal medullary activity, are greater than those imposed on victorious animals; (5) the relationship between adrenocortical activity and relative aggressiveness changes as the dominance order stabilizes; and (6) the role of the pituitary–adrenocortical axis is similar for both injurious and noninjurious forms of aggression.

Acknowledgments

The research reported here was supported in part by NSF Grant GB 8348 to the first author and GB23912 to the second author. The authors thank Drs. Glyn Thomas, Arnold Chamove, Paul Brain, Jack Harclerode, Michael Payne, James Misanin, and Ernest Keen for reading and commenting on an earlier version of this manuscript.

5.   References

Barnett, S. A., 1955, Competition among wild rats, *Nature 175:*126.
Bevan, J. M., Bevan, W., and Williams, B. F., 1958, Spontaneous aggressiveness in young

castrated C3H male mice treated with three dose levels of testosterone, *Physiol. Zool. 31:*284.

Bevan, W., Levy, G. W., Whitehouse, J. M., and Bevan, J. M., 1957, Spontaneous aggressiveness in two strains of mice castrated and treated with one of three androgens, *Physiol. Zool. 30:*341–349.

Brain, P. F., and Nowell, N. W., 1970, Some observations of inter-male aggression testing in albino mice, *Comm. Behav. Biol. 5:*7.

Brain, P. F., Nowell, N. W., and Wouters, A., 1971, Some relationships between adrenal function and the effectiveness of isolation in inducing intermale aggression in albino mice, *Physiol. Behav. 6:*27.

Bronson, F. H., and Desjardins, D., 1970, Neonatal androgen administration and adult aggressiveness in female mice, *Gen. Comp. Endocrinol. 15:*320.

Bronson, F. H., and Eleftheriou, B. E., 1963, Adrenal responses to crowding in *Peromyscus* and C57BL/10J mice, *Physiol. Zool. 36:*161.

Bronson, F. H., and Eleftheriou, B. E., 1965a, Adrenal responses to fighting in mice: Separation of physical and psychological causes, *Science 147:*627.

Bronson, F. H., and Eleftheriou, B. E., 1965b, Relative effects of fighting on bound and unbound corticosterone in mice, *Proc. Soc. Exptl. Biol. Med. 118:*146.

Bullock, L. P., and New, M. I., 1971, Testosterone and cortisol concentration in spermatic adrenal and systemic venous blood in adult male guinea pigs, *Endocrinol. 88:*523.

Candland, D. K., 1970, Changes in heartrate during social organization of the squirrel monkey (*Saimiri sciureus*, Iquitos), *Proc. 3rd. Int. Congr. Primat.*, Zurich *3:*172.

Candland, D. K., Taylor, D. B., Dresdale, L., Leiphardt, J. M., and Solow, S. P., 1969, Heartrate, aggression and dominance in the domestic chicken, *J. Comp. Physiol. Psychol. 67:*70.

Candland, D. K., Bryan, D. C., Nazar, B. L., Kopf, K. J., and Sendor, M., 1970, Squirrel monkey heartrate during formation of status orders, *J. Comp. Physiol. Psychol. 70:*417.

Christian, J. J., and Davis, D. E., 1956, The relation between adrenal weight and population status of urban Norway rats, *J. Mammol. 37:*475.

Cox, G. S., Hodges, J. R., and Vernikos, J., 1958, The effect of adrenalectomy on the circulating level of adrenocorticotrophic hormone in the rat, *J. Endocrinol. 17:*177.

DeWied, D., and Weijnen, J. A. W. M., 1970 *Pituitary, adrenal and brain*, Elsevier, Amsterdam.

Edwards, D. A., 1968, Mice: fighting by neonatally androgenized females, *Science 161:*1027.

Edwards, D. A., 1969, Early androgen stimulation and aggressive behavior in male and female mice. *Physiol. Behav. 4:*333.

Edwards, D. A., 1970, Post-neonatal androgenization and adult aggressive behavior in female mice, *Physiol. Behav. 5:*465.

Harding, C. F., and Leshner, A. I., 1972, The effects of adrenalectomy on the aggressiveness of differently housed mice, *Physiol. Behav. 8:*437.

Hayama, S., 1966, Correlation between adrenal gland weight and dominance rank in caged crab-eating monkeys, *Primates 7:*21.

Leshner, A. I., 1971, The adrenals and the regulatory nature of running wheel activity, *Physiol. Behav. 6:*551.

Leshner, A. I., and Candland, D. K., 1972, Endocrine effects of grouping and dominance rank in squirrel monkeys, *Physiol. Behav. 8:*441.

Levy, J. V., and King, J. A., 1953, The effects of testosterone propionate on fighting behavior in young C57BL/10 mice, *Anat. Rec. 117:*562.

Louch, C. D., and Higginbotham, M., 1967, The relation between social rank and plasma corticosterone levels in mice, *Gen. Comp. Endocrinol. 8:*441.

Ploog, D. W., 1966, Biological bases for instinct and behavior: Studies on the development of social behavior in squirrel monkeys, *Rec. Adv. Biol. Psychiat. 8:*199.

Richter, C. P., 1927, Animal behavior and internal drives, *Quant. Rev. Biol. 2:*307.

Sassenrath, E. N., 1970, Increased adrenal responsiveness related to social stress in Rhesus monkeys, *Horm. Behav. 1:*283.

Scott, J. P., and Fredericson, E., 1951, The causes of fighting in mice and rats, *Physiol. Zool. 24:*273.

Sigg, E. B., Day, C., and Colombo, C., 1966, Endocrine factors in isolated-induced aggressiveness in rodents, *Endocrinol. 78:*679.

Svare, B. B. and Leshner, A. I., 1973, Behavioral correlates of intermale aggression and grouping in mice, *J. Comp. Physiol. Psychol. 85;*203.

Tollman, J., and King, J. A., 1956, The effects of testosterone propionate on aggression in male and female C57BL/10 mice, *Brit. J. Anim. Behav. 4:*147.

Welch, A. S., and Welch, B. L., 1971, Isolation, reactivity and aggression: Evidence for an involvement of brain catecholamines and serotonin, in *The Physiology of Aggression and Defeat*, B. E. Eleftheriou and J. P. Scott, eds., Plenum Press, New York.

Welch, B. L., and Welch, A. S., 1969, Aggression and the biogenic amine neurohumors, in *Aggressive Behaviour*, S. Garattini and E. B. Sigg, eds., John Wiley, New York.

Yen, H. C., Day, C. A., and Sigg, E. B., 1962, Influence of endocrine factors on the development of fighting behaviour in rodents, *Pharmacol 4:*173.

CHAPTER 5

Immunological and Chemical Sympathectomy in the Neonatal Rodent: Effects on Emotional Behavior*

Bruce A. Pappas

Department of Psychology
Carleton University
Ottawa, Canada

1. Introduction

The relevance of visceral responses for emotional behavior or at least subjective states we could define as emotional has been debated since the inception of modern day psychophysiology. This original debate has not yet reached resolution. Its main historical anchor is William James' contention that emotions arise from our perceptions of the central and peripheral (somato-visceral) events which are elicited by a stimulus and the immediate reflexive response it may evoke. James (1894) stated that empirical confirmation of this hypothesis would evolve from demonstrations of reduced affect in subjects with experimental or clinical attenuation of visceral-somatic responsivity. However, as Fehr and Stern (1970) recently pointed out, these demonstrations encountered two difficulties. First, the extent of the reduction in most cases, was incomplete; and secondly, humans can present outward manifestations of emotion in the absence of subjective "feelings" of emotion. The latter difficulty can perhaps be overcome by observation of infrahumans who, we assume, have neither strategy for nor gain from such subterfuge. Despite choice of the infrahuman subject, however, research is still hampered by the inability either to reduce completely visceral responses or selectively to block only the presumedly critical visceral responses.

* This research was supported by research grant number A8267 from the National Research Council of Canada and by Carleton University.

Several modern theorists (see Goldstein, 1968) have assumed visceral events to be important, if not essential, for emotional behavior or feeling. Typically, the critical visceral events are identified as responses mediated primarily by the sympathetic division (SNS) of the autonomic nervous system. This choice is not surprising because of poetic bias which, for example, has coupled the rapidly beating heart and heavy pulse with tenderness or terror, and because the protagonists in the early debate with James, such as Cannon *et al.* (1927, 1929), had attempted to disprove James' theory by experimenting with spinal or surgically sympathec- tomized preparations. Current research typically employs immunological or pharmacological agents to destroy selectively or prevent the development of the SNS (neonatal sympathectomy). This chapter will review recent physiological and behavioral data from experiments in which the development of the sympathetic division has been prevented. Although there will be some discussion of the effects of acute sympathectomy, i.e., the destruction of an already mature SNS, recent and excellent reviews (e.g., Fehr and Stern, 1969) necessitate a limited treatment of this topic.

The effects on emotional behavior of acute and neonatal sympa- thectomy might be expected to differ. In the former instance, visceral responses and their afferent feedback which have typically accompanied emotional behavior are eliminated. In fact if visceral responses are relevant to the behavior, the effects of acute sympathectomy should depend upon the interval between acute sympathectomy and testing since some adapta- tions to the novel physiology might be expected. Even if the visceral event is assumed not to be essential for the behavior, but rather simply a component of the total stimulus complex which elicits or accompanies the behavior, then generalization decrement should be most noticeable im- mediately after sympathectomy. Systematic manipulation of the sympa- thectomy–test interval has not been carried out. In neonatal sympa- thectomy, the organism has only minimally, if ever, experienced the sym- pathetic accompaniments of its emotional behavior. It is entirely possible that what is never there as a relevant stimulus event is therefore never missed or that compensatory physiological or neural adjustments may assume the functional role of the missing event. On the other hand, the lack of experience of the sympathetic response may not mitigate its functional necessity for emotional behavior, and behavioral deficits would then be ex- pected.

Existing data on the effects of acute sympathectomy suggest that be- haviors assumed to be motivated by emotions such as fear are not eliminated, although they may be at least quantitatively different from those seen in normal subjects. For example, Wynne and Solomon in their classic monograph (1955) demonstrated that surgically sympathectomized dogs were capable of learning an avoidance response, although the dogs' responses tended to be somewhat less regular than those typically observed in their laboratory. Several experiments also purport to show that acute pharmacological blockade of autonomic function impairs fear-motivated behavior (e.g., Arbit, 1957, 1958; Auld, 1951), but the side effects of the blocking agents used clearly preclude any conclusions from these demonstrations (Brady, 1953). More recent reports on the tranquilizing effects of the beta-adrenergic blocking agents, propranolol in rats (Bainbridge and Greenwood, 1971) and practolol in human clinical anxieties (Bonn et al., 1972) suggest a reexamination of the role of the SNS in anxiety- or fear-motivated behavior. Whereas propranolol has central as well as peripheral blocking effects, practolol has demonstrably less access to the brain.

This chapter will review some autonomic and concomitant physiological effects, and behavioral effects of neonatal sympathectomy (hereafter simply referred to as sympathectomy) in mice and rats. I intend to point out that although there is some consistency between the behavioral effects of two types of sympathectomy—immunosympathectomy by neonatal injections of nerve growth factor antiserum (NGFA) and chemical sympathectomy by 6-hydroxydopamine (6-OH)—the physiological and neurochemical changes which accompany the latter treatment make it difficult either to compare their behavioral effects or to attribute these effects solely to the arrested growth and/or destruction of the SNS. Furthermore, while neonatal injections of guanethidine may arrest development of the SNS to a degree comparable to that after neonatal 6-OH, they do not appear to also alter neurochemical characteristics of the brain, as do the 6-OH injections. However, the behavioral effects of guanethidine are different from those of 6-OH, and these effects also may differ from those caused by immunosympathectomy.

2.   Immunosympathectomy and 6-OH Sympathectomy*

The antiserum to the sympathetic nerve growth factor was first produced by Cohen (1960). Subsequent research has shown that daily injections of this antiserum in newborn mice for the first 5 days after birth produces a permanently arrested growth and destruction of around 90% of

* For a more extensive introduction to this topic the reader is referred to two recent volumes: *6-Hydroxydopamine and Catecholamine Neurons*, T. Malmfors and H. Thoenen, eds., American Elsevier, New York, 1971, and *Immunosympathectomy*, G. Steiner and E. Schonbaum, eds., American Elsevier, New York, 1972.

the sympathetic nerve cells in the paravertebral sympathetic chain ganglia (Levi-Montalcini and Booker, 1960; Levi-Montalcini and Angeletti, 1966; Angeletti and Levi-Montalcini, 1971). The destructive effects in the rat are somewhat less. Cells in the prevertebral ganglia are more resistant to destruction while noradrenergic ganglia innervating sex organs are highly resistant to destruction.

Marked reduction of norepinephrine (Ne) contents of sympathetically innervated tissues by systemic injections of 6-OH in the adult mouse was reported by Porter et al., in 1963. Subsequent experiments showed that mainly noradrenergic axons were destroyed while the neuronal cell bodies were spared. The time required for regeneration of the axon is dependent upon the frequency and quantity of dose (e.g., Goldman and Jacobowitz, 1971). Angeletti and Levi-Montalcini reported in 1970 that seven daily postnatal injections of 50 $\mu g/g$ of 6-OH in both mice and rats produced a permanent destruction of major portions of the sympathetic nervous system. Unlike injections of 6-OH in the adult rat, which mainly affect noradrenergic terminal axons, neonatal 6-OH, like immunosympathectomy, also destroys noradrenergic cell bodies. As with NGFA, neonatal 6-OH spares sympathetic ganglia innervating the sex organs (Jaim-Etcheverry and Zieher, 1971; Clark et al., 1972).

The mechanisms of action of NGFA and 6-OH are not clear. Presumably the former reacts with the nerve growth factor in the maturing sympathetic cells (Angeletti and Levi-Montalcini, 1971) while the oxidation of 6-OH, after its uptake into Ne-containing bodies, may ultimately produce its destructive effects (Heikkila and Cohen, 1971; Adams et al., 1972).

3.   Neonatal Guanethidine Injections: Sympathectomizing?

Recent research shows that repeated injections of the peripheral catecholamine depleting agent guanethidine produces an almost complete destruction of the SNS in the adult rat (Burnstock et al., 1971; Evans et al., 1972). It has also been noticed that during management of benign essential hypertension with guanethidine, blood pressure is often maintained at normal levels after the patient has been taken off the drug (Burch, 1972). The possibility of permanently damaged sympathetic cardiovascular innervation in these patients has not been examined.

That injections of guanethidine in the neonatal rat might produce a chronic sympathectomy was first suggested by Eränkö and Eränkö (1971a,b). In their experiments, a marked reduction of fluorescence of sympathetic ganglia was observed in 21-day-old rats who had received eight daily injections of guanethidine (20 mg/kg), beginning on the day of birth.

TABLE 1. Ne Contents in Hearts and Spleens of 6-OH,
Guanethidine, and Tyramine Injected Rats[a]

	Heart	Spleen
6-OH	$46.6 \pm 25.3\%$	$14.1 \pm 5.4\%$
Guanethidine	$54.1 \pm 28.3\%$	$62.0 \pm 30.8\%$
Tyramine	$145.8 \pm 58.1\%$	$108.3 \pm 38.5\%$

[a] The data are expressed as mean percent of vehicle control values $\pm$ confidence intervals ($p = 0.05$).

Since the age of sacrifice was not systematically manipulated, there was no indication of the permanence of this effect.

We have conducted an experiment in which newborn rats were administered eight daily injections (s.c.) of either vehicle, 6-OH, guanethidine (25 or 75 mg/kg), or tyramine (100 μg/kg). The latter treatment was included because we were concerned that several behavioral observations of rats injected with 6-OH and guanethidine might be due to the sympathomimetic effects of the drug (by release of endogenous catecholamines) early in life. Tyramine we reasoned, ought to produce somewhat comparable effects and hence would be an appropriate control group for this effect. The rats were sacrificed between 120 and 150 days of age and peripheral organs assayed for endogenous catecholamine contents. Table 1 summarizes these data.

Guanethidine produced a permanent reduction of peripheral endogenous catecholamines which was not quite as marked as that produced by 6-OH. Curiously, tyramine slightly elevated cardiac Ne levels, but these data were extremely variable. Considerably more data need to be collected, particularly from dose and injection frequency manipulations, and measures of residual autonomic functions are also needed, before the degree and extent of this sympathectomizing technique can be clearly assessed. Nevertheless, for reasons that will be more evident when we later discuss the effects of neonatal 6-OH and guanethidine upon brain catecholamines, this treatment may eventually be the most suitable for examining the effects of peripheral neonatal sympathectomy.

4. Some Effects of Immuno- and 6-OH Sympathectomy on Autonomic Reactivity

Neither NGFA (Brody, 1964; Wenzel *et al.*, 1966; Hofer *et al.*, 1971; Thornton and Van-Toller, 1973) nor 6-OH sympathectomy (Pappas and

DiCara, 1973; Pappas *et al.*, 1974) seems to affect basal heart rate. It seems unlikely that basal heart rate is maintained at normal rates in sympathectomized animals by circulating catecholamines from the adrenal medulla. Brody (1966) has found no effect of adrenal demedullation upon heart rates recorded in lightly anesthetized rats who had received either the antiserum or no treatment. Hofer *et al.*, (1971) hypothesized that since the sino-atrial node is innervated several days prior to parturition, its sympathetic connections are spared by the antiserum. Some sparing of the pacemaker may also occur with a 6-OH sympathectomy. However, resting blood pressure in either normotensive or hypertensive (genetic) rats is lowered by both NGFA (e.g., Zaimis, 1965; Clark, 1971) and 6-OH sympathectomy (Pappas and DiCara, 1973; Pappas *et al.*, 1974).

Both the cardiac rate response and the blood pressure response to environmental stimulation have been shown to be altered by sympathectomy. Wenzel *et al.* (1966) found that heart rates of IS mice (Swiss–Webster) exposed for 30 minutes to a novel environment declined over the test interval while rates of control mice remained constant. Furthermore, presentation of a 2-second-duration light shock through floor grids caused a rate elevation in control mice that was significantly higher than their initial basal rates. While IS mice also showed an elevation, the increase was not significantly greater than their initial baseline rates. Furthermore, the decline in rate after shock offset was considerably greater in the IS mice. IS rats also show attenuated cardiac rate responses to transient asphyxia (Hofer *et al.*, 1971) and an inability to learn to either increase or decrease heart rate in order to avoid punishing electric shock while curarized and artificially respirated (Thornton and Van-Toller, 1973).

Alterations in the cardiac rate response to environmental stimulation may be due to at least two mechanisms. First, sympathetic innervation of the heart, as determined by its Ne content, is drastically reduced by both IS (e.g., Visscher *et al.*, 1965) and 6-OH (e.g., Pappas and Sobrian, 1972). Second, the pressor response which may elicit a compensatory cardiac rate adjustment is attenuated by at least 6-OH and presumably also by NGFA. DiCara and I (Pappas and DiCara, 1973) paralyzed 6-OH and vehicle control rats with succinylcholine at about 103 days of age. While blood pressure was being recorded through a previously implanted aortic catheter and heart rate from subcutaneous electrodes, the artificially respirated rats were subjected to a Pavlovian conditioning procedure consisting of 42 light-tone (conditioned stimulus, CS) presentations which were coterminous with a 0.3-second-duration, 0.5-mA shock delivered through electrodes attached to the hind paws. The seventh trial and every eighth trial thereafter were test trials during which only the CS was presented. These test trials permitted assessment in the absence of shock of the development of the conditioned blood pressure and heart rate responses. Half of each of the 6-OH and vehicle subjects were also injected during the course of procedure with atropine sulfate to permit examination of the effects of parasympathetic blockage upon the conditioned responses.

The 6-OH treated rats showed both lower basal systolic blood pressure and attenuated second-to-second blood pressure variability. Atropine had no effect on blood pressure. However, 6-OH rats had basal heart rates equivalent to those of the vehicle group while atropine raised heart rates equally in both the 6-OH and vehicle rats. The upper portion of Fig. 1 shows systolic blood pressure difference scores from pre-CS baselines during the final test trial presentation and for the 3 seconds following CS termination for the four groups in the experiment. The lower portion of the figure shows similarly calculated heart rate difference scores. From the upper portion, it can be seen that 6-OH rats showed a markedly attenuated conditioned pressure increase. Atropine had no effect on the pressor

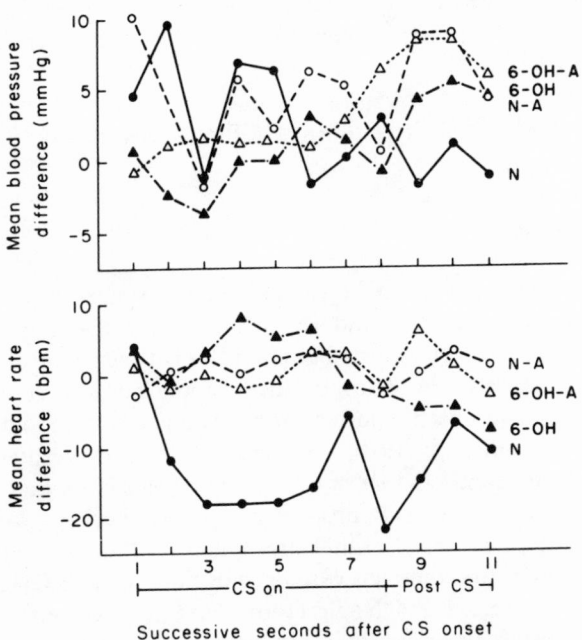

FIG. 1. Systolic blood pressure (upper half) and heart rate (lower half) responses during a conditioned stimulus for footshock and the 3 seconds after CS onset for vehicle–nonatropinized (N), vehicle–atropinized (N–A), 6-OH injected and nonatropinized (6-OH) and 6-OH injected and atropinized (6-OH–A) rats (from Pappas and DiCara, 1973).

response. The lower portion of this figure shows that the vehicle injected, nonatropinized rats showed a marked bradycardia within 2 seconds after CS onset, which was evident until about halfway through the CS presentation. Their rates then increased until CS termination when they again abruptly decelerated. In contrast, the 6-OH injected, nonatropinized rats show an acceleration peaking 4 seconds after CS onset followed by a return to baseline. Atropine also eliminated the deceleration to the CS seen in the vehicle group.

Since 6-OH eliminated the CS-induced bradycardia observed in the nonatropinized control rats, and since this bradycardia was also eliminated by atropine while only 6-OH eliminated the pressor response to the CS, these data suggested to us that conditioned cardiac deceleration in the rat may be a vagal mediated response compensatory to a prior blood pressure increase. This interpretation suggests that differences in heart rate reactivity between control and sympathectomized rats (or mice) to environmental manipulations may be at least partly accounted for by the attenuation of their blood pressure reactivity. When the pressor response is altered, the cardiac rate adjustment through baroreceptor feedback is also affected.

5. Some Additional Physiological Effects of Immuno- and 6-OH Sympathectomy

5.1. Adrenal Function

While weight of the whole adrenals (e.g., Wenzel and Nagle, 1965; Wenzel and Jeffrey, 1967) and the adrenal medullae (e.g., Carpi and Oliverio, 1964) have been reported to not differ between control and IS mice or rats, respectively, hypertrophy in histological sections of adrenal chromaffin tissue has been reported for 6-OH injected mice and rats (Angeletti and Levi-Montalcini, 1970; Angeletti, 1971). However, whole adrenal weights are significantly lighter in 6-OH treated rats (Lew and Quay, 1971; Sachs and Jonsson, 1972; Pappas et al., 1974). Perhaps 6-OH sympathectomy causes hypotrophy of the adrenal cortex? Pituitary–adrenocortical function has not been extensively examined in either IS or 6-OH injected animals, although Wenzel and Nagle (1965) have reported no differences in adrenal corticosteroids or ascorbic acid between IS and control rats. In light of the possible involvement of this axis in fear-motivated behavior (e.g., Di Giusto et al., 1971), further research is warranted.

Both the antiserum (Carpi and Oliverio, 1964; Visscher et al., 1965) and 6-OH (Lew and Quay, 1971; Sachs and Jonsson, 1972) lead to increased adrenal Ne concentrations. Since the epinephrine (E) contents of the gland are reduced by antiserum in mice (Visscher *et al.*, 1965) and rats (Carpi and Oliverio, 1964), this treatment thus increases the adrenal ratio of endogenous Ne to E. We have failed to observe this increased ratio of Ne to E in 6-OH sympathectomized rats. Table 2 shows adrenal concentrations for two rat strains, a normotensive and a hypertensive strain. Both Ne and E contents were found to be elevated by 6-OH in both strains, although the elevation was statistically significant only for Ne. The Ne to E ratios were not found to differ reliably between control and drug-injected rats.

Because of this apparent compensatory adjustment of adrenal function after sympathectomy, adrenal demedullation might be expected to have more profound physiological effects in sympathectomized than in normal subjects. While signs of this have been found, for example, demedullation causes lower rectal temperatures and more attenuated vasoconstrictor responses to a ganglionic stimulant in IS rats (Brody, 1966), IS rats also appear to have remarkable residual capacities for norepinephrine excertion even after demedullation. Amphetamine produces greater urinary Ne excretion in demedullated IS rats than in control demedullated rats (Carpi and Oliverio, 1964), while urinary excretion of Ne is not significantly lowered in demedullated IS rats subjects to extreme cold (Schonbaum *et al.*, 1966). The source of this Ne in IS rats is unknown, but both extra-adrenal chromaffin tissue (Carpi and Oliverio, 1964) and remaining sympathetic neurons which are intact after NGFA (Schonbaum *et al.*, 1966) have been suggested as potential candidates. Whatever the source, the behavioral significance is relatively obscure. Since both IS (Brody, 1964) and 6-OH sympathectomized rats (Clark *et al.*, 1972) show longer lasting vascular responses to exogenous Ne, behavioral comparisons of control subjects with both IS and 6-OH sympathectomized subjects are inevitably confounded with this mechanism unless the subjects are both demedullated and given a peripheral adrenergic blocking agent or simply given the blocking agent.

TABLE 2.   Concentrations of Ne and E (μg/g Tissue) in the Adrenals of Normotensive and Hypertensive Rats (from Pappas *et al.*, 1974)

Strain		Ne	E
Normotensive	control	126.7	199.1
	6-OH	146.9	208.8
Hypertensive	control	103.1	162.3
	6-OH	129.7	184.9

In the two separate laboratory investigations which have combined adrenal demedullation with IS, the combined effects due to IS and demedullation have not been very noticeably different from those due to IS alone (Sampson, 1966; Carson, 1970). Carson reported that, although adrenal medullectomy led to consistently lower heart-rate reactivity in IS mice than in control mice, no additional behavioral effects were noted.

6. Central Neurochemical Effects of Neonatal Sympathectomy

Angeletti (1971), in one of her early reports on 6-OH sympathectomy, reported that Ne contents of whole brains were lower in 6-OH-treated than in vehicle-injected rats. Roughly simultaneously, Jaim-Etcheverry and Zieher (1971) recorded that no changes in Ne levels in the central nervous system were found 3 weeks after neonatal 6-OH treatment. However, shortly thereafter, Lew and Quay (1971) showed that adult rats who had received 7 daily postnatal injections had higher hypothalmic Ne contents than controls. Sobrian and I (Pappas and Sobrian, 1972) failed to observe any effect of the treatment upon hypothalamic Ne—however, we did observe that while cortical Ne was reduced to about 50% in the 6-OH injected rats, brainstem (pons, medulla, and midbrain) Ne was increased to about 150% of control values. Recently, a somewhat different injection schedule (100 μg/g vs. 50 μg/g and weekly for 10 consecutive weeks, as opposed to daily for seven consecutive postnatal days and "booster" injections at 10, 15. and 22 days) has also been shown to reduce prepontine Ne levels while increasing the level in the lower brainstem (Jacks et al., 1972). We have since extended our original findings with one exception, to two different rat strains, a normotensive Wistar strain and the genetically hypertensive strain (Okamoto, 1969). The recent data also reveal an increase in hypothalamic Ne; this finding is consistent with that of Lew and Quay, but apparently inconsistent with our earlier report. Table 3 shows these data. The reason for the variation among the assay results for the hypothalamus is not clear.

The mechanism responsible for the regionally specific altered brain Ne levels is as yet, unclear. Sobrian and I, arguing on the basis of an inverse relationship between blood pressure and brainstem Ne, suggested that the chronic depression of sympathetic activity produced by 6-OH may be responsible for at least the observed Ne increase in the brainstem. This hypothesis rested upon the supposition of an inverse relationship between visceral excitatory afferents, particularly baroreceptor input to the CNS, and brainstem Ne. A more plausible hypothesis is simply that the blood–brain barrier of the immature rat is permeable to 6-OH. Jacks et al.,

(1972) suggest that the permeating 6-OH destroys developing noradrenergic fibers in the anterior brain, and that since the cell bodies of most of these fibers are found in the brainstem, these cell bodies would accumulate the amine in the same manner that proximal catecholamine accumulation occurs in peripheral neurons after axotomy. Dahlstrom and Fuxe (1965) report, however, peak proximal accumulation several days after axotomy followed by a gradual decline. The duration of this peak period is considerably shorter than the time between the 6-OH injection (7–22 days of age) and sacrifice (up to 150 days) used by our laboratory and others (e.g., Lew and Quay, 1971). Perhaps age at time of chemical axotomy may be critical for the duration of accumulation—more cells with increased catecholamine contents after axotomy are observed in young animals than in older animals (Dahlstrom and Fuxe, 1965). At any rate, the observations of decreased Ne levels in the cortex correspond with decreased uptake of radioactively labeled Ne and fluorescent histochemical evidence of disappearance of cortical adrenergic neurons (Sachs and Jonsson, 1972). Sachs and Jonsson also observed uptake to be markedly reduced in the spinal cord while hypothalamic uptake was less severely reduced.

On the other hand, if 6-OH does permeate the infant blood–brain barrier, then its long-term effects on adrenergic systems seem to be quite different from those observed after direct brain injections. Data on regional brain enzyme activity collected by my colleague Dr. David Peters of the University of Ottawa Pharmacology Department indicates that the altered regional levels of Ne are closely matched by regional alterations of activity of the rate-limiting enzyme for the catecholamines, tyrosine hydroxylase. Table 4 shows these data (Pappas et al., 1974).

TABLE 3. Summary of Endogenous Ne Contents for Brain Tissue of 6-OH and Vehicle Injected Normotensive and Hypertensive Rats[a]

	Ne content		
	Cortex	Hypothalamus	Brainstem
Normotensive vehicle	0.59	1.60	0.49
6-OH	0.30	2.08	0.86
Hypertensive vehicle	0.61	1.64	0.51
6-OH	0.33	2.06	0.85

[a] The data are expressed as $\mu g/g$ tissue.

TABLE 4. Tyrosine Hydroxylase Activity in Vehicle and 6-OH
Injected Rats (nmole dopa/hour/gram of tissue)

	Tyrosine hydroxylase activity		
	Cortex	Hypothalamus	Brainstem
Vehicle	2.10 ± 0.10	25.4 ± 1.8	3.80 ± 0.17
6-OH	0.15 ± 0.03	27.3 ± 1.0	5.09 ± 0.15
% vehicle	7%	107%	134%

Not only are these alterations in tyrosine hydroxylase evident in the adult rat, but we also find them in the 9- and 16-day-old rat. These profound changes would be unlikely at this early stage in the rat's existence if in fact they were central manifestations of the effect of chronically reduced peripheral sympathetic tone. Intuitively, one would expect that the latter would be somewhat slow in developing, particularly since sympathetic function does not approach maturity until around the 3rd week of the rat's life. More recently Peters and I have found that neonatal 6-OH not only causes chronic changes in brain catecholamines, but also significantly alters regional brain serotonin turnover and endogenous histamine levels (Peters et al., 1974; Pappas et al., 1974). As Table 5 shows, serotonin turnover (but not serotonin levels) and hypothalamic histamine levels are significantly increased by neonatal 6-OH.

While we have no hypothesis to account for all of these effects of 6-OH upon brain chemistry, we interpret the effects upon catecholamine function as due to selective destruction of the dorsal noradrenergic bundle. This interpretation was originally formulated by Taylor et al. (1972) to account for their observations that brain areas such as the cerebral cortex, cerebellum, and hippocampus, suggested by Ungerstedt (1971) as being innervated by axons from the locus coeruleus, show permanent depletion of catecholamines after neonatal 6-OH. On the other hand, Ne levels in the hypothalamus (Pappas and Sobrian, 1972; Sachs and Jonsson, 1972), thalamus (Taylor et al., 1972), and corpus striatum (Taylor et al., 1972; Sachs and Jonsson, 1972) are not consistently affected by this drug treatment. When we assume Ungerstedt's map, these data suggest that there is no lasting destruction of axons within the ventral noradrenergic system.

This interpretation gains additional credibility from the fact that electrolytic lesions of the locus coeruleus in the adult rat cause decreased Ne contents in the cerebellum, hippocampus, and cortex, but not in the hypothalamus (Thierry *et al.,* 1973). On the other hand, lesions in the area of the pedunculus cerebellus superior, where the axons of the dorsal and ventral systems are adjacent, not only produce regional decreases in Ne similar to those observed after lesioning of the locus coeruleus, but also significantly reduce hypothalamic Ne. In other words, the effects upon regional brain Ne appear to be the same either after electrolytic lesions of the locus coeruleus in the adult rat or after neonatal injections of 6-OH.

The extent to which regional central neurochemical changes occur with immunosympathectomy is not clear. Of the reported data, IS subjects have shown only slightly lower whole-brain noradrenaline (Levi-Montalcini and Angeletti, 1962; Visscher *et al.,* 1965) and 5-HT contents (Klingman, 1969) while Hamberger *et al.* (1964) reported "essentially normal" histochemical fluorescence of the hypothalamus of IS rats. Injecting pregnant mice with NGFA leads to only slightly reduced brainstem Ne contents in the offspring, while Ne levels in the remainder of the brain show only a slight increase (Klingman, 1966).

Neonatal injections of guanethidine, as far as we can determine, have negligible effects upon brain catecholamines. Table 6 summarizes data we have collected on regional brain Ne levels in adult rats who have received guanethidine during infancy. Furthermore, we have also measured tyrosine hydroxylase levels in the brains of 9-day-old rats who had received guanethidine injections in each of the preceding 8 days and have observed no difference between these rats and vehicle controls.

These findings of central neurochemical changes due to neonatal 6-OH raise the question as to whether this treatment is suitable for the determi-

TABLE 5. Effects of Neonatal 6-OH on Various Brain Enzyme and
Amine Levels (% Vehicle Value)

	Levels		
Substance	Cortex	Hypothalamus	Brainstem
Monoamine oxidase	97%	97%	105%
5-Hydroxytryptophan decarboxylase	107%	108%	95%
Tryptophan-5-hydroxylase	110%	130%[a]	145%[a]
Serotonin	—	110%	107%
5-Hydroxyindole acetic acid	—	160%[a]	125%[a]
Tryptophan	—	102%	100%
Histamine	—	116%[a]	—

[a] $p < 0.05$.

TABLE 6. Ne Contents in Various Brain Regions of 6-OH, Guanethidine, and Tyramine Injected Rats[a]

	Ne content			
	Cortex	Hypothalamus	Brainstem	Cerebellum
6-OH	$41.7 \pm 25.3\%$	$118.0 \pm 27.0\%$	$155.2 \pm 23.8\%$	$83.3 \pm 21.5\%$
Guanethidine	$121.7 \pm 53.8\%$	$113.3 \pm 50.1\%$	$108.7 \pm 24.2\%$	$102.1 \pm 36.2\%$
Tyramine	$71.6 \pm 49.5\%$	$116.8 \pm 28.3\%$	$102.4 \pm 34.2\%$	140.8 ± 66.5

[a] The data are expressed as mean percent of vehicle control values $\pm$ confidence intervals ($p = 0.05$).

nation of the role of the sympathetic nervous system in emotional behavior. Rather limited data nominate the antiserum and guanethidine as the manipulations of choice, insofar as the reported brain effects appear negligible, but further research on these effects seems necessary. Furthermore, although it has been generally assumed that systemic injections of 6-OH in the adult rat have only peripheral effects, and therefore that this procedure would produce an acute sympathectomy unconfounded by central effects, recent data indicate that this treatment may in fact have a direct (Sachs and Jonsson, 1973) or at least indirect effect (Clark et al., 1971) upon brain amines. The wisdom of using this procedure for determining the behavioral effects of acute peripheral sympathectomy (e.g., Pappas et al., 1972; DiGuisto, 1972) now seems questionable.

7. Behavioral Effects of Neonatal Sympathectomy

The behavioral effects of neonatal sympathectomy are, at best, obscure. Not only is there inconsistency when the effects of a single technique such as immunosympathectomy are examined (although there are suggestions that inhibitory-avoidance capacity is reduced under some circumstances), but there is no real consistency between the effects of immuno-, 6-OH, and guanethidine sympathectomy. The latter is of course not surprising since 6-OH sympathectomy, as we now know, is accompanied by pervasive effects upon brain chemistry. Most of our research on the behavioral effects of 6-OH sympathectomy was carried out before we were fully aware of these permanent changes in brain amines. In fact, since we had interpreted our first findings showing altered central catecholamine levels as due to feedback effects of the peripheral reduction of sympathetic tone (Pappas and Sobrian, 1972), we assumed that 6-OH sympathectomy provided a sound technique for determining the relevance of visceral responses for emotional behavior. Since it now seems that the brain effects are at least partly independent of the peripheral effects, insofar as the drug has access to the infant brain, this assumption is incorrect. Consequently, we are currently comparing the effects of 6-OH and guanethidine sympathectomy, as our data indicate that the latter's effects may be restricted to the peripheral nervous system.

7.1. Locomotor Activity

The effects of NGFA upon locomotor activity seem to depend upon the apparatus used to measure activity. Comparisons of activity in jiggle cages have consistently failed to yield differences between control and immunosympathectomized (IS) mice (Wenzel and Jeffrey, 1967; Tarpy and Van-Toller, 1972). Durations of tests ranged from 30 minutes (Wenzel and Jeffrey) to 4 hours (Tarpy and Van-Toller). Hofer *et al.* (1971) using EMG and EKG artifacts to measure activity also failed to observe differences between control and IS rats.

The effects of NGFA upon runwheel activity are somewhat equivocal. Only a single experimenter (Sampson, 1966) has subjected her animals (rats) to a multiple-day, controlled light–dark cycle procedure to permit examination of chronic baseline behavior and possible drug-treatment–diurnal interactions. Sampson, running her Charles River rats for 5 days on a 12-hour light-on–light-off cycle found no differences between control and IS males. However, female rats who had been either adrenal demedullated or sham operated were significantly more active than the IS, IS and demedullated, and nonhandled groups. This suggestion of a possible NFGA–sex interaction on runwheel activity has not been further pursued. Wenzel (1968a) gave Swiss–Webster mice access to running wheels for short intervals (15 or 3 minutes) at 85 and 92 days of age, respectively. No differences were found between IS and control mice at either age. However, Tarpy and Van-Toller found IS mice of a heterogeneous strain to be more active than horse serum controls over a 4-hour wheel exposure at either normal room temperature (22.5°C) or in a cold room (3.5°C). Neonatal sympathectomy by 6-OH neither affects runwheel activity measured over 3 days in either a normotensive or a genetically hypertensive strain of rats (Pappas *et al.*, 1974), nor does it alter normal light–dark cycles of activity measured over this same period.

7.2. Positive Reward Procedures

Neonatal sympathectomy apparently does not affect learning or performance motivated by positive reward. Wenzel and Nagle (1965) reported no effect of NGFA on bar press, discrimination performance of Swiss–Webster mice for sweetened milk reward although Wenzel and Jeffrey (1967) found, using a somewhat similar procedure, that both IS mice and their vehicle injected controls barpressed more frequently than handled and nonhandled control groups during both acquisition and extinction periods of a variable interval schedule. However, massed trial runway acquisition and extinction performance for milk reinforcement has also been found to be normal in immunosympathectomized Swiss–Webster mice (Wenzel, 1968a). Saari and I have observed no differences between vehicle and 6-OH injected normotensive and hypertensive rats on a water-rewarded maze learning task (Saari and Pappas, 1973).

7.3. Open-Field Performance

Open-field tests have been used by several different laboratories to assess the effects of neonatal sympathectomy on emotionality. The commonly used indices of performance in this test seem to reflect the operation of several variables, most notably emotionality and exploratory drive. Emotionality seems to be best reflected, at least in the rat, by a combination of high activity and high defecation scores in the initial exposure to the apparatus (Whimbey and Denenberg, 1967, Soubrie, 1971). When we assume this criterion, the data for the effects of neonatal sympathectomy show little consistency.

Immunosympathectomized Swiss–Webster mice when initially tested on the open field have been reported as less active at various ages (Wenzel and Jeffrey, 1967), to defecate more and move less (Wenzel, 1968a), and to be more active (Carson, 1970). Van-Toller (1968) reported that IS mice of an inbred strain were more active than controls. There was indication that they also defecated more in the open field, although they had defecated less frequently when being transported to the apparatus. Furthermore, a significant negative correlation was found between activity and the size of the cervical and thoracic sympathetic ganglia remaining after NGFA.

Sampson (1966) reported that NGFA had no effect on open-field behavior in male Charles River rats while females scored higher on an index comprised of the sum of defecations, urinations, and crouching behaviors. Sobrian and I reported that neonatal 6-OH sympathectomy only slightly reduced the activity of male and female Sprague–Dawley rats tested in the

open field at 43 days of age (Pappas and Sobrian, 1972). Defecation was
unaffected. No effect was also observed for animals first tested at 104 days
of age. This experiment was followed by another (Pappas *et al.,* 1974,
examining the effect of 6-OH sympathectomy on open-field performance in
both a 43-day-old control Wistar strain and a spontaneously hypertensive
Wistar strain (SHR) developed by Okamoto (Okamoto, 1969). The 6-OH
sympathectomy caused a slight, but noticeable, reduction in activity in the
normotensive Wistar rats. However, the same treatment caused an increase
in activity in the hypertensive strain, an increase that when compared only
with the hypertensive vehicle groups, was not statistically reliable.
However, since 6-OH differentially affected the activity of the two strains,
analysis of variance performed on the data produced a statistically significant interaction between drug and strain treatments. Also, 6-OH tended to
reduce rearing behavior in the normotensive strain while increasing rearing
in the hypertensives, although the effect fell just short of statistical reliability. Overall, the hypertensives were considerably more active than the
normotensives. We also found further evidence for drug–strain interactions.
We had made no attempt to cull our litters to a constant size. Consequently, litter sizes were variable. When the rats were later weaned, they
were simply segregated by sex into colony cages until tested at 43 days in
the open field. As a result, the size of the caged groups from weaning until
open-field testing also varied. Table 7 shows rank correlations between
open-field activity scores and both litter size and postweaning, colony cage
group size.

While litter size failed to correlate with activity, group size showed
correlations with activity which varied among the four treatment groups.
The vehicle injected normotensives showed a significant negative correlation between group size and activity, but neonatal sympathectomy
eliminated this correlation. On the other hand, vehicle hypertensive rats
showed no correlation between group size and activity, but the sympathectomy produced a significant positive correlation for this strain. The

TABLE 7. Spearman Rank Correlations Between Open-Field Activity and
Litter Size and Group Size

Correlation	Wistar–Veh	Wistar–6-OH	SHR–veh	SHR–6-OH
Activity–litter size	-0.06	-0.03	0.01	-0.02
Activity–group size	-0.42^a	-0.07	0.12	0.37^b

[a] $p < 0.01$.
[b] $p < 0.05$.

overall effect of the drug treatment for both strains was to produce a more positive correlation between group size and activity scores. While the exact meaning of this interaction between the drug and the pretest social environment is obscure, Sampson (1966) also noted that both immunosympathectomy and adult adrenal demedullation tended to produce decreased open-field emotionality (defecations, urinations, and crouching behavior) when the subjects were tested in the presence of another rat, i.e., these treatments appeared to increase social sensitivity. The lack of further data on the relationship between social variables and neonatal sympathectomy invites experimentation. Our data bearing on this possible relationship in 6-OH treatment rats may of course be due to the direct central effects of the drug or to the peripheral effects.

7.4. Escape–Avoidance Learning

Several different variations of the escape–avoidance procedure have been used to compare the performance of IS and control subjects. No consistent differences have been found with any variation of the procedure, nor are the data from the different procedures in general accord. Wenzel (1968a) trained IS Swiss–Webster mice at either 50 or 64 days of age to traverse a runway to escape or avoid electric grid shock. Acquisition training consisted of five massed trials administered daily for four consecutive days. The IS mice had slower running speeds only on the third acquisition day and were also slower than controls on 10 extinction trials given on days three and four. Wenzel and Jeffrey (1967) using a procedure somewhat similar to that of Wenzel (1968a), with the main difference being an intertrial interval of 20 minutes, found that their IS Swiss–Webster mice made fewer avoidances during acquisition and extinction than control mice. On the other hand, Carson (1970) found no differences between IS and control Swiss–Webster mice trained at 3 months in a similar type runway procedure which was comprised of two exploration and six training days with a "variable" intertrial interval. Van-Toller and Tarpy (1972a) using an alleyway with dimensions nearly the same as those of Wenzel's but permitting a shorter maximum conditioned stimulus (CS)–unconditioned stimulus (UCS) interval (2.85 second, vs. approximately 4 second) and giving a much more intense shock (1 mA vs. 0.25 mA), trained NGFA and horse serum injected mice of a heterogeneous strain on five massed trials for three successive days. Runway training was preceded by confinement of the mice for 2 hours in a temperature-regulated environment of either 3.5°C or 22.5°C. No runway performance differences were found between IS and control mice previously confined in the normal room temperature environment. However, IS mice previously subjected to the cold environment were inferior to their control counterparts. Finally, in a complex experiment in which mice were trained to traverse an inclined runway to avoid intense (1.0-mA) grid shock, with this procedure interpolated between two halves of a Sidman avoidance session, three IS mice were found to have significantly shorter escape–avoidance latencies than three control mice (Van-Toller, 1970).

Wenzel and Nagle (1965) trained NGFA injected and saline injected Swiss–Webster mice at about 3 months on a two-way discriminated avoidance procedure using 0.2-mA grid shock as the UCS. Intertrial interval averaged 2.25 minutes. Over 20 days of acquisition, one extinction session and a retention test about 2 months later, the IS mice did not perform differently from control mice.

Sidman avoidance procedures have also failed to yield convincing differences between normal and sympathectomized mice. Wenzel (1968b) trained IS or gamma globulin injected and handled and nonhandled groups of Swiss–Webster mice to depress a plexiglass ball attached to a lever in order to avoid a 0.25-mA shock. The mice were subjected to 8 daily 20-minute sessions using shock–shock and response–shock intervals of 20 seconds. On the seventh session only, the IS group received significantly more shocks than all three control groups, although the overall tendency across sessions was for the IS group to make fewer responses and to receive more shocks than the other groups. Interpretation of these data is clouded by the fact that unequal numbers of males and females were assigned to the treatment groups, the proportions of males ranging from 6 of 13, 3 of 13, 8 of 18, and 10 of 17 in the NGFA, gamma globulin, handled, and nonhandled groups, respectively. These group differences in distribution of sex were not accounted for in the statistical treatment. Van-Toller (1970) trained three NGFA and three horse serum injected mice of a heterogeneous strain on a barpress Sidman avoidance procedure with response–shock (0.6 mA) and shock–shock intervals of 15 seconds. After hand shaping to lever press and 12 daily training sessions, the following eight Sidman sessions were split into halves with a short runway training procedure separating the halves. Differences between the IS and control mice were found only on the first avoidance session, with the sympathectomized mice displaying significantly shorter inter-response latencies.

Wenzel and Jeffrey (1968) have reported that IS Swiss–Webster mice were slower than controls at escaping both from a water maze and from water immersion. In these experiments, the water-maze procedure consisted of four trials separated by 15 minutes, this procedure administered at 29 and 43 days of age. The sympathectomized mice were slower only at 43 days of age, with the largest difference from the three

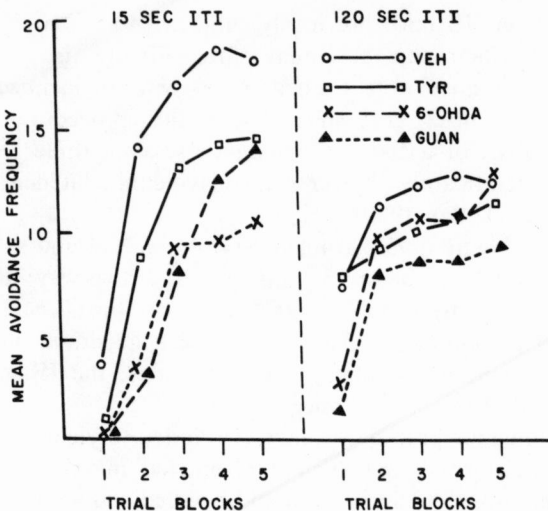

FIG. 2. Mean number of avoidance responses for successive blocks of 20 trials. Rats received neonatal injections of vehicle, tyramine, guanethidine, or 6-OH. Data for the 15- and 120-second ITI's are shown on the left and right panels, respectively.

control groups apparent on the third and fourth trial. On the water escape, administered at 46 days of age, the groups also appeared to differ primarily on the last two trials. Massed presentations (5 second-intertrial-interval) of water-maze trials, on the other hand, did not reveal performance differences between IS and control mice (Wenzel, 1968a). These latter data led Van-Toller and Tarpy (1972) to suggest that the inferior water-escape performance of IS mice reported by Wenzel and Jeffrey (1968) was likely due to the long intertrial interval (15 minutes) used in their experiments which produced more profound hypothermia in the sympathectomized group. It was postulated that the greater hypothermia produces more severe depletion of peripheral catecholamines in IS mice, reducing their capacity for coping with subsequent stress. Van-Toller and Tarpy's demonstration that prior cold exposure severely retards subsequent runway avoidance performance in IS mice is consistent with this interpretation of the water-escape data.

Reports that 6-OH sympathectomy affects neither one-way active avoidance (Pappas and Sobrian, 1972) nor an unspecified type of avoidance learning (Taylor et al., 1972) are difficult to interpret because of the central effects of the drug. Rats sympathectomized in adulthood by systemic injections of 6-OH have been reported to be deficient at two-way avoidance, but equal to controls in one-way avoidance (Diguisto and King, 1972). These data were interpreted as being due to the participation of peripheral sympathetic responses in cueing fear-motivated behavior only when the task is difficult or ambiguous (two-way avoidance) and not when the task is easy and unambiguous (one-way avoidance). However, the possibility of direct central effects of systemic 6-OH, particularly at short time intervals after injection (Clark *et al.*, 1971), render these data difficult to interpret. We have recently attempted to test this interpretation by assessing learning rates in neonatal 6-OH, guanethidine, and tyramine (sympathomimetic control) injected rats (Pappas and Blouin, unpublished data). However, rather than using two-way and one-way avoidance procedures, which require two different types of learning behavioral contingencies (Olton, 1973), we manipulated difficulty within the two-way avoidance procedure by testing the rats under either a short or long intertrial interval. Pilot research had indicated that for our particular apparatus, a short 15-second intertrial interval yielded rapid learning while a longer, 120-second interval yielded slow learning of the avoidance response. The animals were subjected to a single 100-trial session at around 120 days of age.

The results of this experiment, shown in Fig. 2, indicated that while tyramine injected rats learned at about the same rate as vehicle control rats, 6-OH and guanethidine injected rats were somewhat inferior to vehicle controls at both the "easy" and "difficult" intertrial interval. This would

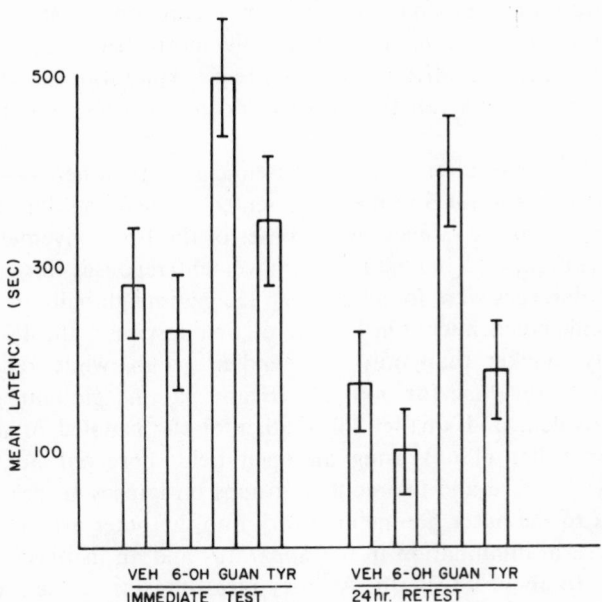

FIG. 3. Mean (±s.e) passive avoidance step-out latencies on immediate and 24-hour retention test for vehicle, 6-OH, guanethidine, and tyramine injected rats.

seem to fit the Diguisto and King interpretation, except that the difference between vehicle control rats and 6-OH and guanethidine sympathectomized rats was most marked at the "easy" intertrial interval. Nevertheless, at face value the data would seemingly indicate that neonatal sympathectomy, whether achieved by guanethidine or 6-OH injections, produces two-way avoidance-learning deficits. However, when we also tested these or similarly treated animals in a simple step-out passive avoidance procedure, there were marked differences between these two types of animal. While 6-OH treated rats were slightly, but not significantly, inferior on an immediate or 24-hour retention test than either vehicle or tyramine controls, Fig. 3 indicates that the guanethidine rats seemed slightly "better" than controls. In fact, the only significant group difference was that between 6-OH and guanethidine-injected rats. This coincided with our impressions that the guanethidine rats seemed very sluggish, although reactive, and that their deficit on two-way avoidance was due more to locomotor lethargy rather than to any effect upon the fear process.

7.5. CER Procedures

Defining a CER procedure as a test situation which examines the suppressive effect of a noxious stimulus or a conditioned stimulus for an aversive event upon either an extrinsically motivated (e.g., barpress for food) or intrinsically motivated response (e.g., exploration or activity), one finds indications that sympathectomized rodents suppress less than control subjects.

Wenzel (1968a), after recording baseline activity of her Swiss–Webster mice in a jiggle cage for 5 minutes, presented a 10-second duration 100-dB tone and observed the latency of the onset of the first movement after the tone presentation, and magnitude of movement reponses during the tone. No clear differences were found between IS, gamma globulin injected, handled, or nonhandled mice. On latency of first response, the IS mice were significantly quicker than only the handled group, while reponse magnitudes during the tone for both the IS and gamma globulin groups appeared equivalent and smaller than either of the handled or nonhandled group. Van-Toller (1968) using an open field, observed no differences between his IS mice and two control groups on latency to cross from the center area to the outer perimeter. Entry into the outer area led to an abrupt increase in illumination in the apparatus and an increase in masking white noise to about 92–94 dB. Activity measures during the 2-minute-duration loud noise presentation showed the IS mice ran further and reared more frequently than the control groups. If we assume that the light and tone were to some extent unpleasant stimuli, then the data may be interpreted as indicating that IS mice suppressed their locomotor activity less during presentation of the stimuli than did control mice.

Using the classical Hunt and Brady (1951) type of CER procedure, Sampson (1966) reported data suggesting that immunosympathectomy attenuates the CER in the rat. Sampson trained her 23-hour-food-deprived rats to barpress for sucrose pellets on a variable interval schedule. After stable baselines were achieved, the rats were given five consecutive daily CER acquisition trials, each trial consisting of the presentation of a 2-minute-duration 16-Hz click (CS) with a brief but intense (1.5-mA) shock presented at CS termination. These five acquisition trials were followed by five consecutive daily extinction trials during which the shock was no longer presented. The IS group showed less overall suppression on the fifth acquisition trial. Detailed group comparisons showed this difference to be attributable primarily to the reduced suppression in the female but not in the male rats. Wenzel (1972) also reports that IS mice show less suppression of barpressing for food or water reward after the termination of warning tone and shock than do horse serum or nonhandled control mice.

Working in my laboratory, Saari (1972) trained vehicle and 6-OH injected rats from both a normotensive strain and the Japanese hypertensive strain to drink their daily water supply in a test environment. Total water volumes consumed and latencies to complete 10 and 20 licks were recorded. Beginning on the 6th day and continuing for the next 5 days, the rats' tenth lick was immediately followed by a 1-second presentation of a 1.0-mA grid shock. The latency of the 20th lick measured, then, the length of time the rat suppressed in response to the shock while on succeeding days, the latency to complete ten licks measured day-to-day retention of the rat's association of the tenth lick with the contingent shock.

Figure 4 shows mean log latencies for the tenth lick for the four groups during adaptation, acquisition, and extinction of this suppression of water-licking procedure. It can be clearly seen that the 6-OH treated rats, both from the normotensive and from the hypertensive strain, showed considerably less suppression during both acquisition and extinction than their appropriate vehicle controls. Interestingly, the SHR rats, which Saari had initially hypothesized might be sympathetically overreactive, suppressed much less than their normotensive counterparts. These group differences were also found in latencies to complete the next ten licks after shock presentations. The decreased suppression in the 6-OH rats does not seem to be due to any direct drug effect upon water ingestion after 23-hour deprivation. Saari demonstrated that latencies to begin licking after either hypertonic saline injections (subcutaneously, s.c.) or varying intervals of water deprivation were equivalent for vehicle- and 6-OH-treated rats.

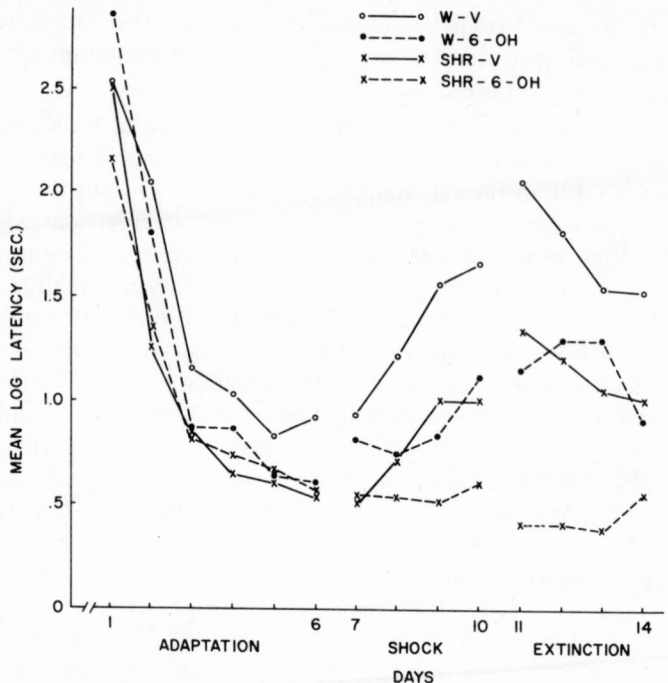

FIG. 4. Mean log latency (sec) for completion of 10 licks by control Wistar
(W–V), 6-OH injected Wistar (W–6-OH), spontaneously hypertensive (SHR–V)
and 6-OH injected, spontaneously hypertensive rats (SHR–6-OH). The data are
plotted for adaptation, tenth-lick-contingent shock, and shock extinction sessions
(from Saari, 1972).

Furthermore, the shock thresholds for eliciting flinch reactions were the
same for these two groups, and they also did not differ in their acquisition
rates for learning a water rewarded Y-maze task. This effect of 6-OH sympathectomy on conditioned and unconditioned lick suppression, while
consistent with the findings of Sampson (1966) and Wenzel (1972) of
reduced suppression in IS rats and mice, may be caused, of course, by
either the peripheral or central effects of the drug.

Given that IS treated rats and mice show reduced suppression in CER
procedures, one would predict deficits in conventional passive avoidance
procedures that do not utilize positive reward to maintain baseline response
rates. Both the CER and these types of passive avoidance procedures elicit
response inhibition. However, passive avoidance behavior is apparently the
same in control and IS mice. Van-Toller (1970) presented 0.3-mA, 0.5-
second-duration shocks to these mice, contingent upon movement between

adjacent metal plates forming the floor of a small rectangular apparatus. The procedure consisted of 2-minute periods of each of adaptation, movement-contingent shock, and no-shock testing. The IS mice did not differ from controls either during the initial session or on retention sessions at varying later intervals and continuing for 8 consecutive days for some of the mice. As mentioned earlier, we have found that guanethidine sympathectomy actually enhances passive avoidance in the rat, although this enhancement is probably due simply to the locomotor lethargy in those rats.

Perhaps it is significant that response-inhibition deficits are observed only in the appetitive, positive-reward baseline procedures. Certainly one would expect that the degree of conflict experienced by the rat would be greater in these types of procedures than in those in which intrinsically motivated repsonses are punished. The behavior of sympathectomized rodents in conflict procedures has not as yet been systematically studied.

8.   Some Concluding Remarks

Obviously, both immuno- and 6-OH sympathectomy drastically alter autonomic reactions elicited by environmental manipulations that are also capable of eliciting emotional behavior. Equally obviously, there seems to be little agreement among data from various behavioral procedures which would definitively indicate alterations in emotional behavior. The highest degree of concordance seems to be derived from the results of experiments involving CER procedures that utilize positive rewards to maintain baseline behavior prior to shock presentations. These results generally indicate attenuated suppression in both immuno- and 6-OH sympathectomized mice and rats. However, as was pointed out, attenuated suppressive behavior could be due either to a reduction of emotionality (fear) or to a rather general impairment in response inhibition. It may be significant that 6-OH sympathectomy causes a permanent depletion of hippocampal Ne (Taylor *et al.*, 1972). Surgical lesions of this area in the rat have been interpreted as impairing inhibitory processes. Douglas (1967), in an extensive review of hippocampal involvement in behavior, concluded that lesioning of the hippocampus produces an inability to withhold propotent responses. This deficit precisely describes the only type of behavioral alteration that we have consistently observed after nonatal 6-OH. Immunosympathectomy does not, however, affect behavior on some procedures such as discriminated, food-rewarded barpress responding and discriminated avoidance (Wenzel and Nagle, 1965), which would be expected to be sensitive to such an impairment. Furthermore, there is no reason to suspect that immunosympathectomy has central chemical effects in any way similar to those observed after 6-OH sympathectomy. Dramatic regional alterations of endogenous brain amine levels are produced by 6-OH. The few data that are available suggest only slight and probably negligible effects after NGFA, although more exhaustive assessments are required.

If neonatal sympathectomy alters the normal autonomic components of the stress response, including adreno-medullary secretions, then relatively chronic stress procedures might be expected to affect the behavioral adaptability of sympathectomized rodents insofar as this adaptability requires mobilization of these components for effective responding. The as-yet small amount of experimentation on this problem agrees with this expectation (Van-Toller and Tarpy, 1972). One interesting and related problem which invites investigation is the degree to which the central nervous system effects of psychological stress, such as changes in catecholamines (e.g., Weiss, Stone and Harrell, 1970) may be altered by manipulation of peripheral autonomic function. Training curarized rats to voluntarily control their heart rate affects endogenous brain catecholamine (DiCara and Stone, 1970). This suggests that peripheral autonomic function may modulate certain aspects of brain catecholamine regulation (or vice versa).

Some further accounting of the behavioral significance of the increased levels of adrenal medullary and extra-adrenal catecholamines in sympathectomized rats is required. Providing these data presents a tricky problem because the effects of demedullation or pharmacologic blockade may be entirely different for normal and sympathectomized rats, and could be due to differing state-dependent effects rather than to differing effects upon a basic emotionality-mediating process. Furthermore, in the case of adrenal demedullation, the interval between surgery and testing might be very critical for either process. For pharmacological blockade, the age of the rat (which is of course directly related to the interval between sympathectomy and testing) may also be critical.

Finally, recent research shows that repeated injections of the peripheral catecholamine depleting agent guanethidine produces an almost total destruction of the SNS in the adult rat. When it is injected into the neonatal rat it also produces a sympathectomy that resembles peripheral sympathectomy by 6-OH in many respects, and that may be very extensive and permanent. Future research with NGFA, 6-OH, and guanethidine certainly ought to permit a final assessment as to the relevance of the SNS for behavior as well as to the mechanisms responsible for the intriguing central neurochemical changes that accompany 6-OH sympathectomy. Furthermore, because guanethidine has sympatholytic effects in both neonatal and adult animals, use of this drug may ultimately reveal the differences or similarities between the behavioral effects of neonatal and adult sympathectomy.

ACKNOWLEDGMENTS

I wish to express my appreciation to the students who helped collect much of the data presented in this chapter and who participated in the shaping of my opinions. The efforts of Sonya Sobrian, Matti Saari, Barbara Drew, and Art Blouin are gratefully acknowledged. I also wish to thank Dr. David Peters of the University of Ottawa Department of Pharmacology for his collaboration and my wife Partricia, who put aside her interests in more provocative literary works to critically review this chapter.

9.   References

Adams, R. N., Murrill, E., McCreery, R., Blank, L., and Karolczak, M., 1972, 6-hydroxydopamine, a new oxidation mechanism, *Europ. J. Pharmacol. 17:*287.

Angeletti, P. U., 1971, Chemical sympathectomy in newborn animals, *Neuropharmacol. 10:*55.

Angeletti, P. U., and Levi-Montalcini, R., 1970, Sympathetic nerve cell destruction in newborn mammals by 6-hydroxydopamine, *Proc. Natl. Acad. Sci. USA 65:*114.

Angelletti, P. U., and Levi-Montalcini, R., 1971, Growth regulation of the sympathetic nervous system: immunosympathectomy and chemical sympathectomy, *Europ. J. Clin. Biol. Res. 16:*866.

Arbit, J., 1957, Skeletal muscle effects of the chemical block of autonomic impulses and the extinction of fear, *J. Comp. Physiol. Psychol. 50:*144.

Arbit, J., 1958, Shock motivated serial discrimination learning and the chemical block of autonomic impulses, *J. Comp. Physiol. Psychol. 51:*199.

Auld, F., 1951, The effects of tetraethylammonium on a habit motivated by fear, *J. Comp. Physiol. Psychol. 44:*565.

Bainbridge, J. G., and Greenwood, D. T., 1971, Tranquilizing effects of propanolol demonstrated in rats, *Neuropharmacol. 10:*453.

Bloom, F. E., Algeri, S., Gropetti, A., Revuelta, A., and Costa, E., 1969, Lesions of central norepinephrine terminals with 6-OH-dopamine: biochemistry and fine structure, *Science 166:*1284.

Bonn, J. A., Turner, P., and Hicks, D. C., 1972, Beta-adrenergic-receptor blockade with practolol in treatment of anxiety, *The Lancet 1* (7755):814.

Brady, J. V., 1953, Does tetraethylammonium reduce fear? *J. Comp. Physiol. Psychol. 46:*307.

Brody, M. J., 1964, Cardiovascular responses following immunological sympathectomy, *Circ. Res. 15:*161.

Brody, M. J., 1966, Effect of adrenal demedullation on vascular responses after immunological sympathectomy, *Am. J. Physiol. 211:*198.

Burch, G. E., 1972, Management of benign essential arterial hypertension, *Am. Heart J. 84:*808.

Burnstock, G., Evans, B., Gannon, B. J., Heath, S. W., and James, U., 1971, A new method of destroying adrenergic nerves in adult animals using guanethidine, *Brit. J. Pharmacol. 43:*295.

Cannon, W. B., Lewis, J. T., and Britton, S. W., 1927, The dispensability of the sympathetic division of the autonomic nervous system, *Boston Med. Surg. J. 197:*314.

Cannon, W. B., Newton, M. F., Bright, E. M., Menkin, V., and Moore, R. M., 1929, Some aspects of the physiology of animals surviving complete exclusion of sympathetic nerve impulses, *Amer. J. Physiol. 89:*84.

Carpi, A., and Oliverio, A., 1964, Urinary excretion of catecholamines in the immunosympathectomized rat—balance phenomena between the adrenergic and the noradrenergic system, *Int. J. Neuropharmacol. 3:*427.

Carson, V. G., 1970, The effect of immunosympathectomy and adrenal medullectomy on telemetred heart rate and foot pad impedance in mice, Unpublished Ph.D. thesis, University of California, Los Angeles.

Clark, D. W. J., 1971, Effects of immunosympathectomy on development of high blood pressure in genetically hypertensive rats, *Circ. Res. 28:*330.

Clark, D. W. J., Laverty, R., and Phelan, E. L., 1972, Long lasting peripheral and central effects of 6-hydroxydopamine in rats, *Brit. J. Pharmacol. 44:*233.

Clark, W. G., Corrodi, H., and Masuoka, D. T., 1971, The effects of peripherally administered 6-hydroxydopamine on rat brain monoamine turnover, *Europ. J. Pharmacol. 15:*41.

Cohen, S., 1960, Purification of a nerve growth promoting protein from the mouse salivary gland and its neurocytotoxic antiserum, *Proc. Natl. Acad. Sci., USA 46:*302.

Dahlstrom, A., and Fuxe, K., 1965, Evidence for the existence of monoamine neurons in the central nervous system. II. Experimentally induced changes in the intraneuronal amine levels of bulbospinal neuron systems, *Acta Physiol. Scand. 64*(Supp. 247):7.

De Champlain, J., and Nadeau, R., 1971, 6-hydroxydopamine, 6-hydroxydopa and degeneration of adrenergic nerves, *Fed. Proc. 30:*877.

DiCara, L. V., and Stone, E. A., 1970, Effect of instrumental heart-rate training on rat cardiac and brain catecholamines, *Psychosom. Med. 32:*359.

DiGuisto, E. L., 1972, Adrenaline or peripheral noradrenaline depletion and passive avoidance in the rat, *Physiol. Behav 8:*1059.

DiGuisto, E. L., and King, M. G., 1972, Chemical sympathectomy and avoidance learning in the rat, *J. Comp. Physiol. Psychol. 81:*491.

DiGiusto, E. L., Cairncross, K., and King, M. G., 1971, Hormonal influences on fear-motivated responses, *Psychol. Bull. 75:*432.

Douglas, R. J., 1967, The hippocampus and behavior, *Psychol. Bull. 67:*416.

Eränkö, O., and Eränkö, L., 1971a, Histochemical evidence of chemical sympathectomy by guanethidine in newborn rats, *Histochem. J. 3:*451.

Eränkö, L., and Eränkö, O., 1971b, Effect of guanethidine on nerve cells and small intensely fluorescent cells in sympathetic ganglia of newborn and adult rats, *Acta. Pharmacol. et. Toxicol. 30:*403.

Evans, B., Gannon, J., Heath, J. W., and Burnstock, G., 1972, Long-lasting damage to the internal male genital organs and their adrenergic innervation in rats following chronic treatment with the antihypertensive drug guanethidine, *Fertility and Sterility 23:*657.

Fehr, F. S., and Stern, J. A., 1970, Peripheral physiological variables and emotion: the James–Lange theory revisited, *Psychol. Bull. 74:*411.

Goldman, H., and Jacobowitz, D., 1971, Correlations of norepinephrine content with observations of adrenergic nerves after single dose of 6-hydroxydopamine in the rat, *J. Pharmacol. Exptl. Ther. 176:*119.

Goldstein, M. L., 1968, Physiological theories of emotion: a critical historical review from the standpoint of behavior theory, *Psychol. Bull. 69:*23.

Hamberger, S., Levi-Montalcini, R., Norberg, K. A., and Sjoquist, F., 1964, Changes in cellular distribution of monoamines induced by immunosympathectomy, *Pharmacologist 6:*173 (abstract).

Heikhila, R., and Cohen, G., 1971, Inhibition of biogenic amine uptake by H_2O_2: mechanism for toxic effects of 6-hydroxydopamine, *Science 172:*1257.

Hofer, M. A., Engel, M., and Weiner, H., 1971, Development of cardiac rate regulation and activity after neonatal immunosympathectomy, *Comm. Behav. Biol. 6:*59.

Hunt, H. F., and Brady, J. V., 1951, Some effects of electroconvulsive shock on a CER ("anxiety"), *J. Comp. Physiol. Psychol. 44:*88.

Jacks, B. R., DeChamplain, J., and Cordeau, J. P., 1972, Effects of 6-hydroxydopamine on putative transmitter substances in the central nervous system, *Europ. J. Pharmacol. 18:*353.

Jaim-Etcheverry, G., and Zieher, L. M., 1971, Permanent depletion of peripheral norepinephrine in rats treated at birth with 6-hydroxydopamine, *Europ. J. Pharmacol. 13:*272.

James, W., 1894, The physiological basis of emotion, *Psychol. Rev. 1:*516.

Klingman, G. I., 1966, In utero immunosympathectomy in mice, *Int. J. Neuropharmacol. 5:*163.

Klingman, G. I., 1969, 5-hydroxytryptamine levels in peripheral organs of immunosympathectomized rats, *Biochem. Pharmacol. 18:*2061.

Levi-Montalcini, R., and Angeletti, P. U., 1962, Noradrenaline and monoamine oxidase content in immunosympathectomized animals, *Int. J. Neuropharmacol. 1:*161.

Levi-Montalcini, R., and Angeletti, P. U., 1966, Immunosympathectomy, *Pharmacol. Rev. 18:*619.

Levi-Montalcini, R., and Booker, B., 1960, Destruction of the sympathetic ganglia in mammals by an antiserum to a nerve growth protein, *Proc. Natl. Acad. Sci., USA 46:*384.

Lew, G. M., and Quay, W. B. 1971, Noradrenaline contents of hypothalamus and adrenal gland increased by postnatal administration of 6-hydroxydopamine, *Res. Comm. Chem. Path. Pharmacol 2:*807.

Okamoto, K., 1969, Spontaneous hypertension in rats, *Int. Rev. Exptl. Pathol. 7:*227.

Olton, D. S., 1973, Shock-motivated avoidance and the analysis of behavior, *Psychol. Bull. 79:*243.

Pappas, B. A., DiCara, L. V., and Miller, N. E., 1972, Acute sympathectomy by 6-hydroxydopamine in the adult rat: effects on cardiovascular conditioning and fear retention, *J. Comp. Physiol. Psychol. 79:*230.

Pappas, B. A., and DiCara, L. V., 1973, Neonatal sympathectomy by 6-hydroxydopamine: cardiovascular responses in the paralyzed rat, *Physiol. Behav. 10:*549.

Pappas, B. A., and Sobrian, S. K., 1972, Neonatal sympathectomy by 6-hydroxdopamine in the rat: no effects on behavior but changes in endogenous brain norepinephrine, *Life Sci.* 11(1):653.

Pappas, B. A., Peters, D. A. V., Saari, M., Sobrian, S. K., and Minch, E., 1974, Neonatal 6-hydroxydopamine sympathectomy in normotensive and spontaneously hypertensive rat. *Pharmacol., Biochem. Behav. 2:*381.

Peters, D. A. V., Mazurkiewicz-Kwilecki, I. M., and Pappas, B. A., 1974, Neonatal 6-hydroxydopamine sympathectomy in the rat: effects on brain serotonin and histamine, *Biochem. Pharmacol.* (in press).

Porter, C. C., Totaro, A., and Stone, C. A., 1963, Effect of 6-OH-DA and some other compounds on the concentration of norepinephrine in the hearts of mice, *J. Pharmacol. Exptl. Ther. 140:*308.

Saari, M. J., 1972, Neonatal sympathectomy by 6-hydroxydopamine: behavioral effects in spontaneously hypertensive and normotensive rats, Unpublished master's thesis, Carleton University.

Saari, M., and Pappas, B. A., 1973, Neonatal 6-hydroxydopamine sympathectomy reduces Goot shock-induced suppression of water-licking in normotensive and hypertensive rats, *Nature (New Biol.) 244:*181.

Sachs, C., and Jonsson, G., 1972, Degeneration of central noradrenaline neurons after 6-hydroxydopamine in newborn animals, *Res. Comm. Chem. Pathol. Pharmacol. 4:*203.

Sachs, C., and Jonsson, G., 1973, Changes in central noradrenaline neurons after systemic 6-hydroxydopamine administration, *J. Neurochem. 21:*1517.

Sampson, P. H., 1966, Sympathetico-adrenomedullary functioning and behavior in the rat: activity, emotionality, and social sensitivity, unpublished Ph.D. thesis, Cornell University.

Schonbaum, E. G., Johnson, E., and Sellers, E. A., 1966, Acclimation to cold and norepinephrine: effects of immunosympathectomy, *Am. J. Physiol. 211:*647.

Soubrie, P., 1971, Open-field chez le rat: inter-relations entre locomotion, exploration et émotivité, *J. Pharmacol.* (Paris) *2:*457.

Tarpy, R. M., and Van-Toller, C., 1972, Relationship between activity and hypothermia in immunosympathectomized mice, *J. Comp. Physiol. Psychol. 81:*108.

Taylor, K. M., Clark, D. W. J., Laverty, R., and Phelan, E. L., 1972, Specific noradrenergic neurons destroyed by 6-hydroxydopamine injection into newborn rats, *Nature (New Biol). 239:*247.

Thierry, A. M., and Sinus, L., Blanc, G., and Glowinski, J., 1973, Some evidence for the existence of dopaminergic neurons in the rat cortex, *Brain Res. 50:*230.

Thornton, E. W., and Van-Toller, C., 1973, Effect of immunosympathectomy on operant heart rate conditioning in the curarized rat, *Physiol. Behav. 10:*197.

Uretsky, N. J., and Iversen, L. L., 1970, Effects of 6-hydroxydopamine on catecholamine containing neurones in the rat brain, *J. Neurochem. 17:*269.

Van-Toller, C., 1968, Immunosympathectomy and open-field behavior in mice, *Physiol. Behav. 3:*365.

Van-Toller, C., 1970, Immunosympathectomy and avoidance behavior in mice, unpublished Ph.D. thesis, University of Durham.

Van-Toller, C. and Tarpy, R. M., 1972, Effect of cold stress on the performance of immunosympathectomized mice, *Physiol. Behav. 8:*515.

Visscher, M. B., Lee, Y. C. P., and Azuma, T., 1965, Catecholamines in organs of immunosympathectomized mice, *Proc. Soc. Exptl. Biol. Med. 119:*1232.

Weiss, J. M., Stone, E. A., and Harrell, N., 1970, Coping behavior and brain norepinephrine level in rats, *J. Comp. Physiol. Psychol. 72:*153.

Wenzel, B. M., 1968a, Behavioral studies of immunosympathectomized mice, *J. Comp. Physiol. Psychol. 66:*354.

Wenzel, B. M., 1968b, Behavior of immunosympathectomized mice in a non-discriminated avoidance task, *Physiol. Behav. 3:*907.

Wenzel, B. M., 1972, Immunosympathectomy and Behavior, in *Immunosympathectomy,* G. Steiner and E. Schonbaum, eds., Elsevier, Amsterdam.

Wenzel, B. M., and Jeffrey, D. W., 1967, The effect of immunosympathectomy on the behavior of mice in aversive situations, *Physiol. Behav. 2:*193.

Wenzel, B. M., and Nagle, B., 1965, The effect of immunological sympathectomy on behavior in mice, *Exptl. Neurol. 12:*399.

Wenzel, B. M., Carson, V., and Chase, K., 1966, Cardiac responses of immunosympathectomized mice, *Percept. Mot. Skills 23:*1009.

Whimbey, A. E., and Denenberg, V. H., 1967, Two independent behavioral dimensions in open-field performance, *J. Comp. Physiol. Psychol. 63:*500.

Wynne, L. C., and Solomon, R. L., 1955, Traumatic avoidance learning: acquisition and extinction in dogs deprived of normal peripheral autonomic functions, *Genet. Psychol. Mon. 52:*241.

Zaimis, E., 1965, The immunosympathectomized animal: a valuable tool in physiological and pharmacological research, *J. Physiol. (London) 177:*350.

CHAPTER 6

The Role of Early Experience in the Development of Autonomic Regulation

Myron A. Hofer

Department of Psychiatry, Albert Einstein College of Medicine
and
Montefiore Hospital, New York, New York

1. Introduction

One of the most striking characteristics of autonomic physiology is the degree to which individuals differ from each other in both resting levels and response magnitude. These differences show stability over time (Lacey and Lacey, 1962), and the patterns described by measurement in multiple systems may provide a kind of physiological fingerprint of the individual (Sargent and Weinman, 1966). Furthermore, certain individuals may show exaggerated or markedly reduced responses in one or another autonomic subsystem which can result in disability, and even in death. One cannot confront such individuals, either as an investigator or a physician, without wondering how they acquired such a characteristic. The usual explanations in terms of aberrant emotional responses and their physiological concomitants have failed to be adequately supported by the evidence, and would fail to answer the question even if a consistent relationship could be demonstrated (Hofer, 1974). Alternately, supposing these individual differences to be due *simply to genetic determinants* ignores the vast body of evidence of developmental biology that even for structural ontogeny, the individual organism (phenotype) is the product of a continuing interaction between the genetic potential (genotype) and its own highly specific environment.

It had been assumed until recently that the relative importance of the environment is minimal in the determination of development in structural and physiological systems, and that only motor behavior and inner experience are importantly affected by environmental factors. Evidence has been published (Miller, 1968), and is discussed elsewhere in this volume, that this is a false dichotomy when applied to instrumental learning, and that at least in the young adult, autonomic physiological changes as well as musculoskeletal responses, under certain conditions, can be learned. There are other ways in which environmental events have recently been shown to shape development in physiological systems, and these will be discussed below. In the area of developmental biology, it has been established that structural modifications (e.g., in the fly's wing) may be predictably caused by a fairly nonspecific disturbance (e.g., heat, agitation, hypertonic solution) occurring at a particular stage in embryological development (Waddingon, 1962). The resulting abnormality closely resembles that produced by the known effects of a single gene. This phenomenon has been called a *phenocopy* and the developmental stage termed a *critical period*. Such findings in the field of embryology, and the theoretical formulations derived from them, have provided impetus and hypotheses to psychologists and others interested in the possible impact of postnatal experience on the infant organism and his subsequent development (King, 1968).

In 1921, Hammett, who was studying the function of the parathyroid glands in rats, was troubled by an 80% mortality rate within 48 hours of the operative procedure of parathyroidectomy. Most of the animals died in tetany. He discovered that rats of the same strain raised by a different animal room technician had considerably better survival. This technician treated his animals like pets and handled them from weaning on, nearly every day. A controlled experiment done on two subcolonies, derived from a single pair, showed that handling after weaning for several generations produced animals whose mortality from parathyroidectomy was 13% as contrasted to 79% mortality in the standard laboratory-raised descendants of the same original pair. This study should have stimulated a flowering of early experience studies, but it was not until 35 years later that Weininger (1953) and J. H. Scott (1955) picked up these earlier findings, and attempted to extend them to more common stressors. At about the same time, Hunt and Otis (1955) had reported increased exploratory and decreased freezing behavior in adult rats that had been handled as infants, suggesting a reduction in emotional behavior as a result of the early experience. Then Levine (1957) found increased survival time and evidence of altered adrenocortical function in stressed adult rats as a result of early handling. Other investigators have replicated and extended these central findings, and Levine and Mullins (1966) have presented further evidence, in a series of studies, which suggests a mechanism for the increased survival of early handled rats under stress. By this hypothesis, early maturation of the hypothalamic–pituitary–adrenocortical response is brought about by the increased stimulation to this system from the early handling. The hypothalamus is exposed to a greater range of corticosterone levels in response to the handling experience at an early age when set points have yet to be established. It is postulated that this endows the developing system with a flexible and wide range of hypothalamic regulatory capacities so that more appropriate and adaptive adrenocortical responses are characteristic of these adults, fitting them better to withstand a variety of imposed stress situations. Recent work in this area has raised doubts about the validity of this appealing hypothesis. Grota and Ader (1972) have shown that the same long-term effects on adrenocortical response to avoidance conditioning are produced whether the animal had its ACTH release blocked by dexamethasone treatment during early stimulation or not. This work suggests that alterations of adrenocortical reactivity in adulthood are mediated by some aspect of early stimulation other than exposure of the immature hypothalamus to a greater range of corticosterone levels. Further work needs to be done to document the blocking effects of dexamethasone as administered to neonatal rats.

Unfortunately, the influence of early experience upon autonomic function has been far less extensively studied. Nevertheless, there is clear evidence that early experience has long-range effects on autonomic responses of the adult. How these effects are brought about, what processes are at work, and how the early experience becomes translated into physiological changes in the young organism are questions which lead us into a consideration of early developmental processes in autonomic regulation.

2.   Long-Term Effects of Early Experience on Autonomic Neural Function

2.1.   Cardiovascular

Henry's original and convincing studies (Henry *et al.*, 1967) on the production of sustained hypertension in mice by exposure to various kinds of psychosocial stimulation contain several examples of how early experience can predispose an adult to pathological cardiovascular changes apparently involving altered autonomic regulation. In his studies, sustained hypertension could be produced by aggregation, repeated exposure to a predator, and by a housing design which elicited persistent territorial conflict. If the mice were separated prematurely from the mother (12 days) and housed singly until 12 weeks of age, more severe increases in blood pressure were produced when they were exposed to stress as adults. An interstitial nephritis (thought to be a complication of advanced hypertensive cardiovascular disease) was present at autopsy which was not observed in other mice similarly stressed in adulthood but without the early isolation experience. Signs of aortic damage and myocardial fibrosis were found in this group, particularly in males.

These studies appear to have created the first successful model of psychosomatic illness and provide, for the first time, the possibility of studying the process and mechanisms of the development of this condition in the laboratory. As in human essential hypertension, the hypertension of these mice could be controlled by reserpine and was more frequently severe in males. Subsequent studies have centered upon the biosynthesis of noradrenaline and adrenaline in these hypertensive mice. Henry, in collaboration with Axelrod and others (Henry et al., 1971), has shown that adrenal tyrosine hydroxylase (the rate-limiting enzyme in catecholamine synthesis) and methyl transferase (the enzyme required for methylation of noradrenaline to adrenaline) are significantly *reduced* under normal laboratory conditions in adult mice which were early weaned and isolated. But when these mice were exposed to the housing system designed to engender repeated social conflict, the levels of these enzymes rose about 150% to levels as high or higher than in mice with normal early experience. These enzyme changes are both neurally (splanchnic sympathetic nerve) and hormonally (ACTH) induced.

These findings raise further interesting questions as to how the early experiences of premature separation from the mother and social isolation exert their effects on the young animal's developing autonomic nervous system. For example, does the isolation reduce turnover of catecholamines in the young mouse, and if so, how is this experience translated into such a biochemical change? What further developmental processes modify the effects of the experience in early life, and how are the biochemical differences related to the development of hypertension?

J. P. Scott's classic experiments on early socialization in the dog (1962) included some interesting observations on cardiac rate in puppies with different rearing experiences. Subsequent studies in rats have obtained generally similar effects, and as a result some tentative generalizations are possible regarding the role of environmental and social stimulation in the development of autonomic cardiac control.

Freedman et al. (1961) working with Scott, raised cocker spaniels outdoors in large fenced pens, bringing different groups in to the laboratory for 1 week only at 2, 3, 5, 7, and 9 weeks of postnatal age. During the week in the laboratory, three times daily, the experimenters exposed the puppies to both active and passive socialization with human handlers. All puppies were replaced in their field area after this early "socialization" experience until 14 weeks of age when they were put through a series of behavioral tests, and heart rate was recorded in reponse to acoustic startle and electric shock. A control group was left in the field until testing. Dogs which had experienced social interaction with human handlers in their seventh postnatal week showed the greatest initial attraction to a handler, ate more readily in a strange situation, and were most active during testing. They also showed the highest peak cardiac responses to stimulation and differed significantly from the second-week socialized and control groups on this and other measures. Second-week socialized and control animals tended to "freeze" and show cardiac deceleratory responses in contrast to the acceleratory responses characteristic of dogs socialized at what Scott terms the "critical period" of 6–8 weeks postnatal age. These studies suggested that the early experience of the animal and the developmental stage at which the experience occurred were important determinants of the autonomic response of the animal to stimulation later in life.

Three studies in rats from different laboratories, published since Scott's early work, have described similar phenomena relating different early experiences to cardiac rate responses in adulthood. Based on all these studies, an hypothesis can be derived which predicts that early experiences which entail decreased levels of stimulation lead to lower heart rates and a tendency for the response to stimulation in adulthood to be deceleratory. Increases in levels of early stimulation would result in a heightened tendency to cardiac acceleration in later life. Two studies (Boyles *et al.*, 1965 and Snowdon *et al.*, 1964) employed periods of social and environmental restriction from weaning to sexual maturity and found decreased heart rates in the open field and deceleratory responses to white noise. One study (Blizard, 1971) utilized handling by the experimenter during the first postnatal week and found increased cardiac rates (in females only) in response to handling in adulthood and higher heart rates in response to white noise and light stimulation. These findings all support the hypothesis and are consistent with Scott's findings in dogs. However, a recent study (Koch and Arnold, 1972) employing incubator rearing of male rat pups from birth, both singly and in groups, found no differences in heart rate responses to noise and electric shock, but baseline heart rates were increased in the isolated animals during the course of the electric shock stimulation. Comparison of the results of this study with the others is complicated by the failure of these last authors to use unrestrained rats and chronic electrode implants for the cardiac rate studies, and by the fact that the incubator-reared animals sustained considerable nutritional deprivation.

These early experience studies demonstrate that an effect exists whereby early experience can alter autonomic cardiac rate responses in adulthood, but raise a host of questions as to how this effect is exerted.

Does the effect of early handling, for example, work through an alteration of the mother–infant interaction, as suggested by Thoman and Levine, (1969), through the effects of temperature regulation as suggested by Hutchings (1963), or through the direct effects of tactile stimulation by the handling itself? How does the autonomic system of the young organism respond to handling or isolation when it first occurs early in development? By what mechanism is this experience translated into physiological change in the young organism with its special physiology?

2.2. Gastrointestinal

Unfortunately, the measures of gastrointestinal function used in early experience studies to date are only indirectly and even questionably related to levels of autonomic function, and therefore will be reviewed briefly as *possible* indicators of autonomic activity.

The most frequently observed measure considered to reflect gastrointestinal autonomic function, defecation rate, is a most indirect measure of parasympathetic tone to the lower bowel. Forced breathing against a semiclosed glottis (as is seen under stress), giving rise to grunting respiration with a prolonged expiratory phase, can increase the likelihood and rate of fecal bolus dropping by increasing intra-abdominal pressure without any alteration in baseline autonomic regulatory control of the bowel. Obviously the level of food intake prior to testing is another determinant of bolus production, independent of autonomic function.

It has been observed consistently that increased handling in early life reduces rats' defecation under stress in later life. In one study (Snowdon *et al.*, 1964), both heart rate and defecatory rate in the "open-field" test were recorded after early environmental and social restriction. The defecatory rate was increased, the heart rate decreased, and there was a statistically significant but low order of negative correlation between the two measures among the individuals ($r = -0.30$).

These data might seem consistent with the interpretation that a state of relative parasympathetic predominance resulted from the early environmental restriction, resulting in vagal bradycardia and increased lower-bowel motility. However, the fact that *mice* that are stimulated early in life show *increased* defecatory rates, (Hall and Whiteman, 1951) raises questions as to the generalizability of this postulated relationship. Moreover, the fact that decreased defecatory rates can be produced in rats by prior handling of the subjects' mothers during pregnancy (Ader and Conklin, 1963) raises questions as to the behavioral and physiological mechanisms which can produce such "early experience effects."

The mechanism for experimental gastric erosions in stressed rats is also poorly understood. However, α-adrenergic blockade has recently been shown to reduce the incidence of restraint-induced gastric erosions in the rat from 90% to 30% (Djahaguiri et al., 1973), a finding which directly implicates sympathetic pathways in the mechanism. Since altered autonomic nervous system (ANS) control over secretion, motility, cell renewal, and vascular flow are likely pathogenic pathways, I will briefly summarize these data which reveal the importance of early experience on this form of adult stress-induced pathology. Early handling of rats has been shown to reduce the incidence of gastric ulcers induced by immobilization, whereas early experience with electric shock does not (Ader, 1965). Handling of the pregnant mothers increased the susceptibility of the offspring to gastric erosions, as did group housing from weaning on (Ader and Plaut, 1968). Early separation from the mother (15 days) also increased susceptibility to shock-avoidance and immobilization-induced ulceration (Erdosova et al., 1967), and the former effect was shown to be limited to males and not to be a result of the nutritional deprivation as consequence of early weaning (Ader, 1971). Here again we very much need more information on how these early experiences become translated into altered ANS regulation under stress in the adult.

2.3. Summary and Perspective

Although present evidence leaves little doubt as to the importance of experience in shaping the development of the autonomic nervous system, there are already inconsistencies and contradictions enough to prevent us from stating even a limited theory capable of explaining how a particular early experience interacts with the developmental characteristics of the organism at a specific age to produce a given long-term effect.

Early experiences which are supposed to involve reduction in levels of ongoing stimulation (such as early separation from the mother, from peers, or from other sources of environmental stimulation) seem to lead to increased blood pressure, lowered cardiac rate, increased inferred gastrointestinal motility, and heightened susceptibility to gastric ulceration under stress in adulthood. Conversely, attempts to increase the level of stimulation through early handling by the experimenter appear to increase cardiac rate, decrease defecation, and reduce susceptibility to gastric ulceration.

It is not at all settled, however, that the common denominator of these classes of experience is in fact the level of sensory stimulation imposed during early development. For instance, increased stimulation with electric shock does not have the same effects as does handling by the experimenter, and increased handling does not have the same effect at different ages. In fact it may not be the direct effect of handling which alters development, but rather indirect effects which this disturbance has upon subsequent mother–infant relationship. Strain and species differences can result in contradictory and opposite results for reasons that remain unexplained by any simple generalization about levels of early stimulation.

Because so much about these early experience phenomena is unknown, it should be worthwhile to examine one autonomic effector system in detail, to gain some understanding of the normal development of autonomic function in that system, and to attempt to analyze how particular experiences affect the autonomic regulation of the young organism at different developmental ages. Then we would like to discover, if possible, how each experience becomes translated into altered autonomic function, both immediately and over the long-term course of development to adulthood.

3. Processes Involved in Early Experience Effects

3.1. A Simple Model System

In order to answer some of the questions raised in the previous section, I would like to turn to some recent work that has been done in my laboratory on a relatively simple model system for studying the interaction of experience and development within the autonomic nervous system. We have developed methods for chronic electrode implantation and recording of cardiac rate along with electrocardiogram, spinal electromyogram, and respiratory rate (by impedenance pneumogram) from freely moving rat pups while they engage in a full range of natural behaviors in their home cage including nursing from their mothers (Hofer and Grabie, 1971).

Figure 1 shows the kind of records we can obtain by these methods, and how we are able to define periods of activity as contrasted with inactivity in order to express heart rate as related to these two states, and to obtain measures of the level of activity (percent time active) of the animal during the recording period. Qualitative observations of behavior are written directly on the polygraph paper.

By administering autonomic neurotransmitters and/or blocking agents, one can infer the relative roles of sympathetic and parasympathetic components of autonomic control over cardiac rate, and the capacity of the immature myocardium to respond to autonomic neurotransmitters at different postnatal ages. The response of the autonomic system to various experiences such as handling, acoustic startle, and separation from the

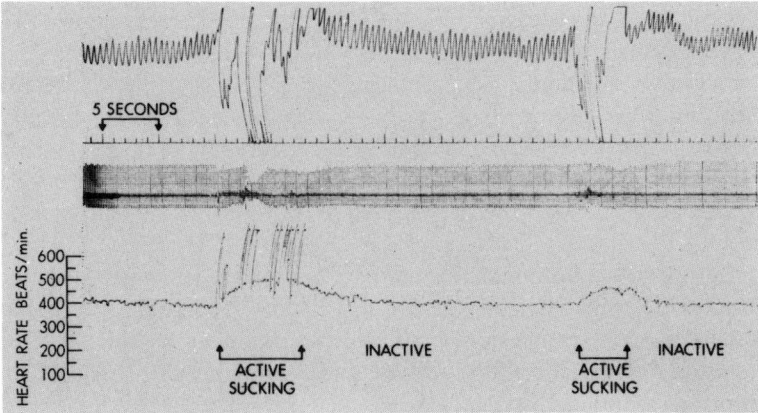

FIG. 1.   Sample polygraph page showing, on the top channel, the impedance pneumograph tracing with both regular quiet respiration and activity artifact during suckling. The second is a time channel; the third channel is electrocardiogram and electromyogram, the latter showing characteristic electromyogram bursts during activity. The bottom channel is the cardiotachometer write-out, with its scale given at the left. Two characteristic rises of heart rate during suckling bursts are shown, the first containing a number of movement artifacts. Paper speed is 5mm/sec. (Reprinted with permission of *Developmental Psychobiology*.)

mother can then be assessed, also at different developmental ages. The behavioral and physiological processes mediating these responses should then be amenable to experimental analysis. At this point, long-term developmental changes resulting from these early experiences can be systematically explored and, finally, understood as a complex process extending over time. Needless to say, we have only been able to make a beginning on this approach, but it has already taught us a good deal.

3.2.   The Normal Development of Autonomic Cardiac Regulation in Laboratory Conditions from Fetus to Adult

The first systematic studies in this area were done by E. F. Adolph (1965), who showed that the fetal rat heart begins to beat at 10 days gestational age and that if the heart is isolated from all extrinsic controls by excision at various fetal and postnatal ages, there is no change in its intrinsic rate. From this we can draw the important conclusion that changes in heart rate with age must be due to altered autonomic neural and hormonal influences or to the capacity of the developing myocardium to respond to these influences. Prior to 15 days gestational age, he found that control of heart rate was dependent primarily on temperature, minimal oxygen supply, and possibly stretch (Adolph 1965). Responses to the parasympathetic neurotransmitter acetylcholine were first found at 13 days and to the sympathetic neurotransmitter norepinephrine at 16 days. Cardiac acceleration in response to cervical sympathetic nerve stimulation was first evident at 20 days gestational age (Adolph 1967), as well as the first evidences of parasympathetic vagal cardiac slowing reflexes. There was little evidence for tonic autonomic drive to the pacemaker prior to birth at approximately 21 days of gestational age. However, in the first postnatal week, a substantial rise in basal heart rates occurred that was almost entirely blocked by propranalol, a β-adrenergic competitive inhibitor, indicating the development of appreciable levels of sympathetic tone early in postnatal development. Adolph found little evidence for parasympathetic tone until after the 2nd postnatal week.

These studies give us much useful information on the development of the physiological *potential* for autonomic regulation in the early life of the rat, but since Adolph's subjects were taped to a board for a half hour prior to cardiac readings and electrodes were acutely placed subcutaneously, no conclusions can be drawn from his data about regulatory patterns occurring in freely moving animals under natural conditions. We do know from his work that cardiac rate can be controlled by the autonomic system from birth onward, since the pacemaker has been shown to respond to both sympathetic and parasympathetic neurotransmitters by that time.

Using the methods described above (Section 3.1), we have recorded heart rates from unrestrained pups adapted to chronically implanted electrodes throughout the period from birth to weaning (Hofer and Reiser, 1969).

As demonstrated in Fig. 2, the resting heart rate of the young rat shows three phases during the first 3 weeks of life. First, an acceleratory phase, gradually raising heart rates from 375 beats per minute (BPM) to 425 BPM occurs in the 1st week. Second, a plateau of high heart rates throughout the 2nd week of postnatal life gives way to increased range in heart rates at 16 days. The third phase begins with a marked fall is resting heart rates from about 425 BPM at 14 days down to 300 BPM at 21 days. Cardiac acceleration with spontaneous bouts of behavioral activity did not become reliably evident until 12 days of postnatal age.

Two interesting phenomena of early cardiac regulation were observed in addition, under natural conditions. During what appeared to be "paradoxical" sleep, sudden bouts of precipitous cardiac slowing occurred, lasting 2–5 seconds. These reached a peak level of occurrence near the end of the 2nd week and were rarely evident in weanling (20-day-old) rats. Secondly, the rather stereotyped behavior sequence of "face-washing" was

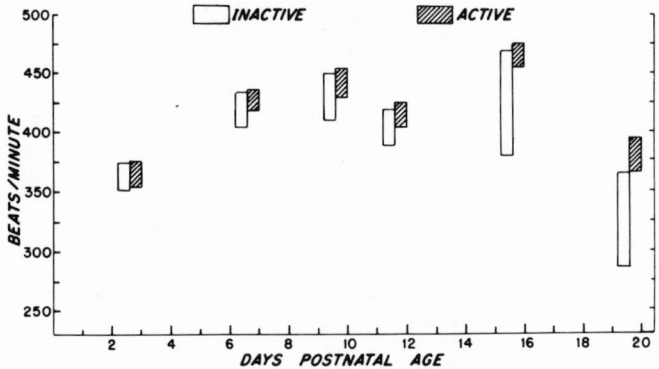

FIG. 2.   Ranges of heart rates recorded from unrestrained rat pups in their home cages during the first three weeks of life. Heart rates were recorded for 10 minutes on eight different pups from two different litters at each age, and the means of the eight pups' minimum and maximum heart rates define the bottom and top of each bar. Mean heart rates were significantly (p < .05) different as follows: 20 days < 3 days < 7, 10, 12, and 16 days. (Reprinted with permission of *Psychosomatic Medicine.*)

accompanied by marked, phasic increases in heart rate to the highest levels recorded under natural conditions, except perhaps during suckling. This behavior developed during the 2nd week and heart rate increases reached a maximum at 3 weeks of age.

As is evident in Fig. 1, bouts of active suckling were regularly associated with increases in heart rate from the baseline rate characteristic of quiet intervals during a period of nursing.

As Fig. 3 indicates, time spent with the mother during nursing was associated with generally higher active heart rates and a gradual increase in resting cardiac rates over the 20 minutes of nursing (Hofer and Grabie, 1971). Similar differences were not found in resting respiratory rate or percent of time spent active. Incidentally, no corresponding increase in heart rates with nursing occurred in the mother rat.

In order to determine the autonomic mechanisms underlying these developmental changes in heart rate, studies with pharmacologic blocking agents were done (Hofer and Reiser 1969). The high plateau of resting heart rates in the 2nd week appeared to be due to high sympathetic tone, since propranalol reduced these heart rates to 20-day-old levels. An increase in parasympathetic tone during the 3rd week was apparently responsible for the fall in heart rates at this period since methyl atropine, which had little or no effect on 2-week-old heart rates, accelerated resting heart rates of 3-week-old pups from 300 BPM to 400 BPM (Hofer,

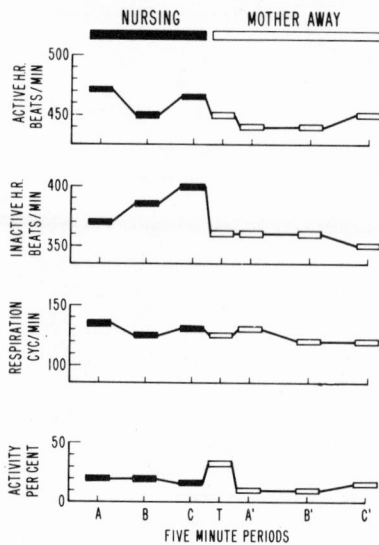

FIG. 3.   Heart rates, respiration, and activity level for a group of nine rat pups aged 12–19 days, each studied over an entire nursing cycle. Nursing periods averaged 26 minutes and mother-away periods, 54 minutes. T: transition periods of disturbance immediately following mothers departure. Nursing active and inactive heart rates significantly ($p < .01$) higher than mother-away rates. Otherwise, only T period of activity significantly different from other periods. (Reprinted with permission of *Developmental Psychobiology*.)

unpublished results). The episodes of transient bradycardia during sleep were also blocked by atropine and cardiac acceleration with activity was found to be absent after sympathetic blockade.

Thus the pattern emerges, that sympathetic cardiac drive increases from birth throughout the 1st week and maintains heart rate at high levels throughout the 2nd week. By the 3rd week parasympathetic tone makes its first appearance and slows the resting heart rate down to levels below those seen in the neonate and to levels characteristic of the adult by the time of weaning (21 days). Data will be presented subsequently that indicate that the high sympathetic tone of the 2-week-old pup is not simply an age-specific characteristic of central regulation, but is dependent on the mother's presence and more particularly on the nutrient she supplies.

3.3.   Autonomic Cardiac Responses to Experience at Different Ages in Early Development

In the studies described in section 2 on long-term effects, there were two main classes of early experiences, early stimulation (e.g., handling) and

early deprivation (e.g., isolation). The following studies examine the ontogeny of the acute cardiac rate responses to 1) being picked up by the experimenter and placed in a plastic box for a few minutes (standard handling
procedure), 2) acoustic startle stimulation, and finally 3) separation from
the mother. The last experience is much more complex than the others, has
been more thoroughly analyzed and has led to some new hypotheses about
the role of the normal mother–infant interaction in early autonomic
development.

Handling. The procedure whereby the experimenter picks a single
young animal out of its natural habitat and holds it in a standard manner
(usually in a plastic box) has traditionally been used as a form of early mild
stimulation. Rat pups respond with increasing degrees of behavioral activation to being placed in a novel environment as their postnatal age
increases, the most rapid increase occurring during the 2nd week (Hofer
and Reiser 1969). Activity recorded over 10-minute samples in the home
cage among littermates does not change over the first 3 weeks. The test box
was temperature controlled at nest temperature for pups younger than 2
weeks.

As can be seen in Fig. 5, the heart rate reponses to handling are markedly different at different postnatal ages. Little or no response occurs in
the youngest pups. However, throughout the 2nd week of life, when resting
rates are high, responses to almost any form of stimulation are deceleratory. This was a highly reliable finding occurring in 15 of 16 pups observed
at this age and taking place during activity as well as during inactivity. At
the end of 6 minutes in the test box heart rate had returned to pre-

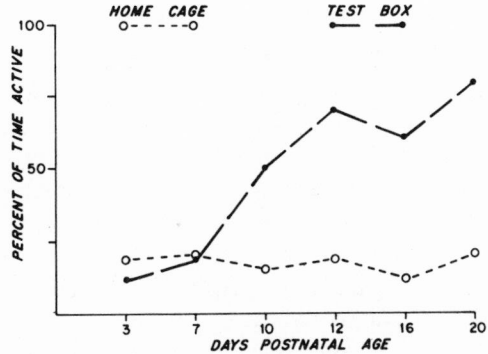

FIG. 4. Activity of rat pups in home cage among littermates and alone in test box at different ages.
(Reprinted with permission of *Psychosomatic Medicine*.)

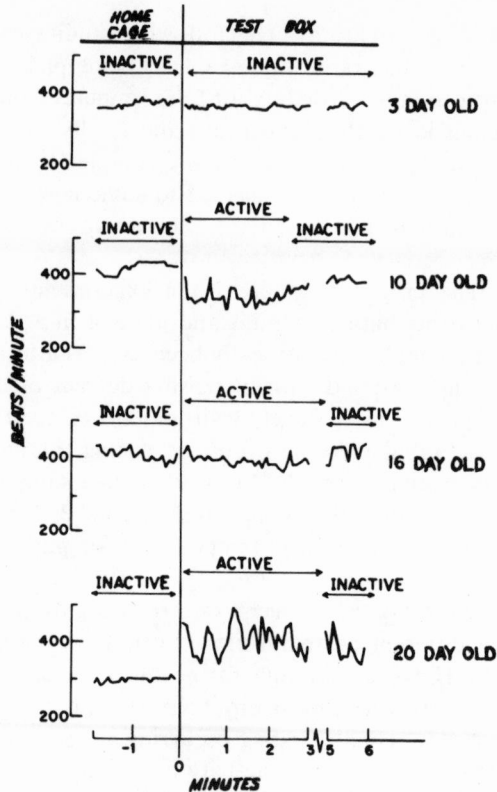

FIG. 5. Examples of typical heart rate recordings at different ages both in home cage and in response to being placed in the test box. Lines connect readings made every 5 seconds on cardiotachometer tracing of a single pup. (Reprinted with permission of *Psychosomatic Medicine*.)

stimulation levels. By 16 days, responses were highly variable, both acceleratory and deceleratory responses occurring and some, as illustrated, showed a balance between the two tendencies. By 3 weeks, the usual adult pattern had become established with low resting rates and cardiac acceleration as the animal became active in response to the handling.

The deceleratory responses were parasympathetic in mechanism and the later, acceleratory ones, sympathetic.

Sudden Auditory and Tactile Stimulation—the Startle Reaction. Figure 6 shows the behavioral and cardiac responses to a sudden click stimulus which was transmitted directly to the floor of the test box as a sharp vibration. In this case, both the behavioral "startle-freeze" response and

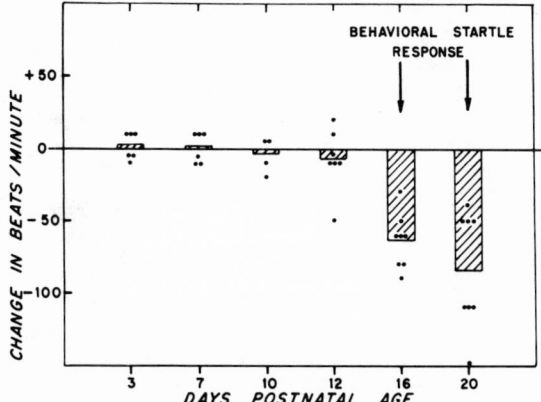

FIG. 6. Cardiac response to startle stimulus at different ages. Shaded bars: mean values, solid circles: individual values. (Reprinted with permission of *Psychosomatic Medicine*.)

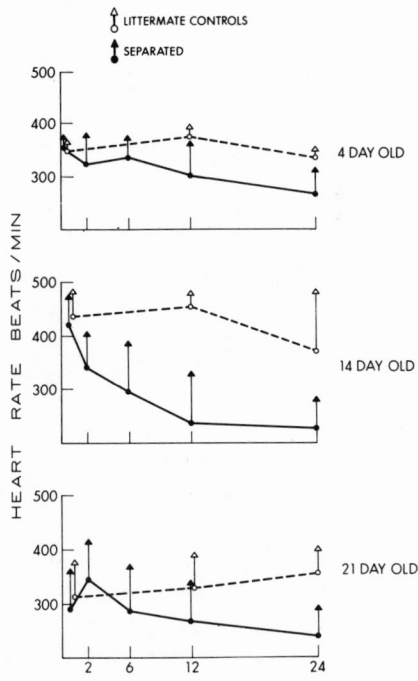

FIG. 7. Cardiac rates during inactivity and activity over 24 hours after separation from mother, compared to littermate controls left with mother. Responses of 4-, 14- and 21-day-old pups are compared (N = 6) animals at each point, total 36). (Reprinted with permission of *Psychosomatic Medicine*.)

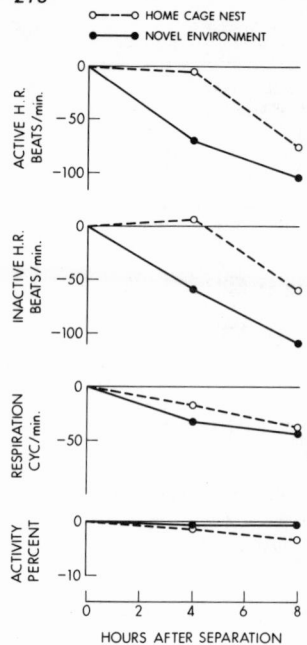

FIG. 8. Onset of physiologic responses to maternal deprivation in 2-week-old rat pups separated in a novel environment, compared to those left in the home cage nest (N = 8 animals at each point, total 16). Differences are significant only for heart rates at 4 hours, p < 0.05 and 8 hours, p < 0.01. (Reprinted with permission of *Psychosomatic Medicine*.)

the cardiac response developed simultaneously. The cardiac response was deceleratory in both 16- and 20-day-olds.

The Acute Autonomic Response to Separation From the Mother. Mothers were removed from young rats at each of the three main developmental stages of cardiac regulation outlined above; littermates were allowed to remain with the mother (Hofer and Weiner, 1971). Body temperature was maintained in separated animals by an incubator or thermostatically regulated heating pad under the cage floor.

The 2-week-old pups were found to have a marked and consistent fall in both active and inactive heart rates over the first 12 hours of separation. This pattern was far less evident in the younger and older pups. There was also a consistent reduction in respiratory rate but no change in activity level in the 3-minute samples recorded for physiologic variables.

Although the separated pups had a supply of home cage shavings, they could have been responding primarily to transfer to a novel environment as in the far shorter experiments cited above. However in those, the bradycardia was transient; heart rates had always returned to home cage levels by the 5th minute in the test box. An experiment to test this proposition directly compared 2-week-old pups left undisturbed in a group in their home cage (heat being supplied through the cage floor) with others transferred to an incubator. The novel environment was found to hasten the onset of the response, but heart rates fell significantly within 8 hours even in the home cage. In another experiment heart rates were found to reach the same low levels in the home cage after 24 hours as in the novel environment (Hofer, 1970).

Since separated pups eat very little and lose weight, we had to know whether the low cardiac rates were simply the result of starvation and a myocardium that was incapable of beating at normal rates due to lack of metabolic substrate. Rat pups were studied under three conditions: fed by tube every 4 hours, intubated only, or left alone for 24 hours (Hofer, 1970). The fed pups all gained some weight and were clearly not dehydrated or starved and yet had identical heart rates to their littermates which lost 2.4 g. However, we had succeeded in achieving a mean weight gain of only 0.9 g in 24 hours, whereas a lactating rat produces increases 2–3 g in pups this age over the same period. Later, we were to find that nutrition *does* have a regulatory influence on cardiac rate within the normal range of weight gain at this age.

We also found that the low heart rates of separated pups were not fixed, but accelerated with stimulation of the pup, to levels characteristic of their preseparation state (Hofer and Weiner, 1971). Vigorous tail pinching drove heart rates of separated pups promptly from 250 to 420 BPM as is shown in Fig. 9.

Figure 9 also summarizes the effects of pharmacologic agents on the heart rates of separated pups. The low heart rates could not have a parasympathetic mechanism since atropine failed to raise heart rates to preseparation levels (although a small but reliable increase was found after atropine). β-adrenergic blockade, in doses sufficient to entirely block the acceleratory response to tail pinching, did not significantly lower the heart

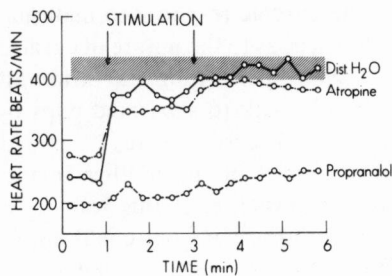

FIG. 9. Heart rate response to stimulation by tail pinching maternally deprived rat pups previously injected intraperitoneally with atropine, propranolol, or distilled water (N = 5 for distilled H$_2$O, 4 for atropine and 5 for propranolol). (Reprinted with permission of *Psychosomatic Medicine.*)

rates of separated pups. We had found previously (see above) that propranolol *does* reduce the high heart rates of *normally* mothered 2-week-old pups to about 300 BPM, a level which we now find is characteristic of separated pups. These results are consistent with the formulation that during the first 12 hours of separation from the mother, a marked fall in sympathetic cardiac tone occurred, aided by a small increase in parasympathetic restraint.

In summary, the data on the development of autonomic cardiac responses further define the three stages which seemed to appear in the data on resting levels. In the first week of postnatal age, while baseline sympathetic drive is slowly increasing, heart rate responds very little to most forms of environmental experience, although the animal reacts vigorously behaviorally. At this age, only specific physiological stimuli such as asphyxia demonstrate intact autonomic reflex pathways. Throughout the second week of life, while resting heart rates are maintained at high levels by sympathetic tone (with little or no resting parasympathetic restraint) the immediate response to most forms of stimulation is parasympathetic deceleration. A much more prolonged and intense bradycardia results from maternal separation in 2-week-old rat pups, apparently produced mainly by a marked reduction in resting sympathetic drive. Acoustic startle response develops both cardiac and behavioral components by 16 days and continues to be deceleratory even at 20 days. By the end of the 3rd week, when resting heart rates are low due to the development of parasympathetic cardiac restraint, cardiac responses to handling and tail pinching have become acceleratory, as in the adult, and mediated by the sympathetic system.

3.4. The Role of the Mother–Infant Interaction in the Early Development of Autonomic Cardiac Regulation

Further analysis of the behavioral and physiological processes involved in the cardiac response to maternal separation have led to some surprising inferences as to the nature of cardiac regulation in early life.

Since preventing starvation and dehydration by giving small amounts of cow's milk to separated pups by stomach tube had not prevented their decrease in cardiac rate, it seemed logical to suppose that the absence of some aspect of the mother–infant behavioral interaction was responsible for the response. If this was so, nonlactating foster mothers, who would stay with the pups but could not supply milk, should maintain heart rates. We found that they did not (Hofer and Weiner, 1971), and although we could not be sure that their behavioral interaction with the pups was normal, the unequivocal results of these experiments turned our attention back to nutritional factors.

First, we wondered if fresh rat's milk might not contain some sympathomimetic hormone or other factor which was responsible for the development and maintenance of high heart rates during the second week of postnatal life. Gradual weaning to other food sources during the 3rd week would allow heart rates to decline, thus explaining several of our observations. Unfortunately, this neat hypothesis did not last long, since fresh rat's milk did not differ from cow's milk in its effect on heart rates of previously separated 2-week-old rat pups (Hofer, unpublished observations). In the course of these experiments, however, we noticed that the larger doses of milk, either rats' or cows', produced rapid, but transient cardiac acceleration.

A controlled study revealed the results shown in Fig. 10 (Hofer, 1971). Bovine milk rapidly reversed the cardiac deceleration which occurred after

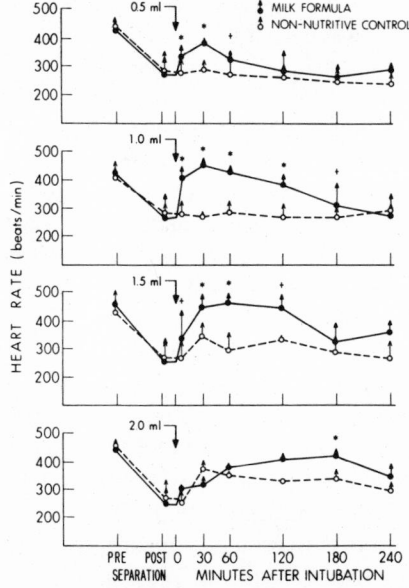

FIG. 10.   Cardiac rates of 2-week-old rats separated from their mothers for 16 hours and given feedings of milk or control fluid in four different volumes. The first points after intubation values are at 5 minutes. Each point represents six pups. Circles indicate median inactive heart rates (solid circles, milk formula; open circles, nonnutritive control); arrow points are median active rates. Statistically significant differences between inactive heart rates of milk-fed and control pups are indicated by asterisk (p < 0.01) or cross (p < 0.05); (Wilcoxon–White two-sample ranks test). (Copyright 1971 by the Am. Assoc. for the Advancement of Science, Science 172:1039-1041, 1971) (Reprinted with permission of American Association for the Advancement of Science.)

separation from the mother. The effect was dose-related, lasted 1–2 hours, and did not occur if the stomach was equally distended with a non-nutritive solution of dilute aluminum hydroxide of similar solute and pH characteristics as milk.

How did the milk exert this effect? The very rapid onset of the response (2–3 minutes) suggested a neural mechanism, and pretreatment with an adrenergic blocking agent prevented the milk effect, implicating β-adrenergic neurotransmission (Hofer, 1971). When the constituents of milk were given separately by stomach tube, both milk carbohydrate (lactose) and milk protein (casein) were equally effective in raising the cardiac rates of separated pups (Hofer 1972). Even vegetable fat was effective, although casein seemed to have the most rapid onset of action. If nutrients were being absorbed from the milk in the stomach and were carried in the general circulation directly to the myocardium (or acted indirectly after an initial effect on the central nervous system), then intravenous injection of lactose or casein hydrolysate should have the most immediate and consistent effects. Miniature jugular cannulas were implanted the day before separation and, after a 20-hour separation, slow infusions of saturated lactose and casein hydrolysate solutions were carried out. No increases in resting heart rates were observed. Even 50% glucose was ineffective. These results suggested that the milk effect on heart rate did not depend on the circulatory transport of absorbed nutrient.

To explore the possibility of a central pathway for the milk effect, spinal cord sections were performed under a dissecting microscope and milk was given by stomach tube after separation (Hofer, 1972). Those pups with sham operations of spinal cord sections at T_8 had normal responses to intragastric milk while those with sections at T_1 showed no milk responses.

It appears that the mechanism for the milk effect does not involve circulatory transport of nutrient, but does involve central neural pathways passing through the junction of cervical and thoracic spinal cord. The efferent limb would appear to be sympathetic (fibers exit from spinal cord $(T_2–T_6)$. But it is not clear whether the afferent limb involves gastric and duodenal chemoreceptors and autonomic afferents via the paravertebral system and spinal cord or, alternately, depends upon the hemodynamic and central neural regulatory consequences of shifts in blood volume to the splanchnic bed during digestion.

The implication of these analytical experiments on the processes involved in the cardiac separation response is that under normal conditions the degree of sympathetic cardiac tone of the young rat may be regulated by the amount of milk supplied by the mother. Long periods of starvation have been shown to have no consistent effects on cardiac rate of *adult* rats, so this relationship would be age-dependent and perhaps unique for the 2nd week of early postnatal development.

Two lines of experimentation support this hypothesis. First, spinal cord section at T_1, when performed on normally mothered rat pups, produced an immediate fall in heart rate to levels characteristic of a 20-hour separation. Section at T_8 had no such effect. This indicates that the high heart rates of normally mothered pups are dependent on intact connections between cervical and thoracic spinal cords, and supports the results of the studies with adrenergic blocking agents which suggested that the high heart rates of 2-week-old pups are the result of high sympathetic tone imposed by central autonomic neural integration. Secondly, if the support for heart rate was primarily through the supplying of milk, then if milk was given artifically in sufficient quantity to separated pups, heart rate should be maintained at preseparation levels without the mothers presence being necessary at all. A constant-rate infusion pump was used in combination with chronically implanted gastric tubes (Hofer, 1973b). Three infusion rates were used as well as noninfused controls with similar chronic gastric tubes. The results were clearcut and showed a pattern in which, at the end of a 24-hour separation, the pups given milk at the highest infusion rate had slightly increased their rates over the previous day, those given the midrange rate declined very slightly while the lowest rate given allowed a decrease in heart rates, but a smaller one than occurred in those given none at all. Thus, heart rates *can* be maintained by intragastric milk infusion in the absence of the mother for at least 24 hours. Moreover, the degree of control exerted by milk intake over heart rate was demonstrated by a rank order correlation of 0.79 between percent weight change and percent change in cardiac rate over all the experimental groups.

3.5. The Relevance of Developmental Data for an Understanding of the Long-Range Effects of Early Experience

What can this information on early autonomic development in a simple model system tell us about how long-term effects resulting from early experience in this system? This is really a premature question, since we have only begun to scratch the surface of our ignorance in this area and are still far from being able to see at all clearly.

What *is* clear is that any eventual understanding will have to include the idea that the functional organization of the autonomic system is quite different at different stages in postnatal development, and in particular that there are fundamental differences in cardiac regulation between a 2-week-old rat pup and an adult (or for that matter, between 2-and 3-week-olds). These facts answer at least one question raised at the end of section 2.1. In 2-week-olds there is a strong sympathetic cardiac drive at rest and acute responses to environmental stimulation are primarily parasympathetic. By

3 weeks of age, and in the adult, the organizational pattern is reversed: sympathetic tone is low at rest with prominent parasympathetic restraint, while environmental stimulation elicits phasic sympathetic bursts.

The implication is that experience is transduced differently in the young organism, that our psychophysiological knowledge, based as it is on adults, may have to be reassessed in the young organism before we can put together meaningful theories relating early experience and long-term effects in the adult. This is more than a critical period concept; it suggests *qualitatively* different and even opposite outcomes from the same experience occurring at different early developmental stages. For example, in long-term studies employing handling as an early experience, the impact of this stimulation in the second week of life may have very different or opposite long-term effects on autonomic development from handling during the 1st or 3rd week when central autonomic regulation is differently organized.

This necessity to understand the behavioral and physiological processes involved in early experiences is perhaps best exemplified by the knowledge we have recently gained on early maternal separation. Without the admittedly incomplete analysis we have done, one would not know that the most important determinant of the dramatic cardiac response to separation is nutritional, and many errors would be made by not properly controlling for this variable, as has already occurred in too many early experience studies. Going one step further, the realization that in early development autonomic regulation is extremely sensitive to the level of nutritional intake via pathways which involve the central nervous system, suggests that early malnutrition may be the early experience to study for its long-term effects on autonomic control in the adult, rather than handling, electric shock, environmental restriction, or even deprivation of behavioral interaction with the mother. This analysis, when completed, will answer the question posed in Section 2.1: "how is the early experience (of maternal deprivation) translated into physiological change."

We have begun to look at the development of cardiac regulation beyond the acute period of 24 hours following separation described above. Preliminary findings indicate that pups eat very little for 1–3 days, low heart rates persist as do low body temperatures, unless heat is applied artificially. Then, often rather suddenly, the pups begin to eat and heart rates rise dramatically. Presumably, the mechanism for nutritional regulation of heart rate described above is responsible for this physiological *rebound*. These pups often gain weight more rapidly than pups left with the mother in the 18–20 day period, and at 21 days have *higher* resting heart rates than normally mothered pups. At 100 days of age, in a small number of subjects, no differences in heart rate responses to handling and a 2-hour adaptation to a novel test box were found between pups permanently separated from their mothers at 15 days as compared to 25 days. These preliminary findings illustrate how developmental processes intervene between an early experience and the long-term expression of its effect in the adult.

All the studies detailed above were concerned with the effects of sudden and prolonged absence of the mother on the infacts remaining in the home cage. One can also enquire what contribution the littermates make to each other. In particular, do the littermates contribute to the development of autonomic regulation of each pup.

Dr. H. Leigh and I (Leigh and Hofer, 1973) removed all but one of a litter from the home cage at various ages and found that prior to 10 days of age the remaining "singleton" invariably died; apparently the mother did not sustain her milk supply. At 12 days' postnatal age, survival was 100%, and curves of weight again did not differ significantly from normal. These young rats were deprived of littermates throughout the socialization period (14–30 days). Active cardiac rates became higher than normal by age 14 days and remained higher until recordings were stopped at day 21. These animals were housed singly after 21 days and tested again in adulthood, 120 days (Leigh and Hofer, 1973). The 12-day singletons were found to have resting heart rates which were identical to controls housed singly from day 21 on and a similar cadiac response to auditory stimulation by an air-blast. However, their cardiac rate response to the presence of a normal adult rat was significantly less than controls housed singly from 21 days until testing. Thus, the experience of premature littermate removal at day 21 affected autonomic responsiveness, but only in a social setting.

We are a long way from understanding the processes underlying the differences in active heart rates we found between day 14 and 20, the absence of some long-range cardiac effects of this early experience, and the presence of other long-range effects. For example, although in adulthood the cardiac response to a rodent intruder was reduced, the behavioral response to the experimenter's hand was increased.

To illustrate how careful we must be in inferring processes underlying early experience affects, it was found that littermate removal at day 12 markedly affected the interaction between the remaining pup and the mother (Leigh and Hofer, 1973). Mothers increased the proportion of time spent with singletons from 30% to 70%, licked the remaining pup much more often and were more often observed in the nursing position over the singleton. The pup, in turn, showed increased stimulation of the mother, self-grooming, and locomotion. The high level of mother–pup contact showed little tendency to decrease from day 12 to day 20.

This unusual experience with the mother may have been even more important for the autonomic development of the singleton than the absence of littermates during the socialization period. In order to reach any understanding of the phenomena involved, we need to know a great deal more about the immediate impact of the various components of these experiences on the developing autonomic regulatory system of the infant.

4. Conclusions and Unknowns

It is relatively easy to study early development and even easier to look for long-range effects of early experiences in adulthood, but it is impossible at this time to bring the two sets of data together within any coherent theoretical framework. For example, if the experience of handling stimulates parasympathetic cardiac responses during the second week of life, will the frequent elicitation of these responses during that week make the animal more or less likely to show parasympathetic responses as an adult? Even more puzzling, how do we understand the long-term effects on heart rate regulation brought about by handling in the first week of life (Blizard 1971), at an age when *no* cardiac responses occur to this stimulation? In other words, the system, although "silent" at the time of the experience, nevertheless shows long-range effects. In the case of handling in the 1st week of life, we have a possible way out of facing this question, since handling probably affects the *subsequent* mother–pup interaction, apparently in the direction of increasing her stimulation of the pups over many hours and days after the actual handling experience (Thoman and Levine, 1969). Alternately, we may suppose that other central neural systems *are* responding to the early stimulation, and if we knew where to record, could observe the acute impact of the experience which is expressed later in heart rate alterations.

As suggested above, we do not even know what circumstances determine whether frequent elicitation of a response in early life *stamps in* the response so that it will be more likely in adulthood (King, 1968) or *damps out* the response by stimulation of sensory filtering, centrifugal inhibition, and the process of habituation (Melzack, 1969). This ignorance is most immediately felt by those working in the area of early "cultural enrichment" programs, for example.

Obviously, elicitation of responses is not the only process involved in early experience effects, as our work on early separation demonstrates. Here again, though, our understanding of long-range effects is complicated by the existence of later developmental processes which may either exaggerate or damp out differences created by any given experience at an earlier age.

Recently we have found that a few hours of maternal separation also effects the behavioral responses of 2-week-old rat pups (Hofer, 1973a,b). Increased levels of locomotor, exploratory, self-grooming, and excretory behavior are found in separated pups observed in an unfamiliar test area. These behavioral changes are *not* related to the level of nutrition artifically supplied and *are* prevented by the presence of a nonlactating foster mother—in contrast to the autonomic and respiratory changes described above. These results indicate that the experience of early maternal separation may become translated into physiological and behavioral changes by separate and different mechanisms.

The findings to date suggest that early experience effects will become understood finally as a complex process involving many fundamental developmental principles which are at present unknown. We know enough already to realize that it is a worthwhile problem and one which promises to add a new and dynamic aspect to our understanding of the autonomic nervous system.

5. References

Ader, R., 1965, Effects of early experience and differential housing on behavior and suscepti-bility to gastric erosions in the rat, *J. Comp. Physiol. Psychol. 60:*233–238.

Ader, R., 1971, Experimentally induced gastric lesions, *Adv. Psychosom. Med. 6:*1–39.

Ader, R., and Conklin, P. M., 1963, Handling of pregnant rats: Effects on emotionality of their offspring, *Science 142:*411–412.

Ader, R., and Plaut, S. M., 1968, Effects of prenatal maternal handling on off-spring emo-tionality, plasms corticosteroid levels and susceptibility to gastric erosions, *Psychosom. Med. 30:*277–286.

Adolph, E. F., 1965, Capacities for regulation of heart rate in fetal, infact and adult rats, *Am. J. Physiol. 209:*1095–1105.

Adolph, E., 1967, Ranges of heart rates and their regulations at various ages, *Am. J. Physiol. 212:*595–602.

Blizard, D., 1971, Individual differences in autonomic responsivity in the adult rat; Neonatal influences, *Psychosom. Med. 33:*445–457.

Boyles, W. R., Black, R. N., and Furchtgott, E., 1965, Early experience and cardiac responsivity in the female albino rat, *J. Comp. Physiol. Psychol. 59:*446–447.

Dijahanguiri, B., Taubin, H. L., and Landsberg, L., 1973, Increased sympathetic activity in the pathogenesis of restraint ulcer in rats. *J. Pharm. Exptl. Therapeut. 184:*163–168.

Erdosova, R., Flandera, V., Krecek, J., and Weiner, P., 1967, The effects of premature weaning on the sensitivity of rats to experimental erosions of the gastric mucosa, *Physiol. Bohemoslov. 16:*400–407.

Freedman, D. G., King, J. A., and Elliott, O., 1961, Critical period in the social development of dogs, *Science 113:*1016–1017.

Grota, L. J., and Ader, R., 1972, Effects of early experience with electric shock and dexa-methazone on avoidance conditioning in adulthood, *Psychon. Sci. 28:*10–12.

Hall, C. S., and Whiteman, P. H., 1951, The effects of infantile stimulation upon later emotional behavior, *J. Comp. Physiol. Psychol. 44:*61–66.

Hammett, F. S., 1921, Studies of the thyroid apparatus, I: the stability of the nervous system as a factor in resistance of albino rats to loss of parathyroid secretion, *Am. J. Physiol. 56:*196–204.

Henry, J. P., Meehan, J. P., and Stephens, P. M. 1967, The use of psychosocial stimuli to induce prolonged systolic hypertension in mice, *Psychosom. Med. 29:*408–432.

Henry, J. P. Stephens, P. M., Axelrod, J., and Mueller, R. A., 1971, Effect of psychosocial stimulation on the enzymes involved in the biosynthesis and metabolism of noradrenaline and adrenaline, *Psychosom. Med. 33:*227–237.

Hofer, M. A., 1970, Physiological responses of infant rats to separation from their mothers, *Science 168:*871–873.

Hofer, M. A., 1971, Regulation of cardiac rate by nutritional factor in young rats, *Science 172:*1039–1041.

Hofer, M. A., 1972, Physiological and behavioral processes in early maternal deprivation, in *Physiology, Emotions and Psychosomatic Illness,* CIBA Symposium, No. 8, Elseiver, Amsterdam.

Hofer, M. A., 1973a, The effect of brief maternal separations on behavior and heart rate of two week old rat pups, *Physiol. Behav. 10:*423–427.

Hofer, M. A., 1973b, The role of nutrition in the physiological and behavioral effects of early maternal separation in infact rats. *Psychosom. Med. 35:*350:359.

Hofer, M. A., 1974, The principles of autonomic function in man and animals, in Vol. IV, *American Handbook of Psychiatry,* Basic Books, New York.

Hofer, M. A., and Grabie, M., 1971, Cardiorespiratory regulation and activity patterns of rat pups studied with their mothers during the nursing cycle, *Develop. Psychobiol. 4:*169–180.

Hofer, M. A., and Reiser, M. F., 1969, The development of cardiac rate regulation in preweanling rats, *Psychosom. Med. 31:*372–388.

Hofer, M. A., and Weiner, H., 1971, The development and mechanisms of cardiorespiratory responses to maternal deprivation in rat pups, *Psychosom. Med. 33:*353–362.

Hunt, H. F., and Otis, L. S., 1955, Restricted experience and timidity in the rat, *Am. J. Psychol. 10:*432–436.

Hutchings, D. E., 1963, Early 'experience' and its effects on later behavioral processes in rats: III Effects of infantile handling and body temperature reduction on later emotionality, *Trans. N.Y. Acad. Sci. 25:*890–901.

King, J. A., 1968, Species specificity and early experience, in *Early Experience and Behavior,* C. C. Thomas, Springfield, Illinois, pp. 42–64.

Koch, M. D., and Arnold, W. J., 1972, Effects of early social deprivation on emotionality in rats, *J. Comp. Physiol. Psychol. 78:*391–399.

Lacey, J. I., and Lacey, B. C., 1962, The law of initial value in the longitudinal study of autonomic constitution: reproducibility of autonomic response and response patterns over a four year interval, *Ann. N.Y. Acad. Sci. 98:*1257–1290.

Leigh, H., and Hofer, M. A., 1973, Behavioral and physiologic effects of littermate removal on the remaining single pup and mother during the preweaning period in rats. *Psychosom. Med. 35:*497–508.

Levine, S., 1957, Infantile experience and resistance to physiological stress, *Science, 126:*405.

Levine, S., and Mullins, R. R., 1966, Hormonal influences on brain organization in infant rats, *Science 152:*1585–1591.

Melzack, R., 1969, The role of early experience in emotional arousal, *Ann. N.Y. Acad., Sci. 159:*721–730.

Miller, N., 1969, Learning of visceral and glandular responses, *Science 163:*439–445.

Sargent, F., and Weinman, K. P., 1966, Physiological individuality, *Ann. N.Y. Acad. Sci. 134:*696–719.

Scott, J. H., 1955, Some effects at maturity of gentling, ignoring or shocking rats during infancy, *J. Abnorm. Soc. Psychol. 51:*412–414.

Scott, J. P., 1962, Critical periods in behavioral development, *Science 138:*949–958.

Snowdon, C. T., Bell, D. D., and Henderson, N. D., 1964, Relationship between heart rate and open field behavior, *J. Comp. Physiol. Psychol. 58:*423–430.

Thoman, E. B., and Levine, S., 1969, Role of maternal disturbance and temperature change in early experience studies, *Physiol. Behav. 4:*143–145.

Waddington, C. H., 1962, *New Patterns in Genetics and Development,* Columbia University Press, New York, pp. 181–182.

Weininger, O., 1953, Mortality of albino rats under stress as a function of early handling, *Canad. J. Psychol. 7:*111–114.

CHAPTER 7

The Neural Pathways and Informational Flow Mediating a Conditioned Autonomic Response*

David H. Cohen

Department of Physiology, School of Medicine
University of Virginia
Charlottesville, Virginia

1. Introduction

Despite a long-standing interest in the mechanisms by which nervous systems store and retrieve information, it is rather disappointing that most fundamental questions regarding long-term storage remain unresolved. For many years the unavailability of methods appropriate for investigating the dynamics of neural activity constituted a major barrier in this regard. Consequently, the advent of electrophysiological methods, and microelectrode techniques in particular, generated considerable optimism that changes in neuronal discharge patterns during development of learned behaviors could be specified, and that this would yield important insights into many basic questions regarding the cellular basis of storage. Unfortunately, such optimism has generally been unfounded. For example, we still cannot answer such fundamental questions as whether all neurons are capable of plastic change or if this capacity is restricted to certain morphologically and/or neurochemically specialized neuronal elements. We remain ignorant of the

* The author's research described here has been generously supported by grants from the National Science Foundation (GB-2767, GB-6850, GB-8008, GB-13816X, and GB-35204X), the Heart Association of Northeast Ohio, and the Benevolent Foundation of Scottish Rite Free Masonary, Northern Jurisdiction, U.S.A. Also, the author held a Research Career Development Award (HL-16579) from the National Heart and Lung Institute during the period much of this work was accomplished.

regions of the neuron which undergo plastic change and, of course, the nature of such change. In fact, in vertebrate brain we have yet to implicate *conclusively* any specific synaptic field in long-term storage.

However, the technology for resolving such questions is probably available, raising the obvious question of what has impeded rapid progress in the field. A possible answer is that we have lacked effective experimental model systems. Partly because long-term *associative* learning may be a property of more complex nervous systems, considerable experimental development is required to establish appropriate models (e.g., Cohen, 1969; Kandel and Spencer, 1968; Thompson and Spencer, 1966), and this has almost certainly constituted a major deterrent.

Important efforts in this direction have most frequently involved "simple" invertebrate systems (e.g., Bullock, 1967; Eisenstein, 1967; Kandel and Spencer, 1968) and to a lesser extent simplified vertebrate systems (e.g., Spencer *et al.* 1966), and the most exciting progress in the field has derived from such efforts. However, these model systems generate various concerns. First, while nonassociative learning phenomena such as habituation have been nicely exploited, these systems have been considerably less effective for investigating the long-term, associative phenomena that are so characteristic of vertebrate learning behavior. In fact, it may not be long before the mechanisms of habituation are understood; however, the mechanisms of long-term associative learning, which may well be quite different, remain elusive and may not be approachable with existing simplified systems. Second, in many "simple" systems only a limited range of questions is admissible. For example, use of a single synapse system does not permit one to ask whether specific regions of the nervous system are specialized for storage, whether sensory pathways are capable of plastic change, whether neurons showing modifications in their discharge patterns as a function of training have unique morphological characteristics, etc. Third, systems presumed "simple" with respect to certain properties, such as neuronal identifiability, size, and number, may well be rather complex in other important respects, such as experimental accessibility of synaptic regions involved in plastic change. Lastly, while invertebrate preparations have provided and will continue to provide important data on information storage, it is possible that the mechanisms could differ from those mediating associative long-term storage in vertebrate brain.

Consequently, when a "simple" system approach to learning is considered, it is necessary to ask "simple" with respect to what properties? That a given system has a limited number of large, identifiable neurons is not sufficient. If, for example, a presumptive "simple" system has plastic changes confined primarily to experimentally inaccessible neuropil, its attractiveness decreases. Moreover, if longer-term associative learning cannot be documented, such a system loses some of its generality. It may also be rather shortsighted to assume that all vertebrate systems are necessarily complex with respect to learning. The possibility cannot be excluded that circuitry participating in storage for a given behavior constitutes a "simple" system embedded in a more complex matrix consisting of many irrelevant elements and highly elaborated sensory and motor pathways which may not participate in storage *per se*.

Such considerations provided the impetus for our effort to develop an effective vertebrate model system, although we recognized that many years of experimental development would be required as a prelude to cellular studies. Important in guiding this effort were certain general criteria that were suggested by Kandel and Spencer (1968) and Cohen (1969). First, the preparation must have a quantifiable behavioral response whose probability of occurrence can be modified with appropriate training conditions, this modification being consistent with established principles of associative learning. This is necessary if one is to be assured that the preparation demonstrates meaningful long-term associative storage. Second, and of paramount importance, the neuroanatomical pathways mediating development of the learned response must be specified in detail, since without such information it is difficult to make statements regarding the meaning, or even the relevance, of changes in neuronal firing patterns occurring during training. Third, it is of great advantage to develop a model system that is as technologically compatible as possible with demands of cellular neurophysiological experiments. Finally, it is desirable to deal with a system that eventually admits experimental study of a broad range of questions, even though development of such a system might require considerable initial effort. Of these four general criteria, the first two are most critical, and few available systems satisfy both (Kandel and Spencer, 1968).

Within this context we have been developing visually conditioned heart-rate change in the pigeon as such a vertebrate model system (Cohen, 1969), and it is this system that constitutes the topic of the present chapter. While a substantial portion of our experimental work has been directed toward a detailed description of the behavioral characteristics of this system, these will be reviewed only briefly. The principal focus, however, will be upon identification of the neural pathways mediating conditioned response development, and this basically will be a discussion of our strategy and progress in attempting to satisfy the second general criterion described above.

2. Summary of the Behavioral Model

As indicated previously, a quantifiable behavioral response is essential for an effective model system. This deserves reemphasis, since the learned behavioral response essentially represents the input–output relation across the entire system, and it is this relation that one hopes to decompose into its components by analysis of the relevant central pathways. Ideally, one would like to specify the input–output relations across each relevant synaptic relay and to reconstruct the behavioral output by a combination of these functions. Viewed in this context, it is clear that an effective system requires not merely verification of the presence of a behavioral response, but also a precise analysis of its dynamics and their stimulus control. More demanding yet is the requirement that this be accomplished in a preparation that is technically compatible with limitations imposed by cellular neurophysiological methods.

As described earlier, we have devoted substantial effort to behavioral development of our specific system. However, the focus in this chapter is upon another critical problem, namely, identification of the anatomical pathways mediating development of the learned response. Consequently, the behavioral features of the system are reviewed in an abbreviated fashion to introduce the four major lines of research comprising this phase of the program and to establish a background for discussing relevant central pathways.

2.1. Basic Paradigm

The behavioral model is visually conditioned heart rate change in the pigeon (*Columba livia*), and the experimental paradigm is of the Pavlovian defensive conditioning type. Although of considerable intrinsic interest, heart rate conditioning was selected primarily because of its compatibility with demands of cellular neurophysiological experiments and the ease with which the response dynamics can be accurately specified. For example, among many methodological advantages of this system are: (1) stable learning occurs within approximately 1 hour and near-asymptotic performance within 3 hours; (2) conditioning can be established in the pharmacologically immobilized animal; (3) the conditioned response is readily quantifiable and in spike train format (R-waves of the electrocardiogram); (4) response dynamics are highly consistent among animals; and (5) long conditioned stimulus presentations are feasible, allowing trial-by-trial analysis of response dynamics (Cohen, 1969).

In investigating this system over the years, we have applied a standardized design involving repeated presentation of a 6.0-second pulse of whole-field retinal illumination (conditioned stimulus) immediately followed by an 0.5-second foot-shock (unconditioned stimulus). The foot-shock invariably elicits marked cardioacceleration (unconditioned response), and after a sufficient number of light–shock pairings retinal illumination itself reliably elicits cardioacceleration with predictable dynamics. This conditioned response develops within 20 pairings and reaches near-asymptotic levels within 40–60 pairings (Cohen in prep. a; Cohen and Durkovic, 1966), the precise rate of development and asymptotic level being a function of such variables as intertrial interval (Cohen and Macdonald, 1971). It might also be pointed out that differential responding is easily established on the basis of such cues as hue and intensity, and once established the conditioned response is highly resistant to extinction (Cohen, 1967; Cohen and Durkovic, 1966). Moreover, control data indicate that orienting and sensitization responses account for only a small proportion of the overall response (Cohen and Durkovic, 1966; Cohen and Macdonald, 1971; Cohen and Pitts, 1968), although this proportion may vary with such parameters as stimulus intensity (Cohen, 1974b).

2.2.   Response Dynamics and Their Development

Regarding the specific response characteristics and their sequential development, early light presentations, independent of foot-shock occurrence, elicit low-magnitude cardioacceleratory orienting responses (Fig. 1A). However, results from animals receiving only light presentations indicate that these orienting responses extinguish or habituate within 10 presentations (Fig. 1B) (Cohen and Durkovic, 1966; Cohen and Macdonald, 1971). The introduction of foot-shock then transforms this monotonic rate increase into a sensitization response with distinctly different dynamics from the orienting response (Fig. 1A), allowing it to be readily distinguished from both orienting and conditioned responses. The sensitization response can be studied in animals receiving unpaired light and shock presentations (Cohen and Macdonald, 1971), and such data show the response extinguishes or habituates within 10 presentations, as does the orienting response (Fig. 1B).

In our paradigm we customarily begin training with systematic light–shock pairings, and results strongly suggest some conditioned response development within the first 10 presentations (Fig. 2) (Cohen, in prep. a). Thus, one might anticipate that during these initial 10 trials there is a confounding of orienting, sensitization, and conditioned responses (Fig.

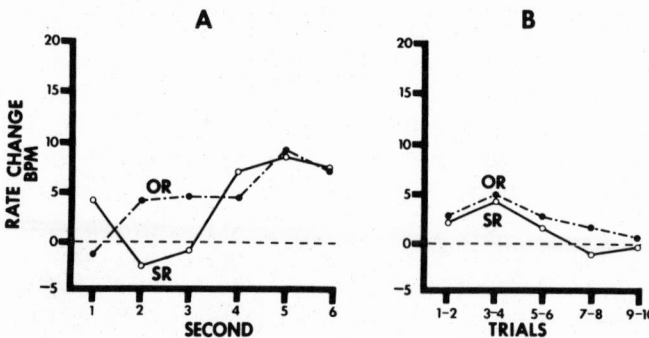

FIG. 1. Panel A illustrates response dynamics for orienting and sensitization responses. The curves show mean heart rate changes from baseline for each succeeding 1-second interval of the light presentation. OR: orienting response, and the curve is the averaged response of over 100 birds to the initial light presentation; SR: sensitization response, and the curve is the averaged response of 20 birds over the first four unpaired light-shock presentations (i.e., response to the light). Panel B illustrates habituation of these responses from the same samples of birds. The curves show mean heart rate changes between the stimulus period and a preceding 6-sec control period averaged over two-trial blocks. BPM: beats/min. (Adapted from Cohen and Macdonald, 1971).

2). However, if orienting and sensitization responses are habituated prior to systematic light–shock pairing, the conditioned response dynamics for the initial 10 pairings do not differ from those of nonhabituated animals. (Compare CR and CR' in Fig. 2.) Consequently, it appears that orienting and sensitization responses have at most a minimal confounding effect in early training, since in some manner the conditioned response development either suppresses these responses or facilitates their extinction.

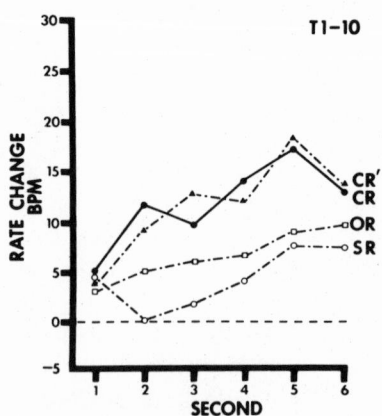

FIG. 2. Illustration of the dynamics of the various responses occurring during the first 10 trials (T1–10). The curves show mean heart rate changes from baseline for each succeeding 1-sec interval of the light presentation averaged over a number of birds. OR: orienting response and indicates the averaged response to 10 light presentations without accompanying foot-shock; SR: sensitization response and indicates the averaged response to 10 light presentations with randomly occurring foot-shocks; CR: conditioned response and indicates the averaged response to 10 light presentations systematically paired with foot-shock; CR: conditioned response of a group in which orienting and sensitization responses were previously habituated, and the curve indicates the averaged response to 10 light presentations systematically paired with foot-shock. BPM: beats/min.

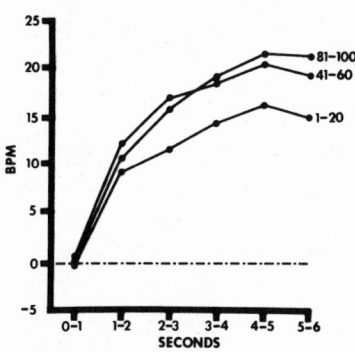

FIG. 3. Illustration of normal response dynamics at various points of training for a group of approximately 200 birds. The curves indicate mean heart rate changes from baseline for each succeeding 1-second interval of the conditioned stimulus presentation, and they show the response dynamics for trial blocks 1–20, 41–60 and 81–100. Note that stable responding occurs in block 1–20 and near-asymptotic performance in block 41–60. BPM: beats/min.

In any case, after these initial 10 training trials, stable and totally un-confounded conditioned responses occur. These are well established by 20 pairings and near-asymptotic by 40–60 (Fig. 3). This conditioned response is a monotonic cardioacceleration with approximately 1.5 second latency and maximal values in the 5th or 6th seconds of the conditioned stimulus period.

As frequently reported in the mammalian literature, the magnitudes of heart rate increases are partially dependent upon baseline rates. We have observed that, within a given bird, trial-to-trial variations in baseline rates are negatively correlated with conditioned response magnitudes (Cohen, 1967; Cohen and Durkovic, 1966; Cohen and Pitts, 1968). Since this inverse relationship is dependent upon the integrity of the vagus nerve (Cohen and Pitts, 1968), in all likelihood it reflects a vagally mediated rate-limiting reflex. However, this baseline dependency has not created analytic problems, since we rarely observe statistically significant baseline trends over the course of training.

2.3. The "Primary" Conditioned Heart Rate Response

Another concern in analyzing the behavioral system regards possible interactions between the heart rate response and concomitantly developing conditioned responses. In any conditioning paradigm, the conditioned stimulus generally elicits an integrated response pattern, and in our model heart rate change is but one component of an organized response ensemble (Cohen, 1969; Cohen and Macdonald, 1974). Certain accompanying responses, such as changes in respiration and arterial blood pressure, may evoke afferent neural activity which feeds back to modify the heart rate response dynamics. This has been of concern in the heart rate conditioning literature for a number of years and has recently been treated at length specifically with respect to our model system (Cohen, 1974a). The critical point is that experimental analysis of such interactions is feasible in this system, and in principle it allows description of the "primary" conditioned heart rate response (Cohen, 1969), that is, the heart rate response free of interactions with concomitantly occurring conditioned responses.

2.4. Variables Affecting the Conditioned Response

Another point concerns the parametric description of variables affecting the rate of development, asymptotic level, and dynamics of the conditioned response. Aside from the value of such studies in generally clarifying factors controlling the response, they are of immense importance with respect to cellular neurophysiological investigations. Microelectrode experiments frequently place restraints upon the specific behavioral paradigm employed, and certain features of a standardized paradigm may require modification to conform to these demands. The concern is that such modifications may alter the conditioned response, and at the extreme may seriously retard or even preclude its development. An obvious illustration is a microelectrode study in which it is extremely difficult to maintain well-isolated single-unit recordings for a period sufficient to establish stable conditioned responses. To overcome this difficulty one might choose to shorten the intertrial interval. However, such a modification could entail some risk without *a priori* information concerning the minimal interval that is free of serious trial massing effects.

For this reason we have maintained a continuing program to explore systematically the effects of parametrically varying the features of our training procedure that might require modification during cellular neurophysiological experiments. For example, this has included investigations of such variables as intertial interval, stereotaxic fixation, and number of pre-exposures to conditioned and unconditioned stimuli (e.g., Cohen and Macdonald, 1971). While in a sense such information is a luxury, it does significantly increase the probability of effective and interpretable cellular studies during conditioning.

2.5. Effective Components of the Conditioned and Unconditioned Stimuli

The final line of behavioral research deals with identifying the specific stimulus components that are most effective in controlling the conditioned response, and it involves the following kinds of questions: What features of the conditioned stimulus are most effective: its onset, termination, duration, total flux, etc.? Does the effectiveness of the various components change over training? At any point in training, do specific stimulus components control specific response components, such that the overall input–output relation can be behaviorally dissected into a set of stimulus–response relations where, for example, stimulus onset may largely control shorter latency response components while total flux may control response magnitude? These are intriguing kinds of questions we are just beginning to broach, and they have important ramifications for analysis of central mechanisms.

In summary, the behavioral phase of our program is itself rather extensive. It consists of (1) detailed specification of the response dynamics in a standardized paradigm, (2) description of these dynamics free of possible interactions with concomitantly developing conditioned responses, (3) determination of the major training variables affecting the conditioned response, and (4) specification of the effective stimulus components. It is important to recognize that the greater the depth of behavioral understanding of the model, the more detailed and rigorous subsequent interpretation of cellular neurophysiological findings. Conversely, information derived from the study of central mechanisms facilitates detailed behavioral investigation.

3. Strategy for Identifying the Relevant Central Pathways

3.1 Introduction

As indicated earlier, the focus of this chapter is upon delineation of the neural pathways mediating conditioned response development in our model system. The availability of a detailed map of the "conditioning pathways" is one of the most essential criteria an effective system must satisfy. Consequently, specifying these pathways has constituted a major phase of our experimental effort, and as discussion develops it will hopefully become evident that this undertaking yields more than merely localization information.

Unfortunately, there have been virtually no systematic attempts to describe the pathways mediating conditioned cardiovascular change. In fact, there have been few efforts to map comprehensively the pathways mediating any learned behavior in vertebrates. More frequently, the inclination has been to focus on a given structure, such as hippocampus or septum, and to manipulate the behavioral task as an approach to elucidating functions of a particular structure. However, even within this context, efforts to specify cell groups and fiber tracts involved in autonomic conditioning have been minimal. For example, with respect to cardio-vascular conditioning most relevant investigations have been concerned with assessing the relative roles of the extrinsic cardiac nerves (recently reviewed by Cohen [1974a]). Studies of central structures have been sporadic and few in number, dealing primarily with possible involvement of hypothalamus, septum, or cortex (e.g., Bloch-Rojas *et al.*, 1964; DiCara *et al.*, 1970; Duncan, 1972; Gantt, 1960; Smith and Nathan, 1964; Smith *et al.*, 1968).

This lack of systematic mapping programs possibly reflects the presumed difficulty of such a task for vertebrate brain, an explanation that may account as well for the emphasis upon invertebrate model systems. Such a bias becomes particularly understandable if one demands more than a simple flow chart of relevant nuclei and fiber tracts and insists, appropriately, upon detailed specification of the precise number, locations, and morphological characteristics of participating neuronal elements. However, there is no reason why this cannot be sought as an ideal in a vertebrate system. Beginning with a flow chart of relevant structures as a first approximation, one could then accumulate more precise information on those specific structures for which preliminary cellular neurophysiological studies suggested involvement in information storage. For example, there is little point in demanding a precise description of the entire set of pathways at the outset, since it could well be that certain implicated cell groups participate exclusively as input or output lines without direct involvement in information storage *per se*.

3.2. General Experimental Approach

3.2.1. Some Underlying Assumptions

Before discussing our general strategy for identifying structures mediating visually conditioned heart rate change, it is important to make explicit certain major assumptions fundamental to our approach. First, a "connectional" bias for information storage processes is weakly assumed, in contrast, for instance, to a "statistical configuration" formulation (e.g., John, 1972). However, it is important to point out that our approach, despite its "connectional" bias, has the potential of evaluating this assumption and without radical alteration could conceivably be redirected for investigating a system that operates on a broader statistical basis. Second, implicit in the present arguments is the postulate that an adequate theory of neural information storage and retrieval must specify the electrophysiological events accompanying these processes. In fact, it could be argued that such electrophysiological events should be specified first, since they may well constitute the stimulus for structural modifications mediating long-term storage. This is not meant to imply, however, that an electrophysiological description is sufficient, but only that electrophysiological events constitute a necessary component of any general formulation. Finally, it is assumed that these electrophysiological events are most effectively specified at the cellular level, clearly a corollary of our connectional assumption.

3.2.2. Subdivision of the Conditioning Pathways into Segments

Early in the development of our program it became evident that systematic mapping of the relevant pathways would require a well-defined framework to assure that analysis would proceed in an orderly manner. Consequently, we made the rather straightforward decision to begin by defining four major segments of the conditioning pathways. These consisted of (1) the visual pathways transmitting the conditioned stimulus information, (2) the somatosensory pathways transmitting the unconditioned stimulus information, (3) the descending or efferent pathways mediating expression of the conditioned response, and (4) the efferent pathways mediating the unconditioned response. (The heuristic value of this is stressed, since we are fully cognizant of the problems in defining more central structures as sensory or motor.) Our approach has been to begin at the periphery of each segment and systematically to trace them centrally. Thus, for conditioned and unconditioned stimulus pathways such analysis starts at the sensory periphery, while for efferent segments it begins with the extrinsic cardiac nerves. The assumption is that a systematic analysis from the periphery centrally along the input and output segments of the system would eventually lead to the sites of convergence of conditioned and unconditioned stimulus pathways as well as the sites of coupling between these pathways and the relevant "cardiomotor" outflow.

3.2.3. An "Algorithm" for Identifying the Relevant Pathways

Our general approach is embarrasingly straightforward and fundamentally brute force in nature. Since its specifics vary for different segments of the system, a detailed presentation is best developed during discussion of each individual segment. Consequently, only the more general features of the approach are given in this section, and they are described in an ordered series of steps for progressing systematically from the periphery centrally.

Simply stated, the initial step entails beginning peripherally at each segment with a view toward (1) determining the peripheral elements involved, and (2) demonstrating that their destruction renders the animal totally incapable of establishing any conditioned heart rate change in our training paradigm. The subsequent step is to describe the entire set of structures to which the relevant elements project, in the case of the sensory segments, or the set of projections upon the relevant structure, in the case of the motor segments. Completion of this would specify the next most central relays that are (1) postsynaptic to the relevant sensory inputs, or (2) presynaptic to the relevant motor outflow. These sets of structures must then include those belonging to the conditioning pathways, and the subsequent task is to determine which are, in fact, involved.

While in specific instances various experimental approaches may facilitate this effort by rapidly eliminating certain structures from consideration, our more general and routinely applied approach is to evaluate the effects of lesions on heart rate conditioning. Of the set of possibly relevant structures, each is individually destroyed in a group of animals which is then trained in order to assess whether such a lesion affects conditioned response development. If it affects the response dynamics in any manner, then that structure is tentatively implicated as a component of the conditioning pathways. However, as analysis progresses centrally it becomes increasingly unlikely that destroying any single cell group or fiber tract will result in a total inability to develop conditioned heart rate change. Consequently, after evaluating the effects of eliminating each individual structure, it is then necessary to determine a combination of lesions that totally precludes conditioned heart rate change. This is demanded if one is to identify the conditioning pathways in their entirety.

The above steps constitute our general approach to identifying the relevant pathways, and its systematic application entails their continued iteration. It should be recognized, however, that this general approach serves primarily as a guideline, and in no sense would we argue that it necessarily represents the optimal strategy. Rather, it is an approach that has evolved over development of the program, and the data generated provide some testimonial to its potential effectiveness. The sections to follow will provide more detailed illustration of its application through what is essentially a progress report of our efforts to map input and output segments of our system.

4.   Pathways Transmitting the Conditioned Stimulus Information

The analysis of visual pathways transmitting the conditioned stimulus information holds particular interest, since, given identification of relevant cell groups and fiber tracts, one may investigate the activity of successively more central neuronal elements until cells are located whose discharge characteristics are modified as a function of training. In principal, this would allow identification of the most peripheral synaptic fields along these pathways that participate in information storage, and as a corollary it would permit determination of whether classically defined sensory pathways participate in information storage or function primarily as input lines.

4.1. Definition of the Conditioned Stimulus

As a prelude to describing the conditioned stimulus pathways, a brief characterization of the conditioned stimulus is in order. As indicated earlier, this stimulus consists of a 6-second pulse of whole-field illumination. The rationale for this choice is that in a classical conditioning paradigm one cannot easily control the specific stimulus features to which the animal responds. Consequently, we have attempted to eliminate or hold constant as many stimulus parameters as possible to minimize the complexity of the conditioned stimulus and thereby facilitate specification of its effective components. Perhaps use of a monochromatic source restricted to a few degrees of visual angle would be even more efficient, and we have considered exploring this alternative in future experiments.

Regarding stimulus presentation, for preliminary assessment of lesion effects involving large samples of animals the presentation has been rather crude and consists of panel-mounted tungsten lamps projecting through a diffuser (e.g., Cohen and Durkovic, 1966). However, for higher-resolution behavioral experiments and for all electrophysiological studies the conditioned stimulus is delivered monocularly by means of an optical system which focuses a light of calibrated intensity upon the retina (e.g., Cohen *et al.*, 1972; Duff and Cohen, in prep. a). This consists of a quartz–iodide source, lens and diaphragm system, calibrated neutral density filters, and an electromagnetic shutter for controlling stimulus duration. The animal's head is rigidly fixed, the pupil dilated with topically administered d-tubocurarine chloride and benzalkonium chloride (Campbell and Smith, 1962), and the cornea fitted with a translucent contact lens of known transmission. This system allows considerable precision in visual stimulus presentation, its major limitation being the inability to control stimulus rise- and fall-times independent of spectral shifts. This is of little concern in most experiments, since only square light pulses are delivered. However, it is a drawback for studies of effective stimulus components, and we have recently overcome it by use of an optoelectronic system employing a PLZT ceramic wafer with a conventional quadratic (Kerr) electro-optic effect. In conjunction with crossed polarizers this system acts as an electro-optic variable density filter, since the birefringence of the wafer, and thus the transmission of the system, is a function of the voltage applied to the ceramic element.

With respect to stimulus intensity, a parametric study of this variable (Cohen, 1974b) indicated that conditioning performance is affected only at relatively high stimulus values, and that these effects are produced by increased sensitization rather than changes in conditioning *per se*. Based on such data we have determined that a stimulus value of approximately 100 ft-L appears optimal from both behavioral and electrophysiological viewpoints. It restricts sensitization to minimal levels (Cohen, 1974b), and yet it is sufficiently intense to activate approximately 95% of the retinal ganglion cells (Duff and Cohen, in prep. a).

4.2. Retinal Output

An important question regarding the visual pathways concerns the quantitative characteristics of retinal ganglion cell responses to the conditioned stimulus, since these define the information available to more central visual structures. Thus, a series of studies was undertaken in which the responses of over 500 single optic tract fibers were characterized during changes in whole-field illumination (Cohen and Duff, in prep.; Duff and Cohen, in prep. a,b; Duff *et al.*, 1972). The pigeon optic nerve contains approximately 2.4 million axons distributed almost unimodally with a mean diameter of somewhat less than 1μ (Binggeli and Paule, 1969), and it is likely that all are myelinated (Cowan, 1970; Duff and Cohen, in prep. a; O'Flaherty, 1971). However, despite the fiber diameter and small size of our sample relative to the total optic nerve population, we have firm reason to believe that the behavior of this sample accurately reflects the spectrum of retinal responses to whole-field illumination (Duff and Cohen, in prep. a Duff *et al.*, in prep.).

To summarize the major findings, most, if not all, retinal ganglion cells in the pigeon respond to increases in whole-field illumination, consistent with recent receptive field descriptions of avian retinal ganglion cells (Holden, 1969; Miles, 1972). At stimulus onset these neurons discharge a burst of spikes whose latency and number are linearly related to log intensity. For example, in the unanesthetized pigeon 100% of the sampled fibers responded to onset of a 600 ft-L stimulus, this percentage falling to 95% and 82% at intensities of 100 and 10 ft-L, respectively. A subset of these neurons also responded with similar latencies but fewer spikes to illumination decreases, and these tended to be units responding more vigorously and at lower threshold to illumination increases. For instance, 72%, 51%, and 20% of fibers responded at termination of 600, 100, and 10 ft-L stimuli, respectively, those not responding gradually resuming their level of spontaneous activity. However, this proportion responding at stimulus termination could be altered by manipulating such stimulus parameters as intensity and duration. It is of interest that analysis of the relationship between "on" and "off" responses indicated that both the probability of occurrence and characteristics of the "off" discharge could be predicted rather reliably from the parameters of the "on" response.

While stimulus onset and termination are effective in activating the ganglion cells, their discharge generally ceases during maintained illumination. Thus, they are primarily sensitive to intensity change rather than sustained illumination, and in many respects they appear analogous to the W-cell system of cat retina (Stone and Hoffman, 1972), a finding consistent with the high ratio of amacrine:bipolar synapses in pigeon (10.8:1) (Dubin, 1970).

Two additional points concern the response variability and the relationship between single-fiber discharges and the optic nerve field potential. First, standard errors of the various response measures are encouragingly small. For example, standard errors of mean latencies to the first spike of the "on" response are 1.85, 1.34, and 1.79 msec for stimulus intensities of 600, 100, and 10 ft-L, respectively. Such low variability is a feature of the system that holds great promise for quantitative analyses of cells postsynaptic to the optic tract. Second, the optic nerve field potential can be reconstructed in detail from single-fiber data. For example, poststimulus

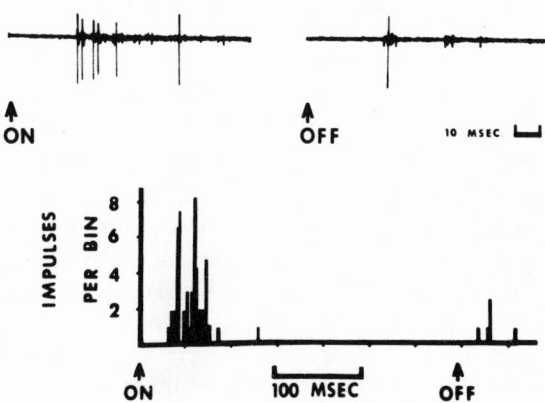

FIG. 4. Illustration of the prototypical response of an optic tract fiber to whole-field illumination (600 ft-L). The upper part of the figure shows the responses at stimulus onset and termination for a single presentation. The lower part of the figure shows a post-stimulus time histogram for 20 stimulus presentations.

time histograms from only 15 randomly selected fibers accurately reflects the field potential. This has the extremely important implication that retinal output in response to the conditioned stimulus can, for many purposes, be reasonably approximated with field potential data, obviating the need for tedious single-fiber experiments.

In summary, the retinal output in this system seems remarkably homogeneous. The prototypical single unit response consists of a short spike-train at stimulus onset, cessation of discharge during sustained illumination, and a short burst at stimulus termination (Fig. 4). Furthermore, the quantitative characteristics of these responses are highly predictable and unimodally distributed. Thus, the absence of evidence that ganglion cells distribute into distinct classes with respect to their responses to whole-field illumination, the extremely low response variability of individual fibers, and the accurate reflection of single-fiber activity by the field potential should all facilitate studies of retinal output during conditioning, as well as quantitative analyses of neurons postsynaptic to the optic tract.

4.3. Relevant Central Visual Structures

Given quantitative characterization of the retinal output in response to changes in whole-field illumination (conditioned stimulus), one might next ask whether complete elimination of this output would totally preclude conditioning. Despite its seeming triviality, sporadic reports of nonretinal photoreceptor mediation of visual learning justifies pursuit of this question. In any case, bilateral enucleation experiments have clearly excluded this possibility (Cohen, in prep. c).

4.3.1. Terminal Fields of Retinal Projections

Once the retinal output has been characterized and the necessity of retinal integrity established, the next goal is to explore each structure receiving a retinal projection for possible involvement in transmitting the conditioned stimulus information. The foundation for this is a precise description of the cell groups immediately postsynaptic to the retina, and such information is available from studies employing silver (Cowan *et al.,* 1961; Hirschberger, 1971; Wall *et al.,* in prep.) and autoradiographic (Wall *et al.,* in prep.) methods. While the details of these results need not be reviewed here, it may be generally stated that the distribution of avian retinal projections is strikingly similar to those of mammalian forms (Cohen and Karten, 1974), and it is summarized in highly schematic form in Fig. 5. Briefly, primary retinal projections terminate contralaterally in the anterior

RETINAL PROJECTIONS

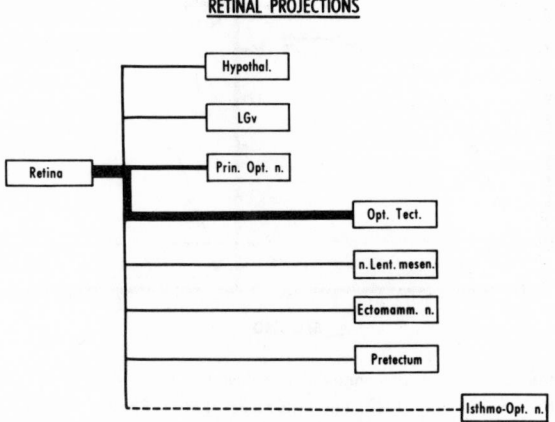

FIG. 5.   A highly schematic illustration of primary retinal projections in the pigeon. Broader lines indicate relatively denser projections, and the broken line indicates a possible, but not established, projection. Ectomamm. n.: ectomammillary nucleus, Hypothal.: hypothalamus, Isthmo-Opt. n.: isthmo-optic nucleus, LGv: ventral geniculate nucleus, n. Lent. mesen.: mesencephalic lentiform nuclei, Opt. Tect.: optic tectum, Prin. Opt. n.: principal optic nucleus of the thalamus.

dorsolateral thalamic complex; this has been denoted as the principal optic nucleus of the thalamus and may well be homologous to the mammalian dorsal lateral geniculate (Karten *et al.*, 1973). The retina also projects contralaterally upon the ventral geniculate nucleus, a complex of small hypothalamic cell groups including nucleus suprachiasmaticus, the posterodorsal pretectal nucleus, the area pretectalis, the ectomammillary nucleus, the mesencephalic lentiform nuclei, and possibly the isthmo-optic nucleus. However, by far the most extensive projection is upon the contralateral optic tectum (superior colliculus) with terminal fields of retinotectal axons being confined primarily to the upper seven tectal laminae.

Establishing the precise boundaries of cell groups receiving primary retinal projections then allows experiments in which each is individually destroyed and the effects on conditioning performance evaluated. In these experiments we bilaterally destroy a given projection region with stereotaxically (Karten and Hodos, 1967) guided electrolytic lesions, generally in a group of 15–25 animals. Following a postoperative recovery period, our standardized conditioning paradigm is applied, and the performance of these birds is compared with that of appropriate control animals.

While this experimental series is still ongoing, analyses of the principal optic nucleus, pretectal region, ectomammillary nucleus, mesencephalic lentiform nuclei, and isthmo-optic nucleus have been completed with no in-

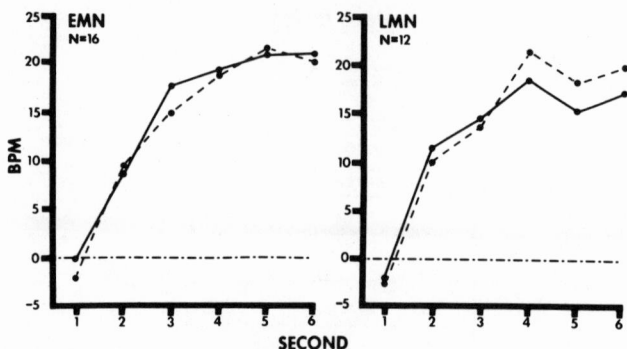

FIG. 6. Illustration of the lack of conditioning deficit following lesions of either the ectomammillary nuclei (EMN) or mesencephalic lentiform nuclei (LMN). Shown are the response dynamics averaged over trials 41–60, the trial block where near-asymptotic performance is reached (see Fig. 3). Solid lines indicate performance of control animals, and broken lines the performance of lesioned animals. BPM: beats/min.

dication of any conditioning deficits. Figure 6 illustrates this by showing response dynamics for two experimental groups during a trial block shortly after attainment of asymptotic performance. Investigations of the remaining terminal fields have not yet progressed sufficiently to permit evaluation, and for reasons that will become evident we have not assessed the effects of bilateral tectal lesions.

The absence of conditioning deficits with destruction of individual structures postsynaptic to the optic tract is perhaps what one should anticipate with whole-field illumination. Most, if not all, cell groups receiving primary retinal projections are capable of responding to such a stimulus, and this provides an opportunity for considerable parallel processing in the transmission of intensity information. In fact, it is unlikely that interruption of any single visual pathway would yield a marked deficit, much less a total inability to establish conditioned heart rate change. As will be discussed shortly, interruption of multiple visual pathways is required to obtain such performance deficits. However, unambiguous interpretation of results from combined lesion experiments relies on a preliminary survey of the effects of individually destroying each cell group, and this has constituted our motivation for pursuing the above experiments on primary retinal projection areas.

4.3.2. Major Ascending Visual Pathways

Concomitant with this survey of optic tract terminal fields, an extended series of studies was undertaken to evaluate the possible involvement of the various central visual pathways. A number of such pathways are well recognized in mammalian brain, and most are undoubtedly capable of transmitting information regarding changes in whole-field illumination. However, since severe deficits in a variety of visual learning tasks have been frequently reported in mammals following interruption of visual pathways ascending to cortex, we arbitrarily chose to initiate our investigations with studies of homologous visual projections to avian telencephalon.

In recent years substantial anatomical, behavioral, and physiological data have accumulated which characterize two such projection systems, the thalamofugal and tectofugal visual pathways. These data further suggest that the thalamofugal and tectofugal pathways of avian brain are homologous, respectively, to the mammalian geniculo-striate and tecto-LP-extrastriate systems. More detailed discussion of these systems and their relationship to mammalian pathways may be found in review articles by Karten (1969), Nauta and Karten (1970), and Cohen and Karten (1974), and they are schematically illustrated in Fig. 7. Briefly, the thalamofugal system consists of a crossed projection to the principal optic nucleus of the thalamus which in the pigeon is composed of several nuclear clusters. Efferents of this nucleus then project upon the telencephalon, terminating most prominently in the granule cell layer of intercalatus hyperstriatum accessorium. This hyperstriate field has been designated the visual Wulst (Karten *et al.*, 1973), and it might also be noted that a smaller number of axons reach homotopic regions of contralateral visual Wulst via the dorsal supraoptic decussation. The tectofugal system consists of a crossed retino-tectal projection, one or more tectal interneurons, and a massive tectal projection through the brachium of the colliculus upon the ipsilateral nucleus

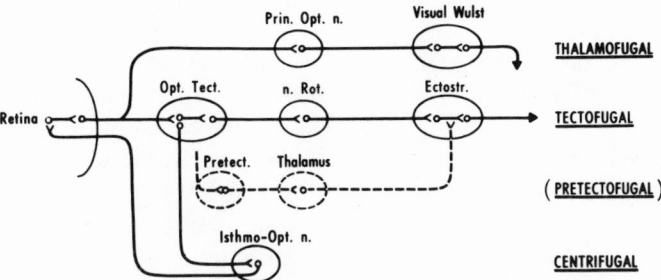

FIG. 7. A stylized illustration of the major ascending visual pathways in the bird, as well as the centrifugal system to the retina. Broken lines showing the pretectofugal pathway indicate its speculative nature. Ectostr.: ectostriatum, Isthmo-Opt. n.: isthmo-optic nucleus, n. Rot.: nucleus rotundus, Opt. Tect.: optic tectum, Pretect.: pretectal region, Prin. Opt. n.: principal optic nucleus of the thalamus.

rotundus of the thalamus. Nucleus rotundus then projects upon a distinct cell mass of the ipsilateral telencephalon, the ectostriatum.

Our initial question regarding these ascending visual pathways was whether interrupting either alone would affect heart rate conditioning. With respect to the thalamofugal system, destruction of its telencephalic (visual Wulst) or thalamic (principal optic nucleus) components does not impair conditioned response development (Fig. 8) (Cohen, 1967; Cohen, in prep. c). Concerning the tectofugal system, destruction of its telencephalic component (ectostriatum) has no effect (Fig. 8), while lesions of its thalamic component (nucleus rotundus) produce only small deficits possibly attributable to peri-rotundal damage (Cohen and Trauner, 1969). These early experiments thus suggested that either thalamofugal and tectofugal pathways do not participate in transmitting the conditioned stimulus information, or a parallel pathway phenomenon occurs. That is, both ascending visual pathways may be capable of transmitting the relevant information, and interruption of either alone leaves an alternate route intact.

In view of this, an electrophysiological study was undertaken to determine whether these ascending systems are even capable of responding to changes in whole-field illumination, since, given the above lesion results, absence of appropriate evoked responses would imply lack of involvement rather than parallel processing. However, microelectrode field potential and single-unit analyses clearly indicated that the telencephalic fields of both thalamofugal and tectofugal systems show highly localized potentials of appropriate latencies in response to increases in whole-field illumination (Cohen and Dooley, in prep.). For example, the visually responsive area of the Wulst is confined primarily to the granule cell layer in a region bounded by anterior 11.75–13.50 and lateral 1.5–3.0 in the stereotaxic coordinate system of Karten and Hodos (1967). Furthermore, field potential analyses indicated preferential responsiveness of both visual Wulst and ectostriatum to onset of illumination, with little activity during sustained illumination or at stimulus termination. Single-unit results generally supported these findings; for example, of 113 (of 315) ectostriatal units responsive to whole-field illumination only 11 responded at stimulus termination.

In any case, details of these electrophysiological results are not of importance here, the principal point being that both the thalamofugal and tectofugal systems are capable of responding to at least some component of the conditioned stimulus. This motivated a return to lesion experiments directed toward evaluating the effects of combined interruption of thalamofugal and tectofugal pathways. The initial study included two experimental groups, one in which both visual Wulst and ectostriatum were ablated and a second in which principal optic nucleus and nucleus rotundus were destroyed (see Fig. 7). Though not fully analyzed, the results suggest

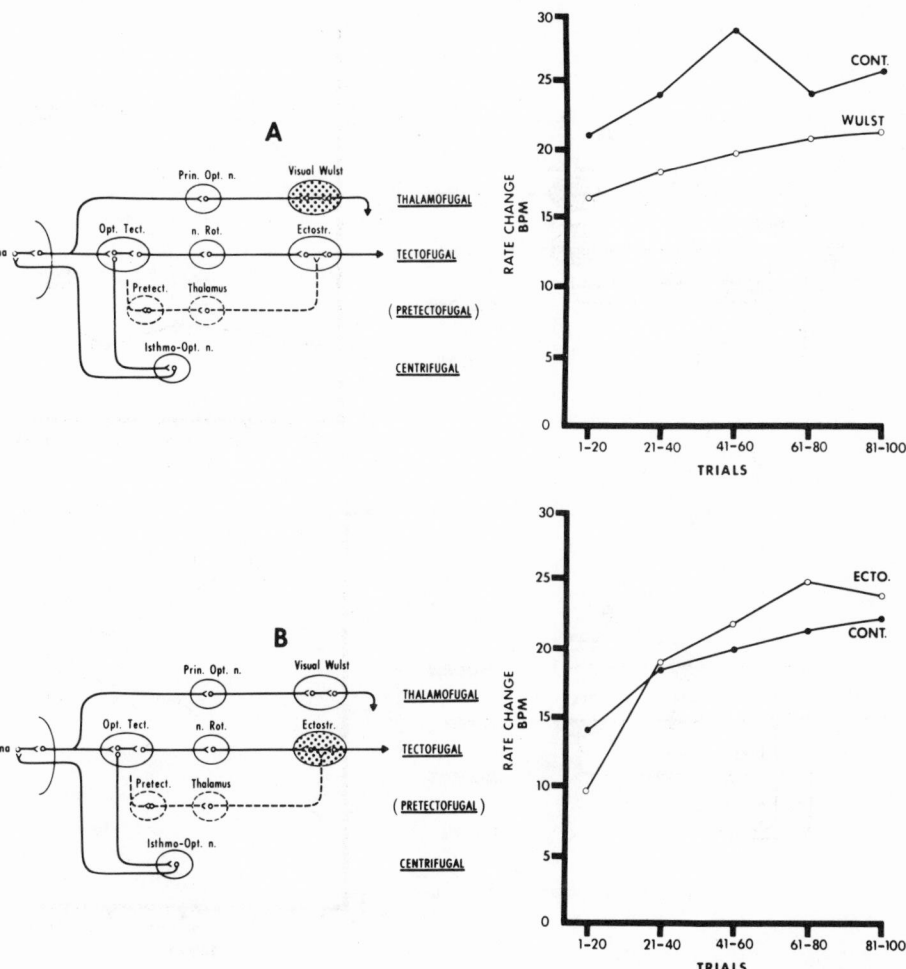

FIG. 8.   Illustration of the effects of interrupting the thalamofugal and tectofugal pathways individually at the telencephalic level by destroying the visual Wulst (Panel A) or ectostriatum (Panel B). The left part of each panel repeats Fig. 7 with the lesioned area stippled. The curves represent mean heart rate changes between conditioned stimulus and preceding control periods. Each point represents a group mean for a block of 20 training trials. CONT.: control curves, ECTO.: ectostriatal lesion group, WULST: visual Wulst lesion group, BPM: beats/min. [Adapted from Cohen (1967) and Cohen and Trauner (1969)].

quite severe, and possibly total, deficits following the combined telencephalic lesion (Fig. 9A) (Cohen, in prep. c). A puzzling finding, however, was that deficits consequent to destruction of the thalamic relay nuclei were only transient, with near-normal responding by the final training block (Fig. 9B).

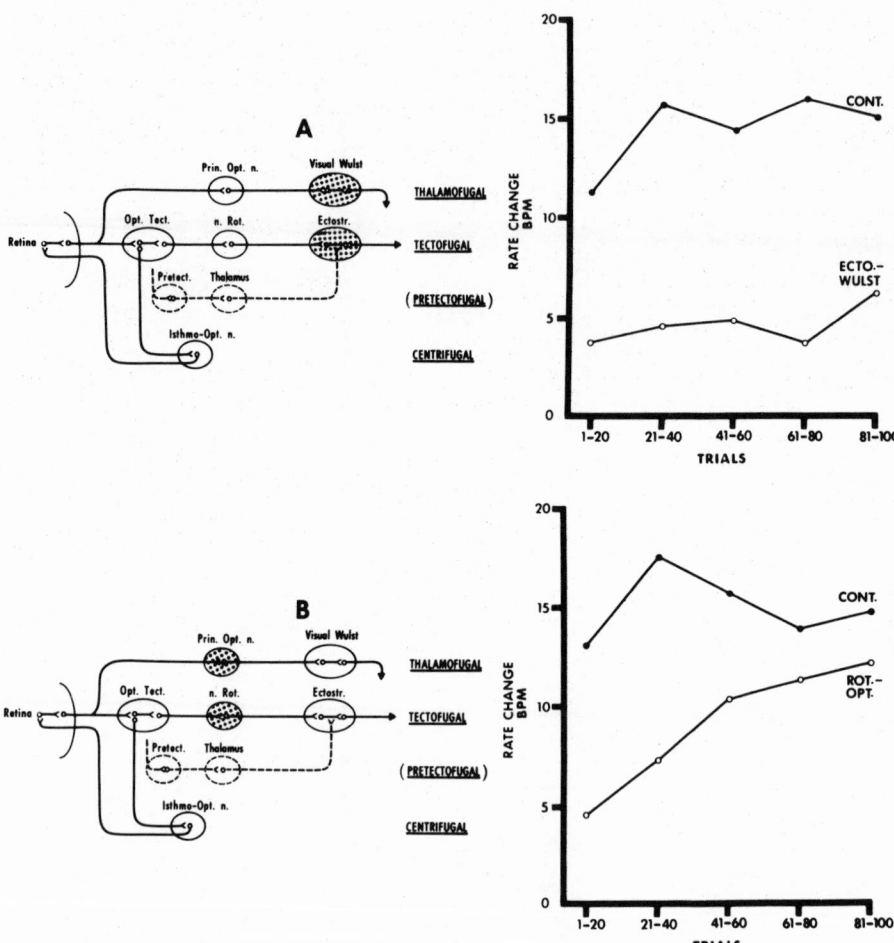

FIG. 9. Illustration of the effects of combined interruption of thalamofugal and tectofugal pathways at telencephalic (Panel A) or thalamic (Panel B) levels. The upper part of each panel repeats Fig. 7 with the lesioned areas stippled. The curves represent mean heart rate changes between conditioned stimulus and preceding control periods. Each point represents a group mean for a block of 20 training trials. CONT.: control curves, ECTO.–WULST: combined ectostriatal and visual Wulst lesion group, ROT–OPT.: combined nucleus rotundus and principal optic nucleus lesion group, BPM: beats/min.

There are two provocative features of these findings. First, deficits following combined destruction of visual Wulst and ectostriatum are sufficiently severe to raise the possibility that *complete* destruction of these regions could effectively produce a *total* conditioning loss. The results illustrated in Fig. 9 are from animals with quite extensive, but not necessarily complete, destruction of these cellular masses, and thus, the possibility of a total loss can be seriously entertained. (It might be noted that a total deficit does not necessarily require *zero* response levels, since, for example, residual response levels could reflect sensitization or the presence of minimal nonvisual cues.) If, however, the deficit is complete, it might imply that transmission of the conditioned stimulus information in our system is mediated entirely by ascending visual pathways with telencephalic terminations in visual Wulst and ectostriatum. It is of interest in this regard that Hodos *et al.* (1973) obtained severe deficits in visual discrimination in pigeons with combined thalamofugal and tectofugal interruption, considerably more severe than found with lesions of either system alone. Moreover, in the shark destruction of a well-circumscribed telencephalic visual area (Cohen *et al.*, 1973) results in complete loss and an inability to relearn a black–white discrimination (Graeber *et al.*, 1972).

A second provocative feature of this combined lesion study is the less severe deficit following thalamic, as opposed to telencephalic, interruption of thalamofugal and tectofugal systems. While it is possible that this discrepancy could be accounted for by lesion extent, an alternative is that there exists another source of visual input to the telencephalon, terminating in either visual Wulst or ectostriatum. Various lines of indirect evidence suggest the latter and, specifically, that another source of visual input converges with the tectofugal pathway upon ectostriatum. This evidence is briefly: (1) certain components of the ectostriatal field-potential response to whole-field illumination are unaffected by destruction of either nucleus rotundus or visual Wulst (Cohen and Dooley, in preparation); (2) a substantially higher percentage of ectostriatal neurons can be activated by natural visual stimulation (Cohen and Dooley, in prep.; Revzin, 1970) than by electrical stimulation of nucleus rotundus (Revzin and Karten, 1967); (3) rotundal neurons characteristically have wide receptive fields (Revzin, 1970), while ectostriatum contains both wide- and narrow-field units (Kimberly *et al.*, 1971). These findings coupled with our lesion results are not definitive but do suggest an unidentified source of visual input to ectostriatum. While there is no direct evidence indicating the nature of this pathway, the generally striking parallel between mammalian and avian visual systems prompts the hypothesis that it may be of pretectal origin, given accumulating evidence for such a pathway in mammals (e.g., Graybiel, 1972). This possibility is speculatively schematized in Fig. 7.

If correct, this hypothesis would imply that combined destruction of principal optic nucleus, nucleus rotundus, *and* the pretectal terminal fields of the optic tract should produce conditioning deficits equivalent to those following combined destruction of visual Wulst and ectostriatum. Preliminary findings from such an experimental group are shown in Fig.

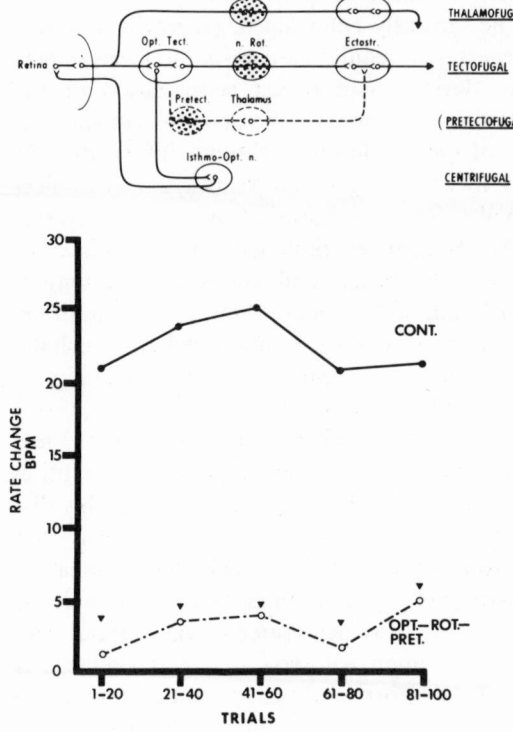

FIG. 10. Illustration of the effects of combined interruption of the principal optic nucleus, nucleus rotundus, and the pretectal terminal field of the optic tract. The upper part of the figure repeats Fig. 7 with the lesioned areas stippled. The curves represent mean heart rate changes between conditioned stimulus and preceding control periods. Each point represents a group mean for a block of 20 training trials. CONT.: control curve; OPT–ROT.–PRET.: lesion group. The solid inverted triangles indicate response levels of birds with a combined ectostriatal and visual Wulst lesion and repeat the lesion group in Figure 9a. BPM: beats/min.

10, and they are remarkably comparable to those of the combined telencephalic lesion (Fig. 9A). This makes us more sanguine about the telencephalic deficit and suggests that visual Wulst and ectostriatum are necessary structures for transmitting the conditioned stimulus information in our system. Furthermore, the hypothesis of involvement of a pretectofugal pathway is strengthened, but by no means definitive. Before such a pathway can be seriously considered further it is essential to demonstrate its existence in avian brain, and we are presently conducting anatomical and electrophysiological studies to assess this possibility.

4.4. Conclusions

To summarize our knowledge regarding the visual pathways transmitting the conditioned stimulus information, we have established that nonretinal photoreceptors do not participate and have characterized in some detail the ganglion cell responses to whole-field illumination. The terminal fields of the retinal projections have been described, and an ongoing survey of the effects of individually destroying each of these fields has yet to demonstrate any conditioning deficit. Similarly, interrupting either thalamofugal or tectofugal visual pathways independently yields no substantial deficits, although both are capable of responding to changes in whole-field illumination. In contrast, combined destruction of the telencephalic terminal fields of these pathways results in severe, and possibly total, deficits. (We would emphasize, however, that this result does not imply the impossibility of establishing some conditioned heart rate change with either prolonged training or modification of the paradigm. The critical point is that in our standardized paradigm near-total loss obtains for at least twice the number of trials required for asymptotic performance in the intact animal. Since we are interested in the pathways normally mediating response development in our specific paradigm, we have not pursued aggressive training regimes to determine if such responses could be forced to occur.)

In view of findings to date, our working hypothesis is that a set of visual pathways ascending to the telencephalon and terminating upon visual Wulst and ectostriatum are necessary and possibly sufficient to transmit the conditioned stimulus information in our system. Moreover, involvement of the thalamofugal pathway appears established, as well as involvement of one or more pathways terminating upon ectostriatum. The immediate task, then, is to determine the relevant pathways to ectostriatum, since this would give a rather complete outline of the conditioned stimulus pathways from retina to telencephalon and would establish a foundation for electrophysiological study of these pathways during conditioning.

5.   Pathways Transmitting the Unconditioned Stimulus Information

5.1.   Introduction

In contrast to other segments of the system we have devoted considerably less effort to delineating the somatosensory pathways transmitting the unconditioned stimulus information provided by the foot-shock. This has been of less immediate interest, since characterization of the conditioned stimulus pathways has more immediate promise for identifying (1) synapses participating in information storage and (2) those synaptic regions where conditioned and unconditioned stimulus information converge. However, it is desirable that the pathways transmitting the unconditioned stimulus information be eventually described, since one can envision systems where these pathways could operate as more than mere input lines, for example, by converging on structures along the conditioned response pathways. Thus, we have pursued this problem, but with less intensity than other segments of the system.

Also in this context, a brief comment upon pathways mediating the unconditioned response is appropriate. Rather than dealing with these pathways independently, for the moment we are treating them primarily in the context of the unconditioned stimulus pathways. The rationale is that nociceptive stimulation reflexly alters cardiovascular activity via pathways at various levels of the nervous system, including at least spino–spinal, spino–bulbo–spinal and spino–ponto–spinal pathways (e.g., Koizumi and Brooks, 1972; Sato and Schmidt, 1973). Thus, there exist numerous routes by which nociceptive stimuli can gain access to structures capable of influencing heart rate, and we tentatively suggest that an effective approach to delineating these routes is through a full description of pathways transmitting the unconditioned stimulus information.

5.2   Definition of the Unconditioned Stimulus

As discussed in the section on the behavioral model, the unconditioned stimulus consists of shock to one foot. More specifically, a 60-cycle, ac current is delivered for 500 msec between a thin metal band around the metatarsal region and a needle electrode inserted in the foot pad of the same leg (Cohen and Durkovic, 1966). At current levels of 0.3–1.5 mA, the unconditioned response is invariably marked cardioacceleration of 350–450 beats/min. Neither constant current nor constant voltage are maintained; rather, stimulus current is continually adjusted to maintain the unconditioned response in this 350- to 450-beat/min range. We would hope at some point to assess the effects of unconditioned stimulus intensity and to evaluate the effects of maintaining constant current, constant voltage, or a constant unconditioned response. Further, it would be of interest to explore the effective components of the unconditioned stimulus in a manner analogous to ongoing studies of conditioned stimulus components.

5.3.   Peripheral Components of the Pathway

Consistent with our general strategy of analyzing each segment of the system from the periphery centrally, our main efforts with respect to the somatosensory pathways began with a determination of which dorsal roots are involved in transmitting the unconditioned stimulus information (Leonard and Cohen, in prep. a). In a series of straightforward experiments, heart rate responses to foot-shock were evaluated after increasingly exten- sive dorsal rhizotomies, and the unconditioned response was considered abolished if after 2 weeks no heart rate change could be elicited with stimu- lating currents up to 10 mA (a stimulus intensity at least five times that re- quired to evoke acceptable unconditioned heart rate increases in the intact bird). Based upon such data we determined that dorsal roots 21–25 [Huber's (1936) notation] must be sectioned to abolish entirely uncondi- tioned heart rate change; this corresponds to roots L1–L5. Furthermore, an independent experiment indicated that birds with dorsal rhizotomies at seg- ments 21–25 do not establish any conditioned heart rate change under our experimental conditions. Given identification of the involved dorsal roots, information provided by the studies of Huber (1936) and Kaiser (1924) then allows one to infer the relevant peripheral nerves and sensory dermatomes, and these are illustrated schematically in Fig. 11. Finally, electrophysio-

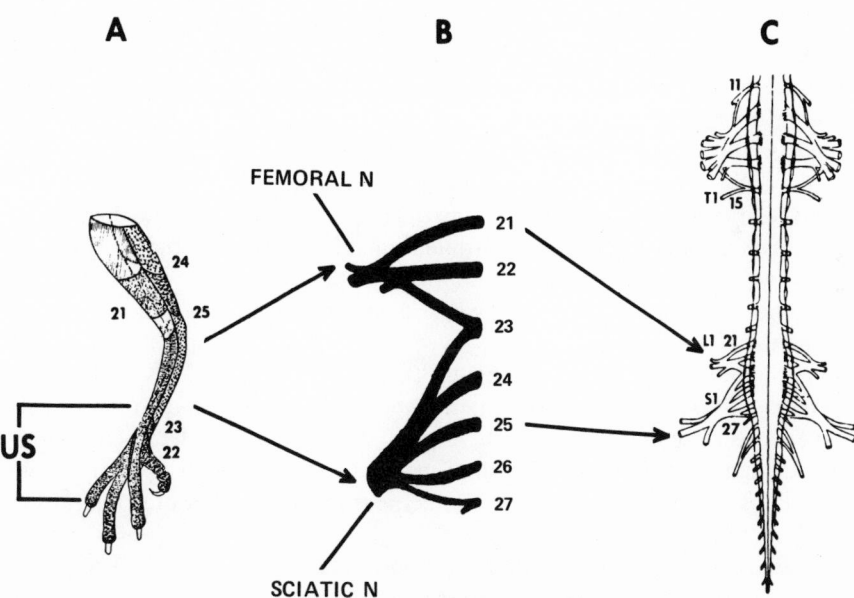

FIG. 11. Schematic illustration of the peripheral components of the unconditioned stimulus path- way. Panel A shows the sensory dermatomes, redrawn from Kaiser (1924), as well as the sites across which the foot-shock (US) is delivered. Panel B, redrawn from Huber (1936), shows an enlargement of dorsal roots 21–27 and their contributions to femoral and sciatic nerves. Both nerves transmit the unconditioned stimulus information. Panel C, redrawn from Huber (1936), schematically illustrates the pigeon spinal cord and shows that the unconditioned stimulus in- formation is transmitted over roots 21–25.

logical experiments have indicated that activation of fibers in the Aδ and C
range is specifically responsible for evoking the reflex heart rate change.

5.4.   Central Pathways

Given this specification of the peripheral components transmitting the
unconditioned stimulus information, it is next necessary to describe the
terminal distributions of the relevant dorsal root fibers, since these define
the alternative possibilities for subsequent synaptic relays. Consequently, a
cytoarchitectonic analysis of the spinal gray of the pigeon was undertaken
to establish a foundation for interpreting results of anterograde
degeneration experiments with dorsal root section. Both the cytoarchitectonic analysis and anterograde degeneration studies have now been completed (Leonard, 1972; Leonard and Cohen, in prep. b,c,d).

At this point we made the tentative working assumption that the
pathways transmitting the unconditioned stimulus information centrally
would constitute a subset of those somatosensory pathways that must be
intact for occurrence of an unconditioned heart rate response. The eventual
validity of this assumption is not critical, since for the moment it guides
one into experiments of unquestionable relevance. In any case, given this
guideline, our first consideration was whether the unconditioned stimulus
could elicit heart rate change via spino–spinal pathways, and, if so, what is
the specific circuitry involved. Consequently, we asked if reflex heart rate
responses could be evoked by stimulation of lumbar Aδ and C fibers in
birds with high spinal transection, since a positive result would indicate
existence of spino–spinal pathways contributing to the unconditioned
response. These experiments clearly demonstrated such spinally mediated
somatic-autonomic coupling, though the trauma of spinal transection demands caution in making statements about the relative magnitude of this
reflex effect (Leonard and Cohen, in prep. d). Preliminary electrophysiological evidence further confirms this finding by indicating that sciatic nerve
stimulation can activate postganglionic neurons at the level of origin of the
cardioaccelerator nerve.

Evidence for a spino–spinal contribution to the unconditioned response
then dictates investigation of the specific circuitry through which lumbar
Aδ and C fibers are able to influence sympathetic neurons controlling heart
rate. In this regard, our first important piece of information derives from
study of the terminal fields of lumbar dorsal root fibers. Specifically, we
observed no direct projections upon the sympathetic preganglionic cell
column (column of Terni), indicating that any spino–spinal pathway to
these neurons is at least disynaptic (Leonard and Cohen, in prep. b). At

present, we are conducting electrophysiological studies in which activity of single pre- and postganglionic neurons is examined during activation of Aδ and C fibers of the relevant lumbar dorsal roots. From these experiments we would hope to obtain some estimate of the number of synapses intervening between lumbar dorsal root fibers and the preganglionic cell column, and possibly to gain some information as to the locations of the relevant propriospinal neurons.

5.5 Conclusions

Our information regarding somatosensory pathways transmitting the unconditioned stimulus information is clearly limited, the most comprehensive data relating to peripheral components of the system. Following the relevant pathways centrally is obviously a tedious task, and we have begun by analyzing the various pathways by which the unconditioned stimulus information gains access to cardiac preganglionic neurons—starting with the spino–spinal circuitry. It may be evident at this point that considerable information on unconditioned response pathways should also emerge from this analysis; in fact, this partially motivated our present approach to the somatosensory segment of the system. Unfortunately, since our analysis is still confined to spinal levels, it is premature to discuss suprasegmental involvement. However, upon description of the relevant spino–spinal circuitry, our plan is to pursue systematically the spino–bulbo–spinal and spino–ponto–spinal pathways that mediate reflex heart rate change to activation of somatic afferents. We anticipate that as this line of investigation develops it would establish the requisite anatomical foundation for subsequently evaluating involvement of these various somatosensory pathways in the actual development of the conditioned response.

6. Descending Pathways Mediating the Conditioned Response

6.1. Introduction

This section describes our efforts to delineate the descending, or motor, pathways mediating expression of the conditioned response. Most properly, only the sympathetic and parasympathetic postganglionic, and perhaps preganglionic, neurons should be designated *cardiomotor*. However, tentatively considering the descending systems as motor has heuristic value and is not necessarily misleading so long as the definitional problems are recognized (Cohen and Macdonald, 1974). As with other segments of the system, our studies began at the periphery and proceeded centrally, but since this involves analysis in a *retrograde* direction a somewhat different strategy is required. Generally stated, the aim has been to delineate these pathways in a caudo-rostral direction with a view toward eventually identifying the sites at which the conditioned stimulus information gains access to the efferent segment of the system. Accomplishing this would be attractive, since it would provide a first approximation to a sequence of structures from the retina to the heart that are necessary and sufficient for conditioned response development. In addition, it would necessarily contribute to our understanding of unconditioned response pathways, since at least at caudal levels these should overlap considerably with conditioned response pathways.

6.2. The Final Common Path

6.2.1. Behavioral Characterization of Sympathetic and Vagal Contributions

Our earliest efforts to describe the efferent pathways involved specifying the final common path (Cohen, 1974a). The initial step in this analysis required evaluation of whether there are any contributions to conditioned heart rate change mediated exclusive of the extrinsic cardiac nerves; as, for instance, from conditioned increases in levels of circulating hormones having chronotropic effects. Based on experiments in which conditioning performance was evaluated following surgical and/or pharmacological elimination of the cardiac innervation, we are reasonably confident that in our system the conditioned response is mediated entirely via the extrinsic cardiac nerves and that these nerves thus constitute the exclusive final common path (Cohen, 1974a; Cohen and Pitts, 1968).

The next important issue was whether the sympathetic and/or vagal cardiac innervations contribute to the conditioned response. This, too, was approached through conditioning studies after various combinations of cardiac denervation and pharmacological blockade (Cohen and Pitts, 1968). Although there are limitations to this approach (Cohen, 1974a), it has proved useful as a preliminary estimate of relative contributions of the different sources of cardiac innervation. In brief summary (Fig. 12), these experiments clearly indicate that conditioned heart rate change includes both vagal and sympathetic components. While the shortest latency component of the response is mediated by release of vagal inhibition, increased cardiac sympathetic outflow is largely responsible for the magnitude of the rate increase. In fact, during early phases of training the vagi

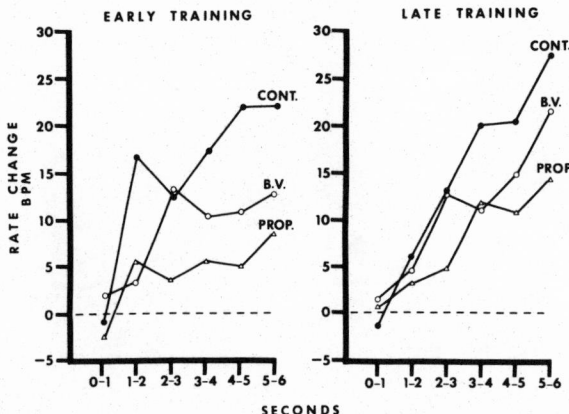

FIG. 12. Illustration of the relative sympathetic and vagal contributions to the conditioned response during early and late phases of training. Shown are mean heart rate changes from baseline for each 1-second interval of the conditioned stimulus period. For EARLY TRAINING each point represents a group mean for trials 11–20. For LATE TRAINING each point represents a group mean for trials 51–60. BPM: beats/min, CONT.: control group, B.V.: bilateral vagotomy group, PROP.: propranolol (β-blockade) group. (From Cohen and Pitts, 1968.)

seem to contribute minimally to overall response magnitude; rather, there is a rapidly developing increase in sympathetic outflow that reaches a plateau early in training and is then maintained throughout the training period. However, the small but consistent increases in response magnitude that occur after early response development appear mediated primarily by release of vagal inhibition.

Regarding the relationship between sympathetic and vagal contributions, analysis of the correlation between baseline heart rate and conditioned response magnitude suggested this relationship is not simply a synergistic one. In the intact bird there is a high negative correlation between baseline rate and response magnitude that is severely attenuated or abolished by bilateral vagotomy (Cohen and Pitts, 1968), suggesting this inverse relationship reflects a rate-limiting reflex. If this is the case, it implies that in a trained animal there are at least two competing influences on vagal cardiac neurons during a conditioned stimulus presentation: (1) inhibitory influences that decrease vagal inhibition of the heart and contribute to conditioned cardioacceleration, and (2) excitatory influences from cardiovascular reflex pathways which perform a rate-limiting function. Hypotheses of this sort, however, can derive only weakly from denervation data and are best evaluated by direct recording.

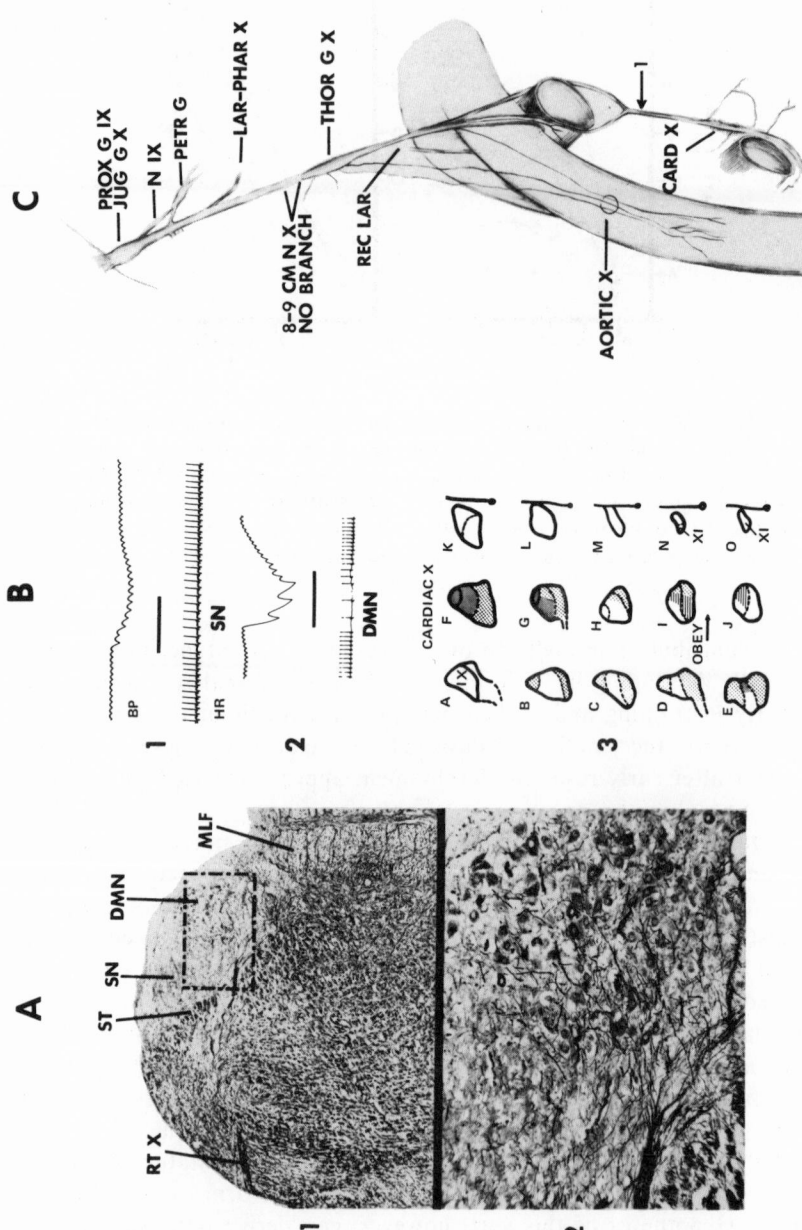

FIG. 13. Schematic illustration of the vagal component of the final common path. Panel A, adapted from Cohen *et al.* (1970), shows low (1) and higher (2) power micrographs of the dorsal motor nucleus of the pigeon. DMN: dorsal motor nucleus of the vagus, MLF: medial longitudinal fasciculus. RT X: vagal rootlets. SN: solitary nucleus. ST.: solitary tract. Panel B (1 and 2) is taken from Cohen and Schnall (1970) and illustrates the effects of stimulating the solitary nucleus (1) and the cardiac portion of the dorsal motor nucleus (2). The horizontal bars indicate stimulus durations. BP: arterial blood pressure. HR: heart rate. Part 3 of Panel B shows the distribution of chromatolytic neurons following cardiac vagotomy and is taken from Cohen *et al.* (1970). It shows a sequential series of schematic sections through the rostrocaudal extent of the dorsal motor nucleus. The cross-hatched regions indicate areas showing chromatolysis following cardiac vagotomy; only the extent and not the density of degenerating neurons is indicated. Horizontal lines indicate regions of questionable retrograde degeneration. Stippling indicates areas in which degeneration was seen in only one case. IX: nucleus of nerve IX, XI: nucleus of nerve XI. Panel C, taken from Cohen *et al.* (1970), schematically illustrates the right vagus nerve based on numerous dissections. This is a dorsal view (with the lung removed) of the right vagus from the medulla through the thoracic region. The distance from the medulla to the break in the illustration is approximately 1 cm. Not shown is 8–9 cm of cervical and upper thoracic vagus from which no branches emerge. The distance from the rostral aspect of the thoracic ganglion to the vagal branch just below the pulmonary vein is approximately 3.5 cm. The segment of the vagus nerve between arrows 1 and 2 courses over the heart, and the fiber network designated as cardiac branches overlies the right atrium in the region of the S–A and A–V nodes. AORTIC X: aortic branches of nerve X, CARD X: efferent cardiac branches of nerve X. JUG G X: jugular ganglion of nerve X. LAR-PHAR X: = laryngeal-pharyngeal branch of nerve X. N IX: nerve IX, PETR G: petrosal ganglion. PROX G IX: proximal ganglion of nerve IX. REC LAR: recurrent laryngeal nerve. THOR G X: thoracic ganglion of nerve X.

6.2.2.   Anatomical Characterization of the Final Common Path

Given that both sympathetic and vagal cardiac innervations participate, our subsequent goal was to describe the peripheral courses of these
nerves and to localize their cells of origin. With respect to the vagus, its peripheral course and the specific location of the cardioinhibitory fibers were
carefully described by combining stimulation and dissection techniques
(Cohen *et al.*, 1970) (Fig. 13). A retrograde degeneration study was then
undertaken in which various vagal branches were sectioned and the
medullary distribution of chromatolytic neurons characterized. The results
indicated a partially inverted topographic representation of the vagus on
the dorsal motor nucleus, and the cells of origin of vagal cardioinhibitory
fibers were specifically localized in the dorsal motor nucleus approximately
0.5–1.0 mm rostral to the obex (Fig. 13) (Cohen *et al.*, 1970). The greatest
density of degenerating neurons was in the more lateral aspects of the nucleus at these rostrocaudal levels, and electrical stimulation indicated that
short latency bradycardia resembling that evoked by vagal nerve
stimulation was elicited from a distribution of sites largely coincident with
the region of maximal degeneration (Cohen and Schnall, 1970). This
restricted localization of cardioinhibitory neurons has since been confirmed
in an independent stimulation study (Macdonald and Cohen, 1973).

In a parallel series of studies we identified the pre- and postganglionic
cardioaccelerator fibers and their cells of origin (Macdonald and Cohen,
1970) (Fig. 14). Based on dissection, stimulation, and retrograde degeneration experiments, preganglionic sympathetic accelerator fibers were
shown to arise from neurons in the column of Terni in spinal segments
14–16 or 17; this is a well-defined cell group just dorsal to the central
canal (Fig. 14). These preganglionic fibers then ramify in the paravertebral
chain and terminate upon postganglionic accelerator neurons in sympathetic ganglia 12–14. As they approach the heart, the postganglionic accelerator fibers anastomose into a single nerve, which is defined as the
cardiac sympathetic nerve. While in all likelihood these postganglionic
cardiac neurons constitute a unique cell population innervating only the
heart, the existence of a unique class of cardiac preganglionic neurons has
yet to be demonstrated, and is a problem we are presently exploring elec-
trophysiologically.

Thus, implication of both extrinsic cardiac nerve supplies and anatomical identification of their cells of origin provide a reasonable delineation of the final output elements of the pathway mediating the conditioned (and unconditioned) response. A basis for microelectrode investigations of the final common path is thus established, and we are presently directing our efforts toward (1) generating electrophysiological criteria for
identifying these neurons under semichronic recording conditions, and (2)

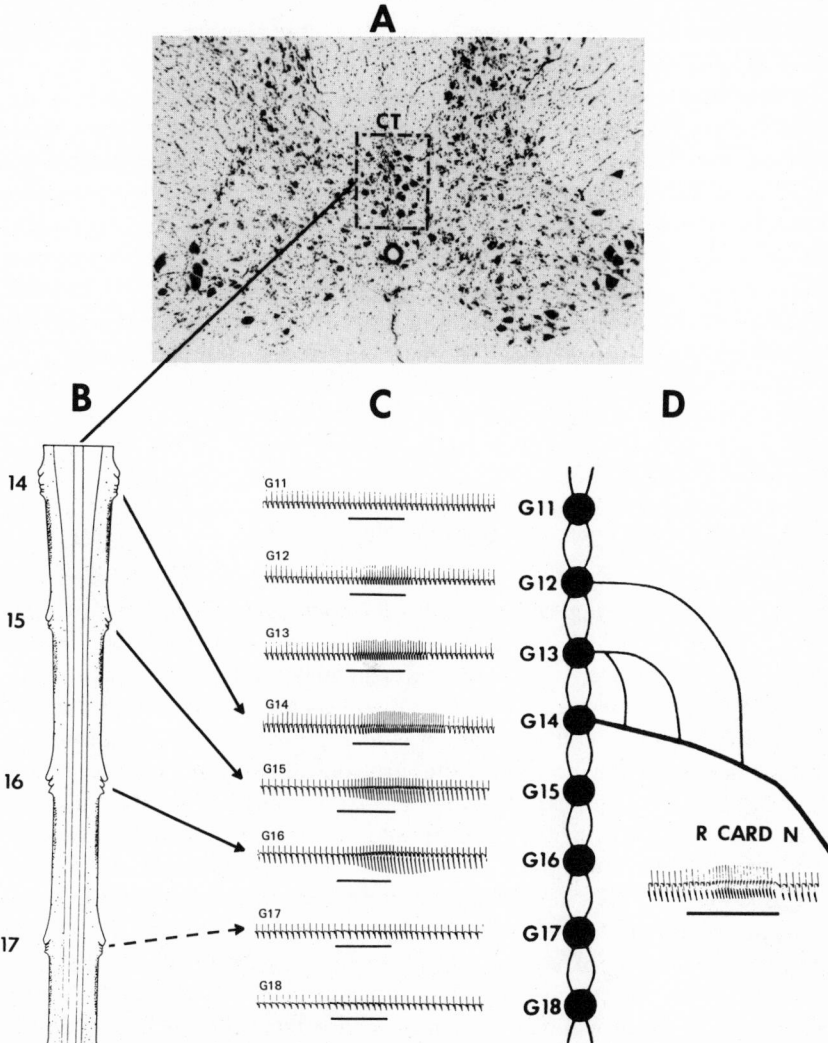

FIG. 14.   Schematic illustration of the sympathetic component of the final common path. Panel A, adapted from Macdonald and Cohen (1970), shows a photomicrograph of a transverse section through segment 15 of a normal spinal cord. The outlined group of neurons dorsal to the central canal is the sympathetic preganglionic cell group, the column of Terni (CT). Panel B, redrawn from Huber (1936), schematically illustrates a horizontal view of the pigeon spinal cord from segments 14–17. Preganglionic fibers from the column of Terni which influence heart rate are shown emerging from 14–16 and sometimes 17. Panel C, from Macdonald and Cohen (1970), shows the heart rate change following stimulation of sympathetic ganglia G11–G18. Horizontal bars indicate stimulation periods. Panel D, from Macdonald and Cohen (1970), shows schematically sympathetic ganglia 11–18 with the branches of the right cardioaccelerator nerve (R CARD N) emerging from ganglia 12–14. Also shown is the effect of stimulating the right cardioaccelerator nerve. For the implications of this figure see the discussion in the text.

describing the relationship between their discharge characteristics and conditioned heart rate change.

As a final point, it might be noted that we have available a rather complete description of the terminal distributions of vagal afferent fibers (Karten *et al.* in prep.). Anterograde degeneration experiments indicate a rather complex distribution of these fibers restricted to the solitary nucleus. Since it is thought that the glossopharyngeal nerve of the pigeon contains no cardiovascular afferents, all such fibers reaching the medulla must travel in the vagus nerve. Consequently, the above information exhaustively identifies the medullary distribution of any baro- or chemoreceptor cardiovascular afferents from cervical, thoracic, and abdominal regions.

6.3.   Central Pathways

6.3.1.   Functionally Defined Central "Cardiovascular Pathways"

Given a description of the final common path, one is confronted with the tasks of identifying central pathways converging upon preganglionic cardiac neurons and of evaluating involvement of these pathways in mediating the conditioned response. Unfortunately, methods for delineating polysynaptic pathways in a *retrograde* direction are less developed than for *orthograde* mapping. Our approach was to apply electrical stimulation as a means for exhaustively describing those regions of the avian nervous system capable of influencing heart rate and/or arterial blood pressure. With such information and existing anatomical data, one could perhaps functionally define the major descending cardiovascular pathways of avian brain (Cohen and Macdonald, 1974). This would establish the entire set of pathways that could potentially participate in mediating the conditioned response, and the specific involvement of each pathway could subsequently be assessed by evaluating conditioning performance after surgical interruption of each. While far from providing a detailed characterization of the relevant descending pathways, this approach does yield an extremely useful first approximation which can rationally guide one to higher resolution studies.

Previous electrical stimulation studies to explore central cardiovascular control in the pigeon indicated the feasibility of this approach (Cohen and Pitts, 1967; Cohen and Schnall, 1970), and thus we undertook an extensive and systematic survey of the entire central nervous system of the pigeon. Using electrodes with tips of approximately $7\,\mu$, it was possible to localize those regions, from forebrain through medulla, from which short-latency, stimulus-locked changes in heart rate and/or blood pressure could be elicited with low stimulating currents (Macdonald and Cohen,

1973). The degree of resolution in these experiments was difficult to evaluate precisely but generally seemed quite good. For example, it was not uncommon for large heart rate increases elicited by medullary stimulation to decrease from 300 to 25 beats/min as the electrode was advanced 250μ at the border of an active area.

The specific details of this study are not necessary here, and the results may be very generally summarized as follows: (1) As in mammals, a pressor–accelerator region exists in the dorsal medulla (Fig. 15C), although an analogue of the mammalian medullary depressor–decelerator area could not be demonstrated. (2) A major pressor–accelerator pathway originates in posteromedial archistriatum (amygdala) (Fig. 15A) and descends to hypothalamus via the tractus occipitomesencephalicus, pars hypothalami. (3) A second prominent pressor–accelerator pathway originates in hypothalamus (Fig. 15A,E) and descends through ventral and ventrolateral brainstem at least to caudal medullary levels (Fig. 15B,C,F,H). (4) As recently demonstrated in the cat, a striking pressor–accelerator pathway arises from the deep medial cerebellar nucleus, leaving cerebellum via the uncinate fasciculus (Fig. 15C,F). (5) Finally, no clear depressor pathway could be located, although hypotension and/or bradycardia could be elicited by stimulation of various isolated regions such as the septum (Fig. 15A) and vagal–solitary complex.

Save for the absence of a depressor–decelerator pathway, in most major respects the general organization of avian cardiovascular pathways is remarkably similar to that of mammalian brain (Cohen and Macdonald, 1974; Macdonald and Cohen, 1973). Further, considering cardiovascular response patterns and the kinds of behaviors occurring during stimulation of the various pathways, one can speculatively associate a more general function with each as has been done in the mammalian literature. For example, the pathway arising from archistriatum may be analogous to the "defense" pathway of mammalian brain, while the ventrolaterally descending pathway of hypothalamic origin and the cerebellar pressor–accelerator pathway may correspond, respectively, to "exercise" and "postural adjustment" pathways (see Cohen and Macdonald, 1974).

In any event, the above experiments have been instrumental in establishing a preliminary outline of the major descending systems capable of influencing heart rate in the pigeon. It is essential to recognize, however, that these are functionally defined systems, and a sound morphological foundation must be established for each. For example, the ventrolaterally descending pathway does not project directly to medulla but cascades caudally in a polysynaptic manner. Thus, while stimulation experiments have outlined the general course of this pathway, its specific synaptic relays are only partially known. Regardless, functional specification of the major

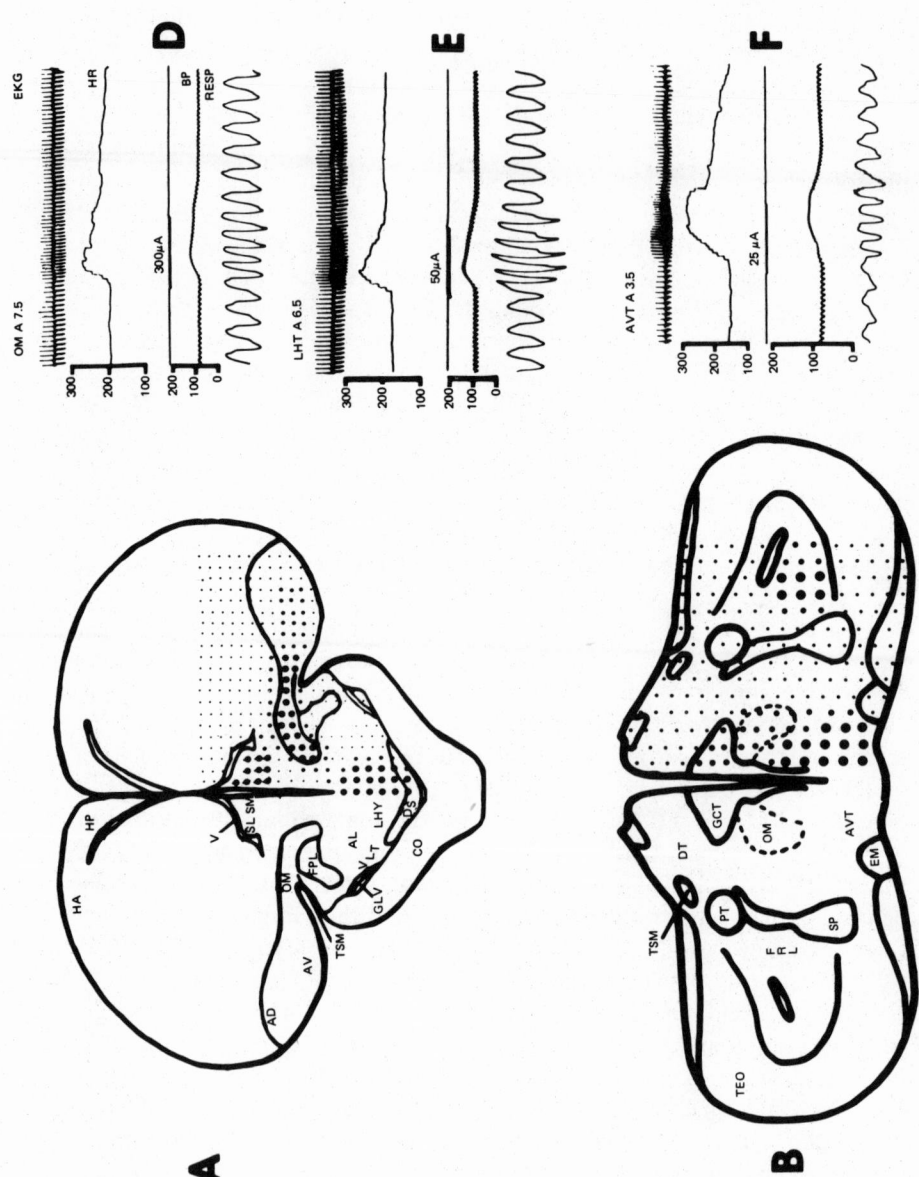

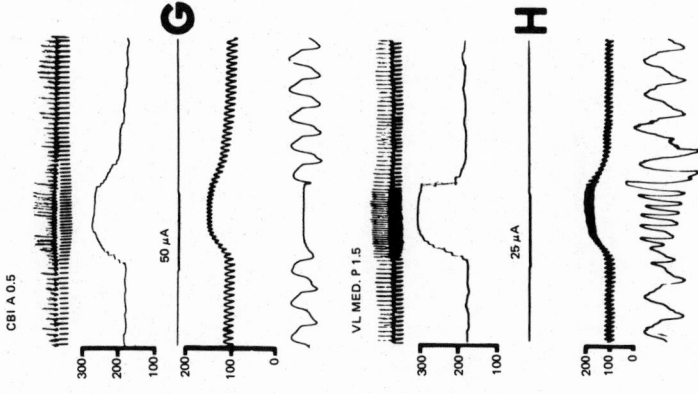

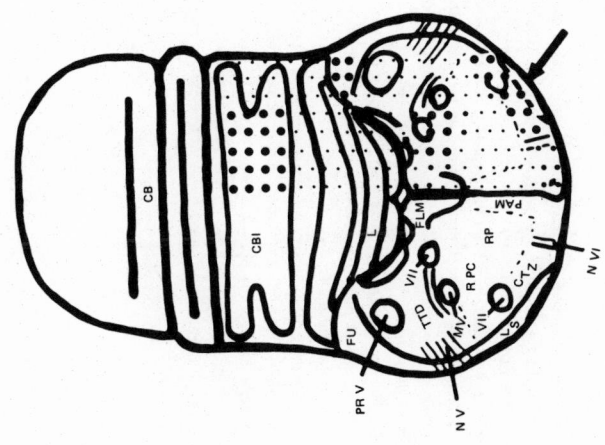

FIG 15. (caption on following page).

FIG. 15. Selective illustrations of cardioactive regions of the pigeon brain; adapted from Macdonald and Cohen (1973). On the left are three schematic tranverse sections which correspond to anterior 7.5 (panel A), anterior 4.5 (panel B), and anterior 0.5 (panel C) in the coordinate system of Karten and Hodos (1967). (Note that these are not scaled relative to each other.) Illustrated on each are indicators of representative heart rate responses elicited on dorsoventral penetrations spaced mediolaterally at approximately 0.5 mm (indicated by small, vertically aligned dots.) Symbols do not represent absolute magnitudes, but magnitudes relative to other responses elicited at the same transverse plane at a given current level. Large solid circles represent *peak* responses at that plane and medium solid circles *intermediate* responses. L indicates delayed tachycardia and small dotted lines either no response or a small response (< 25 beats/min). A key to only selected abbreviations is given, and the reader is referred to Macdonald and Cohen (1973) for a full key. AVT: ventral area of Tsai. CBI: nucleus cerebellus internus. CO: optic chiasm. DT: dorsal thalamus. FLM: medial longitudinal fasciculus. FU: uncinate fasciculus. GCT: central gray. LHY: lateral hypothalamus. N V: fifth (trigeminal) nerve. OM: occipitomesencephalic tract. SM: medial septal nucleus. TE O: optic tectum. VL MED: ventrolateral medulla.

The right side of the figure shows some representative changes in heart rate (HR), arterial blood pressure (BP), and respiration (RESP) elicited by stimulation. The signal mark is 5 seconds in duration and also indicates the stimulating current; the cardiotachograph calibration on the upper left is in beats/min, and the blood pressure calibration on the lower left is in mm Hg. Panel F shows the response elicited by stimulating the ventromedial mesencephalon, the presumed mesencephalic location of the *ventral descending pathway*. The course of this pathway in the rostral medulla may be seen in panel C (arrow), and the effects of stimulating the pathway in the caudal medulla are shown in panel H.

descending systems can at least guide preliminary behavioral investigations of the participation of each in mediating the conditioned response, and such studies can be conducted in parallel with the requisite anatomical experiments.

6.3.2.   Forebrain "Limbic" Structures Involved in Heart Rate Conditioning

Given a functional outline of the major descending systems influencing heart rate, one can then interrupt each at various rostrocaudal levels and evaluate the effects on conditioned response development. The general approach is analogous to that applied in investigating the visual segment of the system, including the eventual need to determine a combination of lesions yielding a total deficit. Such studies have, in fact, been in progress for some time, and following is a review of our findings.

First, consider the pressor–accelerator pathway arising from archistriatum (amygdala) (Fig. 15). In a study exploring this structure initially (Cohen, in prep. b), no lesion effects on conditioning were found. However, these lesions were confined primarily to the anterior two-thirds of archistriatum, and when destruction involved medial or posterior archistriatum sizable deficits followed (Fig. 16). Also included in this study was a large series of lesions interrupting the major archistriatal outflow, the occipitomesencephalic tract, at various levels from telencephalon to caudal pons. A striking finding was that interrupting this pathway at any point from archistriatum to the caudal third of hypothalamus produced severe conditioning deficits, while destruction of the tract at more caudal levels minimally affected heart rate conditioning (Fig. 16).

At this time Zeier and Karten (1971) published an important paper describing nuclear subdivisions of archistriatum having differential afferentation and efferentation. The medial and posterior nuclear groups contain cells of origin of a pathway following the diencephalic course of the occipitomesencephalic tract, but terminating in hypothalamus and no further caudally. In contrast, anterior and intermediate nuclear groups give rise to a pathway following the long descending course of the classically defined occipitomesencephalic tract, but with no hypothalamic terminal field. They thus suggested that posteromedial archistriatum be considered the limbic portion of the structure, possibly homologous to part of mammalian amygdala, and they designated the projection from this region as the hypothalamic component of the occipitomesencephalic tract.

These anatomical findings fit remarkably well with our lesion results, since we obtained conditioning deficits only with destruction of posteromedial, or limbic, archistriatum and its projection to hypothalamus. It might also be noted that the most effective region of archistriatum for

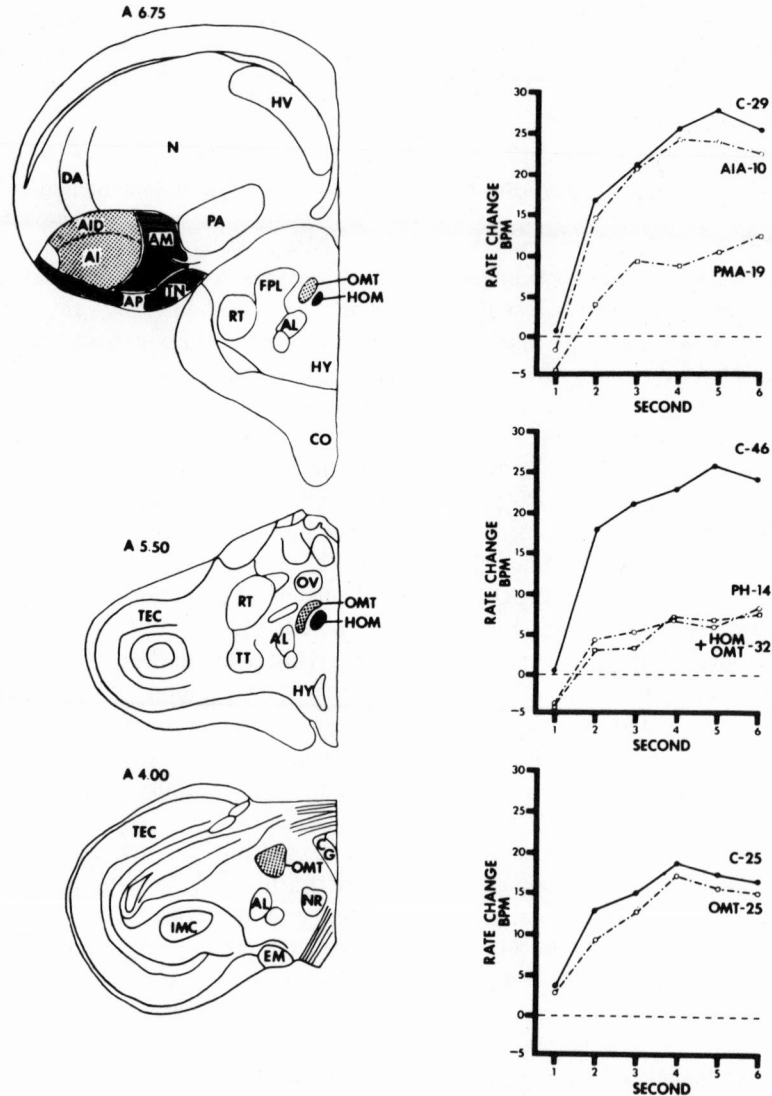

FIG. 16.   Illustration of the effects of lesions in the anterior two-thirds of archistriatum (AIA), posteromedial archistriatum (PMA), posterior hypothalamus (PH), occipitomesencephalic tract caudal
to hypothalamus (OMT), and occipitomesencephalic tract + pars hypothalami rostral to the caudal
third of hypothalamus (HOM + OMT). Accompanying controls (C) are illustrated, and sample sizes
are indicated next to the group abbreviations. The figure shows the response dynamics for each
group averaged over trial blocks 41–60, the training period where near-asymptotic performance is
attained. To the upper left of each schematic section is an indication of its rostrocaudal level in the
Karten and Hodos (1967) coordinate system. The stippled area of archistriatum indicates the region

eliciting cardiovascular responses with electrical stimulation is this postero-medial portion (Fig. 15). In combination, these findings suggest that the pressor–accelerator pathway originating in posteromedial archistriatum is involved in mediating conditioned heart rate change. Moreover, the hypothalamic projection from this region via the tractus occipitomesence-phalicus, pars hypothalami has been implicated as the relevant efferent system from archistriatum (see Fig. 18).

The implication of the avian amygdalar homologue clearly establishes that telencephalic limbic structures participate in mediating conditioned heart rate change, raising the question of possible involvement of other limbic structures of the avian hemisphere. While our anatomical knowledge of such structures in bird is rather limited, in addition to posteromedial ar-chistriatum they primarily include the hippocampus, septum, lobus parolfactorius, and other minor structures associated with the olfactory system. The hippocampus (and entorhinal area) can be eliminated, since only small heart rate changes follow stimulation of this region (Cohen and Pitts, 1967) and no conditioning deficit follows its ablation (Cohen, 1967). In contrast, septal injury may affect conditioning to a limited extent, but these results are preliminary. It is of interest that the cardiovascular response pattern is quite different upon septal as opposed to archistriatal stimulation (Macdonald and Cohen, 1973). Finally, lobus parolfactorius, a large structure contributing substantially to the medial forebrain bundle, is not cardioactive, and preliminary results suggest no lesion effect.

Thus, to date, posteromedial archistriatum and possibly septum have been implicated in mediating the conditioned response, while the remaining major limbic structures of telencephalon can probably be eliminated. It seems clear that the archistriatal contribution is exerted through its hypothalamic projection, but we are unclear as to the direction of in-formation flow from the septum. This could be through modulation of pos-teromedial archistriatum, direct effects on the diencephalon, or both.

Regardless of possible interconnections among relevant telencephalic limbic structures, a nodal point in analyzing the relevant descending

---

from which the occipitomesencephalic tract (also stippled) arises. The blackened area of archi-striatum is the region giving rise to the occipitomesencephalic tract, pars hypothalami (also blackened). AI: archistriatum intermedium, AID: archistriatum intermedium, pars dorsalis, AL: ansa lenticularis, AM: archistriatum mediale, AP: archistriatum posterior, CG: central gray, CO: optic chiasm, DA: dorsal archistriatal tract, EM: ectomammillary nucleus, FPL: lateral forebrain bundle, HOM: tractus occipitomesencephalicus, pars hypothalami, HV: hyperstriatum ventrale, HY: hypothalamus, IMC: nucleus isthmi, pars magnocellularis, N: neostriatum, NR: red nucleus, OMT: tractus occipitomesencephalicus, OV: nucleus ovoidalis, PA: paleostriatum augmentatum, RT: nu-cleus rotundus, TEC: optic tectum, TN: nucleus taeniae, TT: tractus tectothalamicus, BPM: beats/min.

pathways is the hypothalamus, since hemisphere limbic structures gain access to subtelencephalic regions through synaptic contact with or projections through hypothalamus. In fact, it has already been demonstrated that involvement of posteromedial archistriatum is mediated through hypothalamus. Consequently, it is not surprising that hypothalamic lesions result in severe conditioning deficits (Cohen and Macdonald, in prep.). The effects of lesions confined to posterior hypothalamus are shown in Fig. 16, and it can be seen that the deficit is remarkably similar to that following interruption of the hypothalamic component of the occipitomesencephalic tract.

6.3.3. Relevant Structures Caudal to the Diencephalon

Since there is indication that telencephalic limbic structures exert their influence on the conditioned response via hypothalamus, and near-total deficits follow posterior hypothalamic lesions, an obvious question concerns identification of participating cardiovascular pathways caudal to hypothalamus. As described previously, one of the more prominent cardioactive pathways is a pressor–accelerator system probably originating in hypothalamus, traversing ventromedial mesencephalon and then

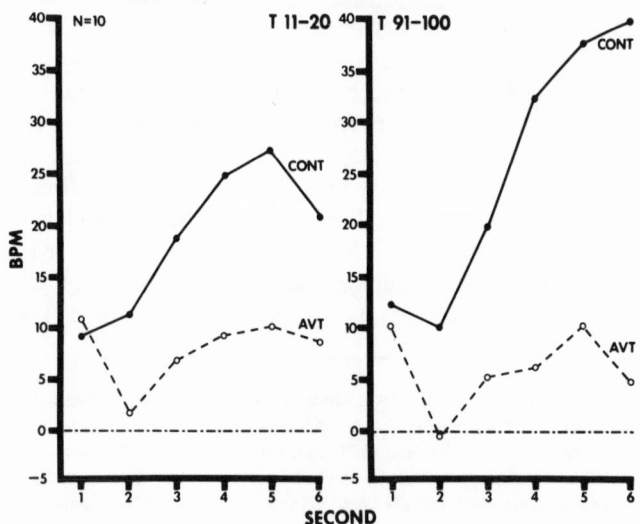

FIG. 17.   Illustration of the response dynamics of animals with ventral area of Tsai lesions (AVT) compared with accompanying controls (CONT). The left side of the figure shows the dynamics averaged over trials 11–20 (T 11–20), while the right shows the dynamics averaged over trials 91–100 (T 91–100). BPM: beats/min.

assuming an increasingly ventrolateral course through pons and medulla (Figs. 15 and 18). While we have not had an opportunity to interrupt this pathway at pontine or medullary levels, ventromedial mesencephalic lesions in the region of the ventral area of Tsai have been shown to produce severe conditioning deficits (Fig. 17) (Durkovic and Cohen, 1969a). In contrast, lesions in central or lateral tegmentum do not yield this result (Durkovic and Cohen, 1969a,b).

The response dynamics of animals sustaining ventral area of Tsai lesions are particularly interesting and differ from those with hypothalamic injury (compare Fig. 16 and 17). The ventromedial midbrain lesion not only prevents conditioned response development, but it may also abolish habituation of the sensitization response (compare Figs. 1A and 17). As described earlier, sensitization and conditioned response dynamics are easily distinguished, and sensitization normally habituates following ten presentations. However, after ventral area of Tsai lesions *sensitization-like* response dynamics persist throughout training. Unfortunately, sensitization control animals were not included in the Durkovic and Cohen (1969a,b) studies, and thus this interpretation must be qualified. However, the results suggest that the heart rate component of the sensitization response may be mediated by a pathway independent of that mediating conditioned heart rate change. Since sensitization-like response dynamics do not follow hypothalamic lesions (Fig. 16), there is the further implication that the presumptive *conditioning* and *sensitization* pathways diverge caudal to hypothalamus, sensitization possibly being mediated by the component of the medial forebrain bundle coursing dorsally to the central gray.

More convincing, though tentative, is the hypothesis that the ventrally descending pathway is critical for mediating the conditioned response and, more generally, any learned modification of heart rate. This pathway and more rostral limbic components are schematically illustrated in part in Fig. 18. It is clear that substantiation of this suggestion will require considerably more effort involving an extensive lesion series (with sensitization controls) in which the ventral pathway is interrupted at many rostro-caudal levels. If the hypothesis is correct, then one would anticipate severe conditioning deficits with comparable response dynamics following lesions at all levels rostral to the point where this descending system relays to gain access to the dorsal motor nucleus. Even then, definitive evidence for such differential mediation would have to include identification of the sensitization pathway and selective elimination of the sensitization response following interruption of that pathway.

Finally, although deficits following hypothalamic and ventromedial mesencephalic lesions are severe, they do not totally eliminate conditioned heart rate change. While residual sensitization could partially account for

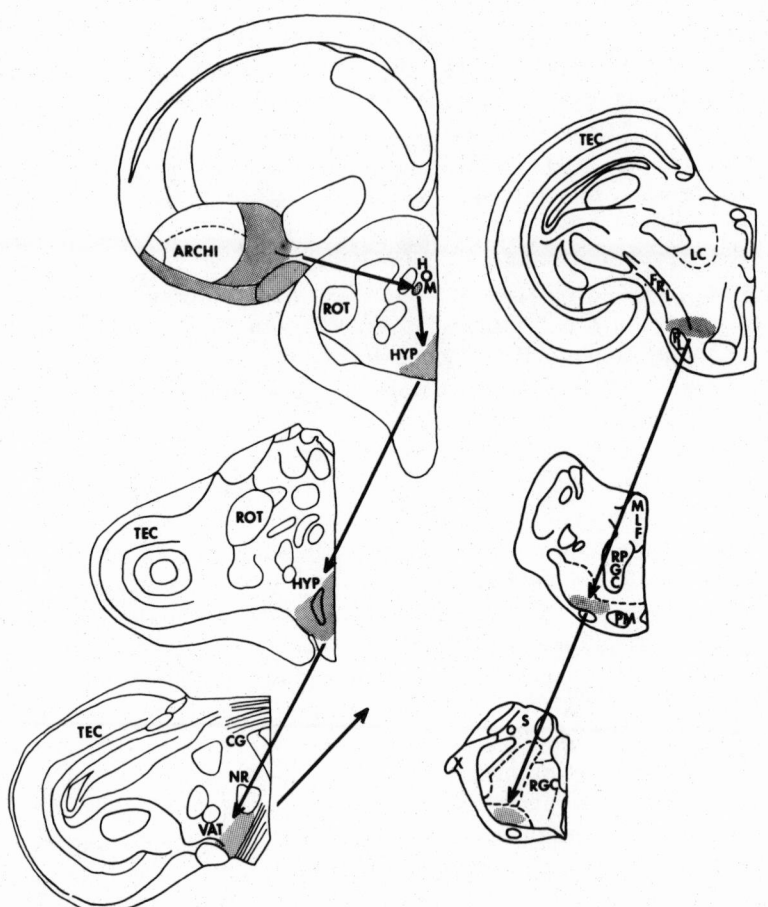

FIG. 18.   Schematic illustration of the major descending pathway hypothesized to mediate the conditioned response. This is shown on schematic sections by the stippled areas joined across increasingly caudal sections by the long arrows. ARCHI: archistriatum, CG: central gray, FRL: lateral reticular formation, HOM: tractus occipitomesencephalicus, pars hypothalami, HYP: hypothalamus, LC: locus ceruleus, MLF: medial longitudinal fasciculus, NR: red nucleus, PL: lateral pontine nucleus, PM: medial pontine nucleus, RGC: nucleus reticularis gigantocellularis, ROT: nucleus rotundus, RPGC: nucleus reticularis pontis caudalis, pars gigantocellularis, S: solitary nucleus, TEC: optic tectum, VAT: ventral area of Tsai, X: vagal rootlets.

this, it must be demonstrated at some point that a total deficit can be obtained by some combination of lesions in the presumed efferent segment of the system. Thus, while it is possible that the ventrally descending pathway is exclusively responsible for mediating the conditioned response, experimental evidence does not yet permit a definitive conclusion.

6.4. Conclusions

Considerable information has been accumulated with respect to more peripheral segments of the pathways mediating the conditioned (and to some extent the unconditioned) response. In fact, the final common path has been characterized sufficiently to allow microelectrode studies of its neuronal elements during conditioning, experiments now in progress.

In contrast to our knowledge of the final common path, information regarding descending systems that influence preganglionic cardiac neurons is still sketchy. However, data obtained from various lines of research are beginning to generate a functional flow chart for certain major components of the relevant descending pathways, and, at the least, have provided important guidelines for subsequent studies on this segment of the system.

Our present working view of these pathways is summarized in highly schematic form in Fig. 18. Of the major cardiovascular pathways of avian brain, the pressor–accelerator system arising from archistriatum has been clearly implicated and appears to exert its effect through hypothalamus. In addition, there is highly suggestive evidence for involvement of the pressor–accelerator pathway descending ventrally and ventrolaterally from hypothalamus. Unfortunately, we have not yet had an opportunity to survey other cardiovascular pathways (see Macdonald and Cohen, 1973).

In concluding this section, two important points merit restatement. First, it must be recognized that our present map of the relevant descending pathways is still primarily a functional one, and a good deal of effort will be required to establish a reasonable morphological foundation for it. Second, these descending systems have been designated as motor only tentatively and primarily for organizational purposes. The designation of such structures as archistriatum and septum as motor is almost certainly inappropriate, but as more information is obtained on the precise functional roles of such structures, an increasingly realistic and rigorous subdivision of the various aspects of the system would hopefully evolve.

7. General Concluding Comments

At the outset of our program some years ago, the single-minded goal was to develop visually conditioned heart rate change in the pigeon as an effective vertebrate system for studying changes in single neuron activity during learning. Before summarizing the model's status in that regard, it is important to mention that, while our interest in such cellular studies has in no way lessened, we have gained an increased appreciation for questions arising at many levels of analysis. At the molar level are exclusively behavioral studies to specify in detail the input–output relation across the entire system and major variables affecting this relation. While direct information on mechanisms does not derive from such studies, they are indispensable in providing the detailed background within which a more structural analysis must operate.

The task of mapping structures mediating conditioned response development turns out to be far from a sterile effort, and generation of a flow chart of relevant structures and their interconnections now represents to us considerably more than an atlas of potential sites for microelectrode penetrations. For example, as delineation of the visual (conditioned stimulus) and descending (conditioned response) pathways progresses, we should be in an excellent position to deal with such problems as how sensory inputs gain access to limbic structures. Furthermore, we find that the mapping task itself provides important indications as to the functional roles of the various relevant structures and thereby establishes a framework for cellular neurophysiological studies of conditioning. Careful examination of the effects of a given lesion on the response dynamics is constituting a powerful source of information. By way of illustration, we have already demonstrated distinct vagal and sympathetic contributions to the response, and these vary at different stages of training. Moreover, there may well be different descending systems mediating such early response components as sensitization. Thus, the response dynamics viewed across the entire system could well represent a composite of contributions from various efferent sources that are partially independent. Taking this line of argument a step further, one could raise the possibility that the different parallel pathways transmitting the conditioned stimulus information have differential access to these various efferent systems. The provocative implication is that there could be a set of at least partially independent stimulus-response pathways with each contributing a specific component to the composite response, being preferentially responsive to specific components of the conditioned stimulus, and varying in effectiveness at different phases of training.While entirely speculative at the moment, concepts of this nature potentially derive from the mapping effort, and they could have important implications for neurophysiological analyses by generating a framework that would be exceedingly difficult to derive exclusively from single cell data. Conversely, single unit data may provide the most rigorous evaluation of such concepts.

Given the appropriate behavioral and functional neuroanatomical information as a substrate, there is then a wealth of data to be gained from cellular neurophysiological studies of conditioning. These add the critical dimension of allowing a dynamic analysis of the system. This not only provides functional information of higher resolution but, importantly, also permits identification of synaptic fields undergoing change as a function of training. It is through such an approach that one can hopefully identify regions of the nervous system actually participating in information storage, and this in turn would allow a broad range of anatomical, chemical, and physiological investigations of information storage. In fact, identification of synaptic regions involved in plastic change may well one of the most important short-term goals in the analysis of a vertebrate model system.

To return to the present status of our program with respect to cellular neurophysiological studies of conditioning, it is important to recognize that with a systematic approach from the periphery centrally it is not necessary that the relevant neuroanatomy be completely specified as a prelude. As the first few synaptic relays are defined for each segment of the system, cellular studies of conditioning can be initiated concomitant with further pathway delineation. For example, we have recently undertaken electrophysiological investigation of the relevant sympathetic pre- and postganglionic neurons and of the more peripheral elements of the relevant visual pathways, and we will shortly begin similar studies on cells of origin of vagal cardioinhibitory fibers. Our guideline in this regard is that, given appropriate behavioral development of the model, a structure can be neurophysiologically studied during conditioning if and only if the following criteria are satisfied: (1) It has been implicated through the mapping program as participating in conditioned response development. (2) Its anatomical connections with the sensory and/or motor periphery of the system are well specified. (3) The response characteristics of relevant neurons presynaptic to the structure for sensory segments and postsynaptic to it for motor segments have been quantitatively described. (4) Sufficient information is available regarding its basic anatomical organization. (5) The response characteristics of neurons in the structure to whole-field illumination have been specified, and, where appropriate, the relationship of the neuronal discharge characteristics to heart rate is known. As these criteria are satisfied for each successive structure along some segment of the pathway, one is able to pursue neurophysiological studies during training systematically centrally. It is such a step-by-step interrogation of each segment of the system that we feel is essential to eventually resolve many of the salient questions regarding mechanisms of information storage and retrieval in vertebrate brain.

8. References

Binggeli, R. L., and Paule, W. J., 1969, The pigeon retina: Quantitative aspects of the optic nerve and ganglion cell layer, *J. Comp. Neurol. 137:*1–18.

Bloch-Rojas, S., Toro, A., and Pinto-Hamuy, T., 1964, Cardiac versus somatomotor conditioned responses in neodecorticate rats, *J. Comp. Physiol. Psychol. 58:*233–236.

Bullock, T. H., 1967, Simple systems for the study of learning mechanisms, in *Neurosciences Research Symposium Summaries, Vol. 2*, F. O. Schmitt, T. Melnechuk, G. C. Quarton, and G. Adelman, eds., The M.I.T. Press, Cambridge, pp. 203–327.

Campbell, H. S., and Smith, J. L., 1962, The pharmacology of the pigeon pupil, *Arch. Opthamol. 67:*141–144.

Cohen, D. H., 1967, The hyperstriatal region of the avian forebrain: A lesion study of possible functions, including its role in cardiac and respiratory conditioning, *J. Comp. Neurol. 131:*559–570.

Cohen, D. H., 1969, Development of a vertebrate experimental model for cellular neurophysiologic studies of learning, *Cond. Ref. 4:*61–80.

Cohen, D. H. 1974a, Analysis of the final common path for heart rate conditioning, in *Cardiovascular Psychophysiology—Current Issues in Response Mechanisms, Biofeedback and Methodology,* P. A. Obrist, A. H. Black, J. Brener, and L. V. DiCara, eds., Aldine-Atherton Press, Chicago (in press).

Cohen, D. H., 1974b, The effect of conditioned stimulus intensity on visually conditioned heart rate change in the pigeon: A sensitization mechanism, *J. Comp. Physiol. Psychol.* (in prep.).

Cohen, D. H., In prep. a, A large sample analysis of the dynamics of conditioned heart rate change in the pigeon, including an analysis of seasonal variation.

Cohen, D. H., In prep. b, Involvement of the avian amygdalar homologue (archistriatum) in defensively conditioned heart rate change.

Cohen, D. H., In prep. c, Avian visual pathways involved in visually conditioned heart rate change.

Cohen, D. H., and Dooley, S., In prep., An electrophysiological analysis of the responsiveness of avian thalamofugal and tectofugal visual pathways to whole field illumination.

Cohen, D. H., and Duff, T. A., In prep., The relationship between "on" and "off" discharges to whole field illumination in single optic tract axons of the pigeon.

Cohen, D. H., Duff, T. A., and Ebbesson, S. O. E., 1973, Electrophysiological identification of a visual area in shark telencephalon, *Science 182:*492–494.

Cohen, D. H., Duff, T. A., and Macdonald, R. L., 1972, Laminar organization of the avian optic tectum: A current-density analysis, *Anat. Rec. 172:*293–294.

Cohen, D. H., and Durkovic, R. G., 1966, Cardiac and respiratory conditioning, differentiation, and extinction in the pigeon, *J. Exptl. Anal. Behav. 9:*681–688.

Cohen, D. H., and Karten, H. J., 1974, The structural organization of avian brain: An overview, in *Birds: Brain and Behavior,* M. W. Schein, and I. J. Goodman, eds., Academic Press, New York (in press).

Cohen, D. H., and Macdonald, R. L., 1971, Some variables affecting orienting and conditioned heart-rate responses in the pigeon, *J. Comp. Physiol. Psychol. 74:*123–133.

Cohen, D. H., and Macdonald, R. L., 1974, A selective review of central neural pathways involved in cardiovascular control, in *Cardiovascular Psychophysiology—Current Issues in Response Mechanisms, Biofeedback and Methodology.* P. A. Obrist, A. H. Black, J. Brener, and L. V. DiCara, eds., Aldine-Atherton Press, Chicago (in press).

Cohen, D. H., and Macdonald, R. L., In prep., The effects of hypothalamic lesions on heart rate conditioning in the pigeon.

Cohen, D. H., and Pitts, L. H., 1967, The hyperstriatal region of the avian forebrain: Somatic and autonomic responses to electrical stimulation, *J. Comp. Neurol. 131:*323–336.

Cohen, D. H., and Pitts, L. H., 1968, Vagal and sympathetic components of conditioned cardioacceleration in the pigeon, *Brain Res. 9:*15–31.

Cohen, D. H., and Schnall, A. M., 1970, Medullary cells of origin of vagal cardioinhibitory fibers in the pigeon. II. Electrical stimulation of the dorsal motor nucleus, *J. Comp. Neurol. 140:*321–342.

Cohen, D. H., Schnall, A. M., Macdonald, R. L., and Pitts, L. H., 1970, Medullary cells of origin of vagal cardioinhibitory fibers in the pigeon. I. Anatomical studies of peripheral vagus nerve and the dorsal motor nucleus, *J. Comp. Neurol. 140:*299–320.

Cohen, D. H., and Trauner, D. A., 1969, Studies of avian visual pathways involved in cardiac conditioning: Nucleus rotundus and ectostriatum, *Exptl. Brain Res. 7:*133–142.

Cowan, W. M., 1970, Centrifugal fibres to the avian retina, *Brit. Med. Bull. 26:*112–118.

Cowan, W. M., Adamson, L., and Powell, T. P. S., 1961, An experimental study of the avian visual system, *J. Anat. 95:*545–563.

DiCara, L. V., Braun, J. J., and Pappas, B. A., 1970, Classical conditioning and instrumental learning of cardiac and gastrointestinal responses following removal of neocortex in the rat, *J. Comp. Physiol. Psychol. 73:*208–216.

Dubin, M. W., 1970, The inner plexiform layer of the vertebrate retina: A quantitative and comparative electron microscopic analysis, *J. Comp. Neurol. 140:*479–505.

Duff, T. A., and Cohen, D. H., In prep. a, Retinal afferents to the pigeon optic tectum: Discharge characteristics in response to whole field illumination.

Duff, T. A., and Cohen, D. H., In prep. b, Responses to whole field illumination of ganglion cell axons in the pigeon optic chiasm.

Duff, T. A., Cohen, D. H., and Macdonald, R. L., 1972, Responses of single optic tract afferents to the pigeon tectum evoked by diffuse retinal illumination, *Arch. Mex. Anat. 13:*14.

Duff, T. A., Cohen, D. H., and Macdonald, R. L., In prep., Laminar organization of the pigeon optic tectum: A current-density analysis.

Duncan, P. M., 1972, Effect of septal area damage and base-line activity levels on conditioned heart-rate response in rats, *J. Comp. Physiol. Psychol. 81:*131–142.

Durkovic, R. G., and Cohen, D. H., 1969a, Effects of rostral midbrain lesions on conditioning of heart- and respiratory-rate responses in pigeons, *J. Comp. Physiol. Psychol. 68:*184–192.

Durkovic, R. G., and Cohen, D. H., 1969b, Effect of caudal midbrain lesions on conditioning of heart- and respiratory-rate responses in the pigeon, *J. Comp. Physiol. Psychol. 69:*329–338.

Eisenstein, E. M., 1967, The use of invertebrate systems for studies on the bases of learning and memory, in *The Neurosciences, A Study Program,* G.C. Quarton, T. Melnechuk, and F. O. Schmitt, eds., The Rockefeller University Press, New York, pp. 653–665.

Gantt, W. H., 1960, Cardiovascular component of the conditional reflex to pain, food and other stimuli, *Physiol. Rev. 40* (Suppl. 4):266–291.

Graeber, R. C., Schroeder, D. M., Jane, J. A., and Ebbesson, S.O.E., 1972, The importance of telencephalic structures in visual discrimination learning in nurse shark, Soc. for Neurosci., 2nd Annual Meeting, Houston.

Graybiel, A. M., 1972, Some extrageniculate visual pathways in the cat, *Inves. Ophthamol. 11:*322–332.

Hirschberger, W., 1971, Vergleichend experimentell- histologisch Untersuchung zur retinalen Repräsentation in den primären visuellen Zentren einiger Vogelarten, Dissertation, Max-Planck-Institut für Hirnforschung Neurobiologische Abteilung, Frankfurt.

Hodos, W., Karten, H. J., and Bonbright, J. C., Jr., 1973, Visual intensity and pattern discrimination after lesions of the thalamofugal visual pathway in pigeons, *J. Comp. Neurol. 148:*447–468.

Holden, A. L., 1969, Receptive properties of retinal cells and tectal cells in the pigeon, *J. Physiol. 201:*56P.

Huber, J. F., 1936, Nerve roots and nuclear groups in the spinal cord in the pigeon, *J. Comp. Neurol. 65:*43–91.

John, E. R., 1972, Switchboard versus statistic theories of learning and memory, *Science* 177:850–864.

Kaiser, L., 1924, L'innervation segmentale de la peau chez le pigeon (*Columba livia var. domestica*), *Arch. Neerl. Physiol.* 9:299–379.

Kandel, E. R., and Spencer, W. A., 1968, Cellular neurophysiological approaches to learning, *Physiol. Rev.* 48:65–134.

Karten, H. J., 1969, The organization of the avian telencephalon and some speculations on the phylogeny of the amniote telencephalon, *Ann. N.Y. Acad. Sci.* 167:164–179.

Karten, H. J., Cohen, D. H., and Macdonald, R. L., In prep., Central projections of the cervical vagus in the pigeon (*Columba livia*): An experimental study.

Karten, H. J., and Hodos, W., 1967, *A Stereotaxic Atlas of the Brain of the Pigeon (Columba livia)*, The Johns Hopkins Press, Baltimore.

Karten, H. J., Hodos, W., Nauta, W. J. H., and Revzin, A. M., 1973, Neural connections of the "visual Wulst" of the avian telencephalon. Experimental studies in the pigeon (*Columba livia*) and owl (*Speotyto cunicularia*), *J. Comp. Neurol.* 150:253–277.

Kimberly, R. P., Holden, A. L., and Bamborough, P., 1971, Response characteristics of pigeon forebrain cells to visual stimulation, *Vision Res.* 11:475–478.

Koizumi, K., and Brooks, C. M., 1972, The integration of autonomic system reactions: A discussion of autonomic reflexes, their control and their association with somatic reactions, *Ergebn. Physiol.* 67:1–67.

Leonard, R. B., 1972, The spinal distribution of lumbar and cervical dorsal roots in the pigeon (*Columba livia*), *Anat. Rec.* 172:354.

Leonard, R. B., and Cohen, D. H., In prep. a, Peripheral unconditioned stimulus pathways in a conditioning model system: Defensively conditioned heart rate change in the pigeon.

Leonard, R. B., and Cohen, D. H., In prep. b, The spinal distribution of lumbar dorsal roots in the pigeon (*Columbia livia*).

Leonard, R. B., and Cohen, D. H., In prep. c, The spinal distribution of cervical dorsal roots in the pigeon (*Columba livia*).

Leonard, R. B., and Cohen, D. H., In prep. d, Circuitry mediating spino–spinal somatosympathetic reflexes in the pigeon.

Macdonald, R. L., and Cohen, D. H., 1973, Heart rate and blood pressure responses to electrical stimulation of the central nervous system in the pigeon (*Columba livia*), *J. Comp. Neurol.* 150:109–136.

Miles, F. A., 1972, Centrifugal control of the avian retina. I. Receptive field properties of retinal ganglion cells, *Brain Res.* 48:65–92.

Nauta, W. J. H., and Karten, H. J., 1970, A general profile of the vertebrate brain, with sidelights on the ancestry of cerebral cortex, in *The Neurosciences: Second Study Program*, G. C. Quarton, T. Melnechuk, and F. O. Schmitt, eds., The M.I.T. Press, Cambridge, pp. 7–26.

O'Flaherty, J. J., 1971, The optic nerve of the Mallard duck: Fiber-diameter frequency distribution and physiological properties, *J. Comp. Neurol.* 143:17–24.

Revzin, A. M., 1970, Some characteristics of wide-field units in the brain of the pigeon, *Brain Behav. Evol.* 3:195–204.

Revzin, A. M., and Karten, H. J., 1967, Rostral projections of the optic tectum and nucleus rotundus in the pigeon, *Brain Res.* 5:264–276.

Sato, A., and Schmidt, R. F., 1973, Somatosympathetic reflexes: Afferent fibers, central pathways, discharge characteristics, *Physiol. Rev.* 53:916–947.

Smith, O. A., Jr., and Nathan, M. A., 1964, Effect of hypothalamic and prefrontal cortical lesions on conditioned cardiovascular responses, *The Physiol.* 7:259.

Smith, O. A., Jr., Nathan, M. A., and Clarke, N. P., 1968, Central nervous system pathways mediating blood pressure changes, *Hypertension* 16:9–22.

Spencer, W. A., Thompson, R. F., and Nielson, D. R., 1966, Response decrement of the flexion reflex in the acute spinal cat and transient restoration by strong stimuli, *J. Neurophysiol. 29:*221–239.

Stone, J., and Hoffman, K.-P., 1972, Very slow-conducting ganglion cells in the cat's retina: a major new functional type?, *Brain Res. 43:*610–616.

Thompson, R. F., and Spencer, W. A., 1966, Habituation: A model phenomenon for the study of neuronal substrates of behavior, *Psychol. Rev. 73:*16–43.

Wall, S. M., Ebbesson, S. O. E., and Cohen, D. H., In preparation, Retinal projections in the pigeon described by silver and autoradiographic methods.

Zeier, H., and Karten, H. J., 1971, The archistriatum of the pigeon: organization of afferent and efferent connections, *Brain Res. 31:*313–326.

CHAPTER 8

CNS Integration of Learned Cardiovascular Behavior*

Neil Schneiderman, James Francis, Larry D. Sampson, and
James S. Schwaber

Department of Psychology
University of Miami
Coral Gables, Florida

1. Introduction

The intent of the present chapter is to review what is currently known about the involvement of the CNS in learned cardiovascular activity. Although separate, but extensive bodies of literature exist describing conditioning on the one hand and CNS control of the circulatory system on the other, relatively little is known about the CNS integration of learned cardiovascular responses. This is because important information is lacking about (1) cardiovascular dynamics during conditioning, (2) pathways mediating learned responses, and (3) the role of learned cardiovascular respones as biological adjustments.

Historically, most studies of cardiovascular conditioning monitored only heart rate. In some instances this occurred because the heart rate measure was merely used as a convenient index of conditioning. In other instances, the heart rate measure was used as an index of conditioned arousal, conditioned fear or some other learned motivational–emotional state. The widespread use of a single measure of cardiovascular conditioning also reflects the fact that relatively little effort has been made to characterize the major cardiovascular events occurring during conditioning. The relative contributions of cardiac output and total peripheral resistance

* The research from our laboratory described in this chapter was primarily supported by research grants GB-5307, GB-7944, and GB-24713 from the National Science Foundation and by a grant from the Florida Heart Association and its affiliate chapters.

to various conditioned responses is largely unknown. Furthermore, effects such as baroreceptor modulation and regional shunting of the blood flow have been largely ignored in the cardiovascular conditioning literature.

Another difficulty that has handicapped serious study of the CNS integration of learned cardiovascular responses is that the pathways mediating conditioned responses are still unknown. This is true not only with respect to the cardiovascular system, but with respect to all other response systems as well. Although various structures such as the hippocampus have been implicated in the learning process, most of our information is fragmentary, and few investigators have had the patience to systematically explore input–output relationships. A conspicuous exception to this has been the work of David Cohen and his associates, described in Chapter 7 of this volume.

A final obstacle that has limited comprehension of the CNS integration of learned cardiovascular responses is that these responses are still poorly understood as biological adjustments. Relatively few studies have focused upon learned cardiovascular changes as part of the normal cardiovascular regulatory activity of the organism. If learned cardiovascular responses are to be understood as biological adjustments, several things must be done. First, we must recognize that the cardiovascular system is closely tied to our metabolic needs. Therefore, other stimuli besides peripheral electric shock are needed to elicit cardiovascular responses in conditioning situations. These might include use of a treadmill or intracranial stimulation as the unconditioned stimulus (US). Second, comparisons must be made between learned and unlearned cardiovascular responses. Third, the neural bases of learned and unlearned cardiovascular adjustments need to be compared, and integrated into a general theory of cardiovascular regulation.

Since the learned aspects of cardiovascular regulation are a part of the normal activity of the circulatory system, a general description of the nervous control of the circulation precedes our discussion of (1) CNS involvement in learned cardiovascular activity, (2) the pathways mediating cardiovascular responses, and (3) the relationship of learned and unlearned cardiovascular adjustments.

2. Preliminary Considerations

Central regulation of the cardiovascular system involves neural integration at virtually every level of the CNS from the cortex to the spinal cord. It was once believed that medullary centers in the dorsal reticular formation exerted almost exclusive control over both vascular tone and reflexive cardiovascular adjustments, but this view has long since been modified. The essential role of the bulbar reticular formation in central cardiovascular regulation is still recognized, but some of its eminence is now shared with supramedullary integrative mechanisms. Interactions between supramedullary and medullary levels of integration play an important role in contemporary conceptualizations of CNS control over the circulatory system.

The involvement of the CNS in cardiovascular regulation has been under scrutiny since Claude Bernard (1852) transected the spinal cord and observed a marked fall in blood pressure. Subsequently, Owsjannikow (1871) and Dittmar (1873) discovered the bulbar vasomotor area while working in Ludwig's laboratory in Leipzig. They observed that successively lower transections of the brainstem in cats and rabbits caused a pronounced fall in blood pressure only when the section was caudal to the inferior colliculi. Progressively lower transections resulted in further decreases in pressure until maximum hypotension occurred after section of the medulla. Central stimulation of the sciatic nerve caused a reflexive rise in pressure after the medulla was separated from more anterior structures, but this reflexive pressor response was abolished following transection of the medulla. The experiments at Leipzig demonstrated that the medulla contains mechanisms which are essential for both the maintenance of a normal blood pressure level and for reflexive increases in pressure.

The characteristics of the bulbar vasomotor area were further elucidated by Ranson and Billingsley (1916) using punctate electrical stimulation to explore the floor of the 4th ventricle. They found one small area in which a rise in arterial pressure was obtained, and another small area in which only a fall in pressure was observed. Subsequent experiments have shown that the pressor area maintains tonic arterial blood pressure at a normal level by means of sympathetically induced vasoconstriction, and that vasodilation induced by stimulation of the depressor area is primarily due to an inhibition of vasoconstrictor tone (e.g., Lindgren and Uvnäs, 1953; 1954).

Cardiovascular integration within the medulla of the intact animal involves a bilaterally represented cardioinhibitory area as well as the pressor and depressor zones. Unlike the vasomotor areas, which primarily act via the sympathetic nervous system, the cardioinhibitory area has a parasympathetic outflow to the heart by means of the vagus nerves. As early as 1845 Weber and Weber determined that the vagus nerves depress the heart. Subsequent histological analyses indicated that the cells of origin for the cardiac vagus originate in the nucleus ambiguus (Bunzl-Federn, 1889) and/or the dorsal motor nucleus (Kohnstamm, 1901) of the medulla. Stimulation of the dorsal motor nucleus produced a strong cardioinhibitory effect (Miller and Bowman, 1916).

The medulla plays an essential role in the neural integration of cardiovascular activity. This integration depends upon neural inputs from inside and outside of the circulatory system. Some of these neural inputs are considered to be intrinsic, because they originate within the circulatory system. Receptors in the walls of the carotid sinus, for instance, send impulses to the medulla that may lead to cardiovascular adjustments. Other neural inputs leading to cardiovascular adjustments, however, are considered to be extrinsic, because they originate from outside of the circulation. Stimulation of a peripheral nerve, for example, may lead to cardiovascular changes even though the source of stimulation is extrinsic to the circulation. An adequate theory dealing with the learned aspects of cardiovascular regulation must depend upon a thorough comprehension of both intrinsic and extrinsic cardiovascular adjustments.

Before turning to an examination of the intrinsic and extrinsic neural adjustments of the circulation, it would be well to note that circulatory adjustments are mediated by local mechanisms within tissues as well as by the CNS. Within specific tissues, for example, blood flow appears to adjust to local metabolic activity. In addition, changes in arterial blood pressure at constant levels of tissue metabolism encounter vascular resistance changes that tend to maintain a constant blood flow. This phenomenon is referred to as autoregulation of the blood flow (e.g., Berne and Levy, 1972). Most of our concern in the present chapter will be directed to neural control of the circulation, but it should be kept in mind that neural and nonneural adjustments interact with one another.

3. Intrinsic and Extrinsic Neural Adjustments

Intrinsic cardiovascular adjustments have their origins in the responses of chemoreceptors and mechanoreceptors located within the circulatory system. Information about respiratory performance is provided by arterial chemoreceptors located in the aortic and carotid bodies. Information about mean pressure and about changes in pressure occurring in different portions of the cardiovascular system are provided by arterial, pulmonary, atrial, and ventricular mechanoreceptors.

Mechanoreceptors sensitive to arterial pressure are known as baroreceptors. The major groups of arterial baroreceptors lie within the walls of the carotid sinus and aortic arch, although some receptors are located along the thoracic aorta as well as the subclavian, common carotid, and mesenteric arteries (e.g., Green, 1967). The baroreceptors are stretch receptors that are stimulated by deformation of the arterial wall. Study of the baroreceptors located in the wall of the carotid sinus indicates that pulsatility and mean arterial pressure jointly determine receptor output (Heymans and Neil, 1958).

Efferents from the carotid sinus and aortic arch reach the medulla via the glossopharyngeal and vagus nerves, respectively. Section of these nerves causes a rapid rise in arterial pressure indicating that the nerves are tonically active.

An increase in baroreceptor stimulation leads to a pronounced reflexive decrease in heart rate and a diminution in blood pressure unless the reflex is gated within the CNS. The reflexive bradycardia or slowing of heart rate is mediated by the vagus nerves. Systemic injections of atropine that blockade the vagus and abolish the bradycardia do not eliminate the systemic hypotension. This suggests that the diminution in pressure is largely due to an inhibition of vasoconstrictor activity.

At one time the arterial baroreceptor reflex was conceptualized as a simple pressure regulator that minimized generalized disturbance of the circulation (e.g., Koch, 1931). More recent formulations have emphasized that it is the interaction of the intrinsic baroreceptor inputs with those of extrinsic influences that determines the neural control of the systemic circulation (e.g., Korner, 1971).

Extrinsic neural adjustments of the circulation consist of those neurally mediated adjustments that are not initiated by receptors within the cardiovascular system. They may originate from sensory receptors in the periphery or they may originate within the CNS. Electrical stimulation of the nerves in a limb will produce increases or decreases in arterial pressure depending upon the characteristics of the stimulus. Low-frequency, low-intensity stimulation of long duration, for example, may cause a depressor response; whereas high-frequency, high-intensity stimulation of short duration may cause an increase in arterial pressure. The extrinsically induced increase in pressure may in turn elicit an intrinsically induced baroreceptor reflex.

The influence of the anterior hypothalamus and preoptic region during temperature regulation provides another example of extrinsic neural involvement in the circulation. Cooling of the blood perfusing the hypothalamus causes the vessels of the skin to constrict, whereas localized heating of the blood perfusing the hypothalamus results in cutaneous vasodilation (e.g, Hardy, 1961).

The unconditioned (e.g., peripheral electric shock) and conditioned (e.g., tones) stimuli of conditioning experiments initiate extrinsic cardiovascular changes. These in turn may interact with intrinsic cardiovascular adjustments such as the baroreceptor reflex. The initial interactions between intrinsic and extrinsic adjustments may be influenced further by both supramedullary mechanisms and by autoregulation of the blood flow.

Recent evidence, for example, indicates that baroreceptor influences may be modulated upward and downward by hypothalamic mechanisms (e.g., Gebber and Synder, 1970; Hilton and Spyer, 1971; Hockman and Talesnik, 1971). Other supramedullary mechanisms exert a tonic inhibitory influence upon the modulation of the baroreceptors (e.g., Korner et al., 1969; Reis and Cuenod, 1965) and play an important role in the redistribution of blood flow to different vascular beds (e.g., Eliasson et al., 1951; Green and Hoff, 1937; Schramm and Bignall, 1971).

4.   Supramedullary Mechanisms of Integration

Afferent projections from the glossopharyngeal (9th) and vagus (10th) cranial nerves convey information from the baroreceptors. The projections travel in the main ascending pathways from the medial bulbar reticular formation (Brodal, 1957; Dell, 1952). Some of these pathways pass through the midbrain, synapse in the hypothalamus, and send fibers to the septum and amygdala. Other pathways traverse the midbrain and thalamic reticular formations and project to the temporal and orbital-frontal cortices.

The efferents from the orbitofrontal cortex project to the hypothalamus (e.g., Hirata, 1965). Some fibers from the temporal cortex descend through the hypothalamus, but others travel over a more direct temporal–tegemental–bulbar pathway (Wall and Davis, 1951). Cells originating in the septal region and amygdala also synapse in the hypothalamus (e.g., Dreifuss and Murphy, 1968). Although some pathways descend through the hypothalamus, a new pathway also appears to arise within the medial posterior region of the hypothalamus (Enoch and Kerr, 1967a,b). Neurons descending from the hypothalamus traverse several different pathways through the midbrain tegmentum and central gray. Most fibers synapse, and then travel to the cardiovascular centers of the medulla. Some fibers, however, bypass the cardiovascular centers and terminate directly in the spinal cord (e.g., Schramm and Bignall, 1971).

Cardiovascular changes can be elicited from the preceding pathways by means of electrical stimulation of the brain. Although the responses obtained are dependent upon such factors as anesthetization and the parameter values of stimulation, many useful observations have arisen from stimulation experiments. In most instances, for example, stimulation of the orbitofrontal cortex has evoked a reduction of blood pressure and a decrease in heart rate. These changes have been traced to a reduction of vasoconstrictor tone, an augmentation of vagal tone, and an inhibition of catecholamine secretion by the adrenals (e.g., Euler and Folkow, 1958; Goldfein and Ganong, 1962; Kaada et al., 1949). Depressor responses have also been elicited from the temporal cortex, pyriform lobe, septal region, and regions of the amygdala (e.g., Ban, 1966; Reis and Oliphant, 1964; Wall and Davis, 1951).

Electrical stimulation of the anterior hypothalamus also elicits bradycardia and a depressor response (e.g., Folkow *et al.*, 1964; Gellhorn, 1964; Hilton and Spyer, 1971). These responses are in part due to descending influences upon the hypothalamus since they are diminished by degeneration of corticofugal fibers from the frontal lobe (Magoun, 1938). Korner *et al.* (1969) and others, however, have shown that vagally mediated inhibition of heart rate can occur in thalamic animals. In addition, several investigators (e.g., Gellhorn, 1957; Hilton and Spyer, 1971; Klevans and Gebber, 1970) have provided evidence that the anterior hypothalamus potentiates the effects of baroreceptor afferent stimulation.

Increases in heart rate and/or blood pressure have also been observed following electrical stimulation of the brain. Hoff and Green (1936), for example, obtained pressor and cardioaccelerator responses following stimulation of the motor cortex in cats and monkeys. Similar changes as well as increased secretion of adrenal catecholamines have been observed following stimulation of parts of the amygdala and hypothalamus (e.g., Fang and Wang, 1962; Goldfein and Ganong, 1962; Hilton and Zbrozyna, 1963; Reis and Oliphant, 1964). It would thus appear that different patterns of cardiovascular responses can be obtained from various supramedullary regions.

The suprabulbar neurons involved in cardiovascular regulation can in part be regarded as integrative interneurons interposed between the afferent projections of the 9th and 10th cranial nerve and the efferent neurons innervating the heart and blood vessels. They must also be understood, however, as loci for interactions with integrative neuronal groups involved in other physiological activities such as temperature regulation, movement, sex, and feeding. Some integrative groups of cardiovascular interneurons provide for the relative distributions of blood flow among different vascular networks. Others are responsible for modulating the intrinsic cardiovascular afferents. The manner in which these adjustments take place has long been studied, but is just beginning to be understood.

4.1. The Regional Distribution of Blood Flow

Green and Hoff (1937) pointed out that a change in arterial pressure occurs as a result of a variety of different vascular changes occurring concomitantly in different portions of the body. They observed that following stimulation of the motor cortex in cats and monkeys, cardiovascular responses included renal vasoconstriction accompanied by vasodilation within the muscular portions of the limb. This shunting is similar to that which occurs during muscular exercise. The experiment by Green and Hoff therefore suggests that CNS mechanisms related to the concomitant control of cardiovascular and muscle activity are involved in the shunting of regional blood flow. This shunting of blood to muscle is facilitated by a sympathetic vasodilator nerve supply to skeletal muscle.

Although the changes in arterial pressure mediated by the vasomotor center are due to changes in adrenergic vasoconstrictor activity, the existence of a sympathetic vasodilator nerve supply to the skeletal muscles of the dog and cat has long been known (Bülbring and Burn, 1935; Folkow and Uvnäs, 1950). Experimental evidence indicates that the sympathetic vasodilator pathway descends from the motor cortex and runs through the hypothalamus, midbrain tegmentum and ventrolateral medulla to the spinal cord (e.g., Abrahams *et al.*, 1960; Eliasson *et al.*, 1951; Lindgren *et al.*, 1956). According to Schramm and Bignall (1971) the sympathetic vasodilator pathway sends a branch to the dorsal mesencephalon, but descends through the ventral mesencephalon and continues caudally on a course which is cospatial, but not dependent upon, the medial lemniscal, spinothalamic, and spinotectal pathways. In the medulla it bypasses the cardiovascular centers in the reticular formation and travels in a pathway that is cospatial with the spinothalamic tract.

Several procedures have been used to detect evidence of neurally mediated vasodilation in muscles following sympathetic stimulation. One method involves abolishing vasoconstrictor activity by use of an alpha-adrenergic blocking agent or by depleting normal stores of norepinephrine by prior treatment with reserpine. Stimulation then results in active vasodilation, which in dogs and cats can be blocked by administration of atropine (e.g., Uvnäs, 1967). A more common method of examining sympathetic cholinergic vasodilation in cats and dogs is to monitor blood flow through a deep femoral vein or artery after circulation below the ankle is occluded by a tight ligature. This provides a reasonable estimate of the blood supply to the skeletal muscles of the limb. Following sympathetic stimulation large increases in blood flow occur in the deep femoral vein or artery. The short-latency component, but not the long-latency component of the response can be blocked by systemic injection of atropine (e.g., Djojosugito *et al.*, 1970; Schramm and Bignall, 1971).

Although sympathetic vasodilation that is sensitive to atropine has been demonstrated in carnivores such as cats, dogs, jackals, and foxes, it has not been possible to demonstrate the phenomena in noncarnivores such as the rabbit or monkey (Bolme *et al.*, 1970, Uvnäs, 1967). Schramm *et al.* (1971), however, have argued that atropine sensitivity may not be an adequate defining criterion for making interspecies comparisons of sympathetic vasodilation. They point out that atropine may block sympathetic vasodilation at ganglionic sites rather than at the autonomic, myoneural junction (e.g., Brown, 1969; Honig and Myers, 1968), and that atropine sensitivity at the ganglia may simply differ among species.

Schramm et al. (1971) examined the possibility of obtaining sympathetic vasodilation in the squirrel monkey. They observed a system in the monkey which was entirely homologous in its CNS organization to the sympathetic vasodilator system of the cat. They found, for example, that lesions of the spinothalamic tract that blocked sympathetic vasodilation induced by supramedullary stimulation in cats also blocked the response in the monkey. Destruction of the vasomotor centers in the bulbar reticular formation failed to abolish vasodilation either in the cat or in the monkey. In both the dog (Honig and Myers, 1968) and the monkey, sympathetic vasodilation was blocked by the beta-adrenergic blocking agent propranolol. The Schramm et al. experiment therefore suggests that the resistance vessels of the sympathetic vasodilator system may contain beta-adrenergic receptors, and that anatomical criteria rather than atropine sensitivity is more useful in assessing evidence of sympathetic vasodilation in various species.

4.2. Modulation of the Baroreceptor Reflex

Electrical stimulation of several supramedullary areas including the anterior hypothalamus produces a fall in arterial pressure and bradycardia. In contrast, stimulation of other supramedullary regions including the posterolateral hypothalamus produces an increase in arterial pressure and tachycardia. The results of several studies suggest that some of the cardiovascular changes induced by hypothalamic stimulation are related to the modulation of responses to baroreceptor stimulation.

Gellhorn (1957) observed that elevations in arterial pressure potentiated the vasodepressor response obtained to electrical stimulation of the anterior hypothalamus. Subsequently, Klevans and Gebber (1970) potentiated the vagal bradycardia resulting from baroreceptor afferent stimulation by concomitantly stimulating the anterior hypothalamus. Hilton and Spyer (1969, 1971) further found that the responses elicited by stimulation of the anterior hypothalamus were indistinguishable from those obtained by baroreceptor afferent stimulation. The responses included parasympathetic activation of the vagus nerves and sympathetic inhibition of vasoconstrictor tone.

Afferents from the baroreceptors project to the nucleus of the solitary tract (e.g., Biscoe and Sampson, 1970; Cottle, 1964; Crill and Reis, 1968; Ramon y Cajal, 1909). Hilton and Spyer (1971) found that either bilateral destruction of the anterior hypothalamus or lesions in the medullary depressor area that spared the nucleus of the solitary tract, reduced but did not abolish the baroreceptor reflex. Combination of both lesions abolished the reflex.

The pattern of responses obtained by stimulation of the anterior hypothalamus or medullary depressor area can also be obtained from intermediate areas of the brainstem. Since the anterior hypothalamus is known to receive sympathoinhibitory input from paleocortex (e.g., Löfving, 1961) and cardioinhibitory input from the neocortex (e.g., Achari et al., 1968) it appears possible that the entire brainstem depressor area constitutes a functional unit that integrates the responses to baroreceptor afferent stimulation with those from other sources of stimulation impinging upon the CNS.

In contrast to stimulation of the anterior hypothalamus, which elicits depressor responses and cardioacceleration, electrical stimulation of the posterolateral hypothalamus elicits a pattern of cardiovascular responses including an increase in heart rate and blood pressure accompanied by active sympathetic vasodilation in skeletal muscle (e.g., Djojosugito et al., 1970; Hilton, 1963; Humphreys et al., 1971; Kylstra and Lisander, 1970). These changes closely resemble normal physiological reactions occurring during muscular exercise (e.g., Rushmer, 1959; Rushmer and Smith 1959; Wilson et al., 1961) or locomotion and food intake in dogs (Antal, 1963).

Increases in pulse and mean systemic pressures ordinarily elicit baroreceptor reflexes. The finding that stimulation of the posterior hypothalamus induced neither a reflexive decrease in blood pressure nor reflexive bradycardia led Hilton (1963) to suggest that the baroreceptor reflexes may be suppressed during such stimulation of the hypothalamus. Subsequent experiments (e.g., Gebber and Snyder, 1970; Humphreys et al., 1971; Kylstra and Lisander, 1970) have fully confirmed Hilton's hypothesis as it pertains to the inhibition of reflexive bradycardia, but have failed to confirm the inhibition of reflexive hypotension. In these experiments stimulation of the posterior hypothalamus has been shown to block the bradycardia evoked by increased sinus pressure or carotid sinus stretch, but has not altered the accompanying depressor response. Kylstra and Lisander (1970) have shown that this suppression of reflexive bradycardia in conjunction with the persistence of the reflexive hypotension has considerable functional significance. Thus, cardiac output increases without a proportional increase in cardiac workload, and the increased output selectively favors increased blood flow to muscles.

The cardiovascular changes induced by stimulation of the posterior hypothalamus in lightly anesthetized animals closely resemble the physiological reactions occurring during muscular exercise (e.g., Rushmer and Smith 1959; Wilson et al., 1961). These include vasoconstriction in the splanchnic and cutaneous regions, vasodilation in skeletal muscle, as well as increases in heart rate and blood pressure (e.g., Eliasson et al., 1951). The hypothalamic regions from which these cardiovascular responses have been elicited appear to be closely related to the areas in which Hess and Brügger (1943) elicited so-called defense reactions in conscious cats. Defense reactions induced by hypothalamic stimulation frequently begin with an orienting response and then culminate in fight or flight behavior.

Abrahams et al. (1960) sought to determine the relationship between autonomic responses in anesthetized and behavioral responses in unanesthetized cats following intracranial stimulation. Stimulating electrodes were therefore implanted in the posterior hypothalamus, midbrain tegmentum, and central gray. Autonomic responses in anesthetized and behavioral responses in unanesthetized cats were then examined following stimulation through the same electrodes at identical parameter values. Abrahams et al. (1960) observed that stimulation at identical placements in the posterior hypothalamus elicited defensive reactions in unanesthetized cats and cardiovascular responses including increases in heart rate and blood pressure as well as atropine-sensitive vasodilation of skeletal muscle in anesthetized cats. They therefore concluded that the region of the posterior hypothalamus from which vasodilation in skeletal muscle was obtained constituted part of a reflex center that coordinates the autonomic and behavioral responses comprising the defense reaction. Subsequent investigators, examining atropine-sensitive vasodilation elicited by stimulation of the posterior hypothalamus in anesthetized preparations, have typically referred to the site of stimulation as the defense area (e.g., Djojosugito et al., 1970; Humphreys et al., 1971).

The intensities of intracranial stimulation used by Abrahams et al., (1960) were considerably above the threshold required to elicit autonomic responses. Using relatively less-intense stimulation, Abrahams et al., (1964) working with cats and Uvnäs (1967) and his collaborators working with dogs have elicited atropine-sensitive vasodilation accompanied by orienting, but not defensive behavior. This has led both groups of investigators to suggest that the constellation of behavioral and autonomic responses associated with moderate intensities of posterior hypothalamic stimulation, constitute a preparatory pattern that normally occurs immediately prior to muscular exertion. Similar views have been expressed by Rushmer (1962) and by Folkow et al., (1965). The examination of cardiovascular changes as preparatory adjustments has been studied in conditioning experiments.

5. Conditioning of Cardiovascular Responses

Abrahams et al., (1964) paired tone as a conditioned stimulus (CS) with peripheral electric shock as the unconditioned stimulus (US) in unanesthetized cats. The constellation of conditioned responses (CRs) included vasodilation in skeletal muscle. Since moderate intensities of stimulation in the posterior hypothalamus elicited similar responses, Abrahams et al. (1964) suggested that both the CRs and the responses to hypothalamic stimulation were preparatory reactions.

Bolme and Novotny (1969) also examined the hypothesis that sympathetic vasodilation in skeletal muscle is a preparatory response. They classically conditioned dogs using tone as the CS and either peripheral electric shock or movement of a treadmill as the US. The CRs and unconditioned responses (URs) under both conditions consisted of increases in heart rate, blood pressure, and muscle blood flow in the hind limb. The finding that exercise on a treadmill as well as peripheral shock can induce conditioned increases in heart rate, blood pressure, and sympathetic vasodilation in skeletal muscle is consistent with the notion that this pattern of responses is preparatory to reactions requiring increased blood flow in skeletal muscle.

Bolme and Novotny (1969) observed that blood flow CRs, but not URs, were abolished by injection of atropine. This suggests that sympathetic vasodilation of muscle is probably most important just before or at the onset of exercise. Once exercise has commenced for several seconds, however, regulation of the muscle blood supply appears to be more heavily influenced by metabolic vasodilator influences than by sympathetic vasodilation (e.g., Berne and Levy, 1972).

The observation that injections of atropine that abolished vasodilation CRs did not abolish blood pressure CRs suggests that the loss of the vasodilation CR was not due to the central influence of atropine upon the CNS. This is an important consideration in interpreting the results of Bolme and Novotny (1969), because injection of atropine has been shown to have CNS effects that can interfere with classical conditioning performance (Downs et al., 1972).

In the Abrahams et al. (1964) and Bolme and Novotny (1969) experiments the cardiovascular CRs resembled the URs. Adams et al., (1968), however, have challenged the view that organisms necessarily anticipate situations that elicit strong emotion or exertion by making preparatory cardiovascular changes similar to those elicited by the emotion or exertion. In their experiments, Adams et al. observed that cats made very different cardiovascular changes during fighting than they did in the period during which a snarling, hissing cat was viewed. Cardiovascular responses during fighting included increases in heart rate, blood pressure, and cardiac output as well as vasodilation in skeletal muscle. In contrast, during the period in which the hissing, snarling cat was presented, the subjects' cardiovascular responses included bradycardia, decreased cardiac output, and vasoconstriction in skeletal muscle.

We have observed some experimental situations in our own laboratory in which cardiovascular CRs and URs were similar to each other, and other situations in which they were not. Thus, for example, when tone was used as the CS and peripheral electric shock was the US, the CRs and URs of monkeys both included increases in heart rate and blood pressure (Augenstein, 1974; Klose, 1974); whereas, the cardiovascular CRs and URs of rabbits were quite different from one another (e.g., Schneiderman et al., 1969; Yehle et al., 1967). The cardiovascular URs in rabbits reflected sympathetic activation and included changes in blood pressure and heart rate. In contrast, the cardiovascular CRs were primarily parasympathetic, and included bradycardia unaccompanied by changes in pressure.

The conditioning studies just cited suggest that the cardiovascular CR is not necessarily a replica of the UR. Therefore, the CNS integration of learned as well as unlearned cardiovascular responses needs to be studied. During the past several years, several studies using lesioning techniques or electrical stimulation of the brain have attempted to examine the CNS integration of learned cardiovascular responses. These studies have begun to clarify some of the relationships between learned and unlearned cardiovascular responses.

5.1. The CNS Integration of Learned Cardiovascular Responses

5.1.1. Lesion Studies

Several experiments have examined the effects of lesions upon cardiovascular conditioning. Classical conditioning of heart rate has been demonstrated in rats with up to 90% of the neocortex removed (Bloch-Rojas, et al., 1964; DiCara et al., 1970). In contrast, DiCara et al., (1970) were unable to demonstrate instrumental conditioning of heart rate in neodecorticated rats. Since neodecorticated rats made heart rate adjustments in the classical conditioning situation, the response deficit in the instrumental situation was apparently not due to the rat's inability to make heart rate adjustments. Even after decerebration, animals reveal relatively few changes in either resting arterial pressure or cardiovascular responsivity to baroreceptor stimulation (e.g., Bacelli et al., 1965; Korner et al., 1969). The data of the DiCara et al. (1970) experiment, however, do suggest that important elements of the cardiovascular integration of instrumental autonomic responses may require cortical involvement.

Smith et al., (1968) classically conditioned squirrel monkeys using a light CS paired with peripheral electric shock as the US. The classical conditioning procedure was superimposed upon a situation in which the monkeys barpressed to secure a food reward. The CRs included increases in heart rate and aortic blood flow as well as a decrease in barpressing. Smith et al. (1968) observed that destruction of the frontal cortex in conjunction with lesions of the lateral hypothalamus eliminated the cardiovascular CRs without affecting the barpress suppression. The results suggest that when a light CS is paired with peripheral shock as the US, the integration of classically conditioned cardiovascular CRs occurs at least as far rostral as the diencephalon.

Durkovic and Cohen (1969) conducted an experiment in pigeons which has helped to relate heart rate CRs and URs to the central integration of cardiovascular responses. In this experiment light was the CS and peripheral electric shock was the US. Prior to conditioning, lesions were made bilaterally either in the (1) central tegmentum, (2) dorsolateral tegmentum at the level of the oculomotor nucleus, or (3) ventromedial tegmentum at the caudal level of the interpeduncular nucleus.

The CRs in a control group included increases in heart rate and breathing rate. Lesions of the central tegmentum influenced the development of neither the heart rate nor the breathing rate CR. In contrast, injury of the dorsolateral tegmentum produced a deficit in heart rate but not breathing rate CRs; and lesions in the ventromedial tegmentum enhanced the magnitude of the heart rate CR without influencing the respiratory CR. The dissociation of the heart rate and breathing rate CRs suggests that the lesions disrupted cardiovascular pathways rather than influencing other mechanisms involved in conditioning.

The results of the Durkovic and Cohen (1969) study suggest that the lesions may have influenced descending cardiovascular pathways. Destruction of the dorsolateral tegmentum disrupted heart rate CRs. Electrical stimulation of the same region had previously been found to increase heart rate and blood pressure (e.g., Enoch and Kerr, 1967a,b). Bilateral destruction of the ventromedial tegmentum enhanced the heart rate CR. Electrical stimulation of this region would be likely to activate a pathway homologous to the depressor–decelerator circuit previously described in cats (e.g., Chai and Wang, 1962; Enoch and Kerr, 1967a,b). Consequently, the lesions of the ventromedial tegmentum may have interrupted a decelerator pathway normally exerting a rate-limiting influence upon cardioacceleration. The results of the experiment were consistent with the hypothesis that the lesions interfered with descending cardiovascular pathways. They did not, however, rule out the alternative or supplementary possibilities that the heart rate changes may have been importantly influenced by either interruption of afferent cardiovascular pathways or other factors.

In summary, the lesion studies suggest that instrumental conditioning of cardiovascular responses may require an intact cortex and that the integration of cardiovascular changes during classical conditioning involve structures as far rostral as the hypothalamus. They also suggest that in conjunction with other methods (e.g., histology, electrical stimulation of the brain, extracellular recording), lesion techniques can provide an important tool for studying the cardiovascular pathways involved in learned cardiovascular adjustments.

5.1.2. Electrical Stimulation of the Brain

Several investigators have used electrical stimulation of structures in the midbrain, hypothalamus, or septal region as the US in order to examine cardiovascular changes during classical conditioning. The CRs have included changes in heart rate, blood pressure, blood sugar level, and leukocyte count (e.g., Ban and Shinoda, 1961; Elster et al., 1970; Lico et al., 1968; Magnitskii, 1953; Malmo, 1965; VanDercar et al., 1970).

Magnitskii (1953) used electrical stimulation of the posterior hypothalamus in rabbits and observed conditioned increases in blood pressure. Subsequently, Ban and Shinoda (1961) used electrical stimulation of the lateral or ventromedial hypothalamus in rabbits as the US. They reported that lateral hypothalamic stimulation induced conditioned decreases and ventromedial hypothalamic stimulation induced conditioned increases in both blood sugar level and leukocyte count. Malmo (1965) working with conscious rats, and Lico et al. (1968) working with anesthetized rabbits have used septal stimulation as the US. Malmo observed conditioned bradycardia, and Lico et al. found both conditioned and unconditioned decreases in blood pressure.

The major contribution of the Ban and Shinoda (1961), Magnitskii (1953), Malmo (1965) and Lico et al. (1968) studies is that they demonstrated that various circulatory changes could be conditioned using electrical stimulation of the brain as the US. The results are also more or less consistent with the functional mapping studies of Hess (1957) and Ban (1966). According to Ban, for example, the septal region and parts of the lateral hypothalamus are essentially parasympathetic regions, whereas, the ventromedial hypothalamus is part of a sympathetic zone. Although the results are consistent with the findings of Ban and of Hess, they also are in agreement with the formulation that stimulation of the anterior and posterolateral hypothalamus activate neuronal mechanisms involved in the regulation of baroreceptor reflexes. What is presently needed, then, is a comprehensive series of studies that will distinguish between alternative formulations, clarify the various relationships between cardiovascular CRs and URs, and relate learned circulatory adjustments to the known facts of cardiovascular integration.

Initially, in our laboratory we used intracranial stimulation as a tool for examining the behavioral and physiological relationships between cardiovascular CRs and URs in rabbits. This strategy subsequently led to our present research program in which we are beginning to examine the neural integration of cardiovascular CRs and URs with a view toward relating these adjustments to their anatomical substrates.

Prior to our using brain stimulation as a US to induce conditioning, we noted that by merely adjusting current intensity of hypothalamic stimulation in rabbits, the direction of heart rate changes and somatic activity could be readily and reliably divided into two distinct classes. One class consisted of increases in heart rate accompanied by overt movement; the other consisted of heart rate decreases unaccompanied by movement. These findings led Elster *et al.* (1970) to examine the relationship between movement or lack of movement on the one hand, and the topography of heart rate URs and CRs on the other.

Elster *et al.* (1970) used a differential conditioning procedure in loosely restrained rabbits. One CS (designated CS+) was immediately followed by intracranial stimulation as the US, whereas, another CS (designated CS−) was never followed by the US. Differentiation is considered to have occurred when the organism learns to respond to the CS+, and does not respond or makes only a small response to the CS−. In the Elster *et al.* study, the US inducing this differentiation consisted of short pulse-train stimulation of the midbrain central gray, subthalamus, or various regions of the hypothalamus.

Elster *et al.* (1970) found that differential conditioning was induced by midbrain, subthalamic, or hypothalamic USs. Greater differential conditioning was induced by diencephalic (subthalamic, hypothalamic) than by midbrain stimulation as the US. Diencephalic stimulation in particular induced a strong positive relationship between diffuse movement and cardioaccelerative CRs and URs.

We observed that cardiodecelerative CRs occurred in instances in which US stimulation elicited a decrease in heart rate and an absence or inhibition of pronounced movement. Conversely, cardioaccelerative CRs occurred in animals in which US stimulation elicited an increase in heart rate accompanied by diffuse somatic activity. The Elster *et al.* (1970) findings therefore indicated that a firm coupling of cardiac and somatic responses occurs when short pulse-train electrical stimulation of the diencephalon is used as the US. Several investigators (e.g., Eliasson *et al.*, 1952; Hess, 1957; Kaada, 1960) have emphasized that the hypothalamus and other limbic system structures are involved in the concomitant regulation of somatic and cardiovascular changes. The nature of cardiac–somatic coupling has also been examined with regard to exercise (e.g., Rushmer, 1962; Rushmer and Smith, 1959) and conditioning (e.g., Obrist, 1965; Obrist and Webb, 1967; Obrist *et al.*, 1972).

The absence of concomitant cardiovascular measures in the Elster *et al.* (1970) experiment precluded an analysis of the autonomic relationships involved in heart rate classical conditioning induced by the intracranial US. Therefore, in our next experiment, VanDercar *et al.* (1970) concomitantly examined heart rate and blood pressure changes during differential classical conditioning induced by US stimulation of the hypothalamus or septal region. In order to examine heart rate conditioning in the absence of gross movement, the US intensity was kept below the threshold for eliciting gross somatic activity.

VanDercar *et al.* (1970) found that differential conditioning developed readily between CS+ and CS−, but no conditioned blood pressure changes were observed. The heart rate CRs and URs both consisted of bradycardia, and the blood pressure UR consisted of a pressor response. Latencies of the blood pressure URs were invariably shorter than those of the heart rate URs. The same patterns of URs and CRs were obtained regardless of the site of the US electrode within the hypothalamus or septal region. Current intensities required to elicit similar URs, however, were considerably greater in the septal region than in the hypothalamus.

Many animals, including the rabbit, initially respond to fear-arousing stimuli by "freezing" (i.e., inhibiting their somatic activity). During instances in which blood pressure increases occur in the absence of movement, a reflexive bradycardia occurs (e.g., Schneiderman *et al.*, 1969). The possibility that the heart rate UR in the VanDercar *et al.* (1970) experiment was a reflexive response to an increase in blood pressure is of interest, because the heart rate CR, which also consisted of bradycardia, occurred in the absence of a blood pressure CR. This indicates that the heart rate CR was not a reflexive response to a change in pressure. Consequently, it seemed to us that the CR and UR might be controlled by different CNS mechanisms. In order to investigate this possibility we conducted a series of investigations in which cardiovascular CRs and/or URs were selectively abolished by various adrenergic blockades.

Since the sympathetic innervation of the arterioles, which control peripheral vasoconstriction, is predominantly alpha-adrenergic, we used the alpha-adrenergic blocking agent, phentolamine, to antagonize sympathetic vascular tone. In contrast to the sympathetic innervation of the arterioles in the skin and mucosa, which is alpha-adrenergic, the sympathetic innervation of the heart is primarily beta-adrenergic. Therefore, we used the beta-blocking agent, propranolol, to antagonize the sympathetic innervation of the heart. Because parasympathetic (vagal) innervation of the heart is cholinergic, atropinic drugs were used to block the vagal innervation. We used methylatropine as well as atropine sulfate in our experiments, because methylatropine passes the blood–brain barrier more slowly than atropine sulfate, and hence has fewer central effects (e.g., Carlton, 1962; Downs et al., 1972; Giarman and Pepeu, 1964).

In our initial study examining the effects of autonomic blockades upon cardiovascular responses to intracranial stimulation, Powell et al., (1972) assessed the effects of pharmacological blockades on URs. Unanesthetized rabbits received high-frequency, short (1.0-second) pulse-train stimulation of the septal region or hypothalamus at current intensities not producing obvious gross movement. Dose-response and time-response effects were observed for heart rate and blood pressure changes following intracranial stimulation under alpha-adrenergic (phentolamine), beta-adrenergic (propranolol), and cholinergic (methylatropine, atropine sulfate) blocking agents.

Intracranial stimulation elicited an increase in arterial blood pressure accompanied by a decrease in heart rate. Both of these cardiovascular changes showed dose-dependent attenuation or abolition following systemic injection of phentolamine. Since phentolamine blocks the innervation of the arterioles rather than the heart, the results indicated that the bradycardia following stimulation in nonblockaded animals was a compensatory baroreceptor response that was secondary to the initial pressor response. We used injection of propranolol and the atropine drugs to examine the reflexive bradycardia. Propranolol, which blocks the sympathetic innervation of the heart, augmented the bradycardia. In contrast, the atropinic drugs converted the heart rate decrease into a reliable acceleration. These results indicate that following stimulation in the nonblockaded rabbit, the sympathetic and parasympathetic innervations of the heart actively opposed one another and that the parasympathetic activity predominated.

Fredericks et al. (1974) conducted two experiments in which autonomic blocking agents were used to compare the physiological bases of heart rate CRs and URs in unanesthetized rabbits. As in the Powell et al. (1972) study, the US consisted of high-frequency, short pulse-train stimulation of the hypothalamus or septal region.

In the first experiment, differential conditioning was established and then during separate sessions the rabbits were injected with phentolamine, propranolol, atropine sulfate, and methylatropine. Because we specifically wanted to compare the effects of the blockades on CRs and URs, each session included US alone as well as CS+ and CS− trials. The changes that occurred in both baseline heart rate and the heart rate URs after administration of the blocking agents were consistent with the known pharmacological properties of the drugs as well as with our previous findings (i.e., Powell *et al.*, 1972).

Our major finding was that phentolamine severely attenuated the heart rate UR, but had little effect upon the heart rate CR. Thus, in most instances the heart rate UR was totally abolished by phentolamine, but on temporally adjacent trials HR CRs continued to occur. Since the baselines were similar on the CS+ trials and on those using the US alone, the diminution of the heart rate UR cannot be attributed to a change in the HR baseline. The results emphasize that while the heart rate UR to short pulse-train stimulation is a reflexive response to a sympathetically induced change in blood pressure, the heart rate CR is not.

In the second experiment of this study, we differentially conditioned rabbits injected with either saline or phentolamine. The phentolamine injected rabbits never made blood pressure or heart rate URs, but nevertheless developed decelerative heart rate CRs. This indicates that the development of decelerative heart rate CRs was not dependent upon baroreceptor feedback to the CNS following US stimulation.

In our initial studies using intracranial stimulation as the US we were primarily interested in the relationship between cardiovascular CRs and URs in situations resembling those observed in rabbits using peripheral shock or other emotionally arousing stimuli. Since we received a similar UR constellation following stimulation at electrode sites throughout the hypothalamus and septal region, we worried about the possibility that our results might be due to some nonspecific, aversive effect such as the stimulation of pain fibers associated with cerebral vessels. We were also very interested in the general relationship between motivation and cardiovascular responses. Consequently, Sideroff *et al.* (1972) examined cardiovascular classical conditioning using appetitive or aversive hypothalamic stimulation as the US. As in our previous studies using intracranial stimulation, the US consisted of short (1.0-second) pulse-trains.

Rabbits were implanted with stimulating electrodes in either the lateral or ventromedial hypothalamus. Upon recovery each animal was tested to determine if it would bar-press to receive stimulation. A day later each rabbit was tested in a shuttle-box preference situation in which the subject received or did not receive stimulation by being on the appropriate side of the box. Then, each animal received differential conditioning. The US consisted of the medial or lateral hypothalamic stimulation received during the previous operant conditioning tests. Current intensity and other parameter values within the pulse-train of the US were identical with those used in the operant conditioning tests.

We found that the rabbits having access to lateral hypothalamic stimulation barpressed to receive stimulation and made approach responses in the shuttle-box. In contrast, the rabbits having access to medial hypothalamic stimulation did not barpress and made escape responses in the shuttlebox. As in our previous studies, the cardiovascular URs of all rabbits consisted of a pressor response and bradycardia; whereas, the CRs consisted only of bradycardia. Thus, while medial and lateral hypothalamic stimulation had very different motivational properties, both provided effective USs for eliciting heart rate CRs. Therefore, it would appear that the directionality and topography of heart rate and blood pressure changes are not necessarily influenced directly by whether a US is appetitive or aversive.

The cardiovascular responses we observed to intracranial stimulation appear to be part of an important constellation of responses used by the aroused rabbit, and cannot be attributed to nonspecific, pain-producing properties of the US. Since the same constellation of cardiovascular URs is elicited throughout the hypothalamus and septal region, however, this precluded our relating the URs to more specific anatomical substrates within these regions. For this reason, it seemed profitable to examine the role that structures such as the anterior and posterolateral hypothalamus play in learned cardiovascular behavior using parameter values permitting URs to be related to an anatomical substrate. In order to develop USs eliciting these diverse patterns of cardiovascular response in the rabbit, Francis *et al.* (1973) examined the effects of anesthetization and changes in pulse-frequency, pulse-train duration, and current intensity upon the heart rate and blood pressure responses of chronically prepared rabbits.

We observed that when 1.0-second trains of stimulation were used, neither anesthetization nor changes in pulse frequency or current intensity induced divergent patterns of cardiovascular responses in various hypothalamic or septal region locations. In contrast, when 10-second pulse trains were used, various patterns of cardiovascular responses could be related to different brain locations. This appeared to be due at least in part to the lower intensities of stimulation required to elicit cardiovascular responses when long pulse-train durations were used. An alternative explanation for the disparity in the kind of cardiovascular responses obtained following short versus long pulse trains is that the long pulse trains may have activated neuronal systems capable of modifying the original cardiovascular responses to stimulation. Thus, the original response to stimulation of the hypothalamus or septal region may be a pressor response accompanied by a reflexive bradycardia, and prolonged stimulation at various brain locations such as the anterior and posterolateral hypothalamus may differentially modulate the original response. At present we are testing this hypothesis.

The finding that long pulse-train stimulation in various parts of the septal region and hypothalamus leads to different patterns of cardiovascular response has been important for the development of our research program. Because we can now use intracranial stimulation to relate various cardiovascular response patterns to specific anatomical substrates, our experimental preparation lends itself to a variety of important behavioral and physiological interventions.

In one set of experiments, for example, we are using long pulse trains of microstimulation to further map the anatomical substrates from which various cardiovascular changes are elicited by stimulation in the hypothalamus and various limbic areas. We are also using long pulse trains of stimulation in the anterior or posterolateral hypothalamus as the US to induce classical conditioning. When used in conjunction with baroreceptor afferent stimulation, these studies should permit us to relate both conditioned and unconditioned cardiovascular responses to CNS induced baroreceptor modulation. Thus, we are now in a position to determine whether presentation of a CS that comes to elicit heart rate and blood pressure increases because it was paired with a particular central US, can then gate the cardiovascular changes induced by stimulation of the aortic depressor nerve. Our use of intracranial stimulation as the US in classical conditioning is therefore allowing us to study the bases of learned cardiovascular regulation in a way that could not be accomplished if we arbitrarily restricted our US to peripheral electric shock.

6. The Analysis of Single Unit Activity

In the previous section we described the manner in which CNS lesions and intracranial stimulation have been used as tools to examine some of the supramedullary structures and mechanisms involved in cardiovascular conditioning. Although interesting and informative, these studies provided relatively little information about the CNS integration of learned cardiovascular responses at the neuronal level. It is apparent from the results of these studies that further analyses of the CNS mechanisms involved in cardiovascular conditioning, as well as a delineation of the pathways mediating cardiovascular CRs and URs, require the use of additional techniques. These include the concomitant recording of cardiovascular activity and the extracellular discharge patterns of individual neurons.

One of the first tasks we faced in initiating such research was the development of a minimally stressed, conscious, nonparalyzed preparation from which stable unit recordings could be obtained over the course of several experimental sessions (Schneiderman et al., 1974; Schwaber, 1973; Schwaber and Schneiderman, 1974). In these experiments recordings were made from the dorsal motor nucleus, nucleus solitarius, and anterior and posterolateral hypothalamus. Spontaneous unit activity was examined as well as discharge patterns to electrical stimulation of the aortic and vagus nerves, and septal and caudate nuclei. Blood pressure and heart rate were monitored and related to the recordings of single-unit activity.

These were the first experiments to document unit recordings from bulbar cardioinhibitory neurons. In order to be classified as cardioinhibitory neurons, the units had to be antidromically activated by stimulation of the vagus nerve and synaptically activated by stimulation of the aortic depressor nerve. The cardioinhibitory neurons were localized in the region of the dorsal motor nucleus within 0.6 mm anterior of obex. Activation of these cardioinhibitory units by stimulation of the septal region or caudate nucleus was also demonstrated.

Several interesting types of units were observed in the nucleus solitarius. Among these were units whose firing rate was correlated with the cardiac rhythm. Some of these units fired in synchrony with the R wave of the electrocardiogram. The activity of these units was apparently closely related to that of the pressure pulse. Units in nucleus solitarius were found that were responsive to aortic and/or vagus nerve stimulation. These units appear to be higher-order baroreceptor afferents, and were of several types. Activation and inhibition of these units by septal region and caudate nucleus stimulation was also demonstrated.

Besides recording unit activity from the medulla, unit activity was recorded in anterior and posterolateral hypothalamus. This activity was responsive to septal region and caudate nucleus stimulation. Several of the hypothalamic units revealed short-latency activation following ipsilateral stimulation. This indicates that fairly direct connections exist between the caudate nucleus and hypothalamus and between the septal region and hypothalamus.

Following train stimulation of the caudate nucleus and/or septal region several hypothalamic units revealed changes in firing rate that covaried with changes in cardiovascular activity. The findings that some of these units showed consistent variations in firing rate approximately 1 second before detectable changes in heart rate or blood pressure occurred, suggest that the connections between the caudate nucleus and hypothalamus and between the septal region and hypothalamus form part of the cardiovascular control system. The finding that behavioral manipulations such as snout tapping concomitantly influenced the hypothalamic units and cardiovascular activity suggests that these units normally play a role in cardiovascular regulation.

Since the septal region and caudate nucleus have been implicated in behavioral suppression and the inhibition of movement (e.g., Brady and Nauta, 1953; Doty, 1969; Ellen and Powell, 1962) it is conceivable that impulses conveyed from these regions to the hypothalamus provide information concerning movement to the cardiovascular control system. Numerous studies have previously related cardiodecelerations to behavioral suppression and/or an inhibition of movement (e.g., Obrist et al., 1972). The results of our extracellular recording study, in which the activity of hypothalamic unit responses to caudate nucleus and septal region stimulation was related to cardiovascular changes, are consistent with the notion that at least part of the integration between movement and cardiovascular activity takes place within the hypothalamus.

Another important finding of our extracellular recording study was that major differences in unit activity occurred between cardiovascular-related neurons in the anterior and posterolateral hypothalamus following telencephalic stimulation. Thus, for example, a distinctive *cardiovascular bursting unit* observed in the posterolateral hypothalamus was never observed in the anterior hypothalamus. Following a single pulse of caudate nucleus or septal region stimulation, these units showed a complex pattern consisting of short-latency (4-msec) activation, followed by strong inhibition, then further long-lasting phase-locked activation. The characteristics of these neurons are unique in vertebrates for several reasons: (1) The effect of a single pulse, as brief as 0.01 msec., produced up to 3 seconds of effect. (2) The effect was absolutely regular with each stimulus pulse triggering off the same activity pattern of activation–inhibition. (3) Behavioral manipulations such as snout tapping produced unit activity closely correlated with concomitant changes in cardiovascular activity. (4) The activity of these neurons was closely related to spontaneously occurring changes in cardiovascular activity.

Many of the findings of our unit study seem relevant to an understanding of the supramedullary CNS integration of learned cardiovascular responses. Medullary units, for instance, were recorded that responded to telencephalic as well as to aortic nerve stimulation. The units were activated in the same manner by telencephalic as by aortic nerve stimulation although activation by telencephalic stimulation was less pronounced and occurred at substantially longer latencies. In addition, it was observed that stimulation of the caudate nucleus or septal region produced cardiovascular effects similar to those produced by stimulation of the medullary areas examined in the present study although the thresholds in the medullary areas were much lower. The results of our extracellular recording experiment are therefore consistent with the notion that the caudate nucleus, septal region, and hypothalamus are critically involved in cardiovascular response selection, and that cardioinhibition, when selected, is mediated by cardioinhibitory interneurons and motor (vagal) neurons within the medulla.

The results of our single unit recording experiment were consistent with the hypothesis that impulses from the extrapyramidal and limbic system activate cardiovascular-related neurons in the hypothalamus and thereby integrate cardiovascular and somatic activities. If this notion is correct, and response selection does indeed occur within the hypothalamus, then the hypothalamus would appear to be an ideal place to begin looking at the neural integration of learned cardiovascular responses. Furthermore, the presence of distinctive cardiovascular-related neurons such as the cardiovascular bursting unit of the posterolateral hypothalamus should facilitate this investigation. Consequently, in our first conditioning study using extracellular recording techniques, we are examining the activity of hypothalamic units during cardiovascular classical conditioning.

Another promising lead stems from our finding of close connections between neurons in the caudate nucleus and cardiovascular-related neurons in the hypothalamus. The caudate nucleus contains many units that respond to stimulation of more than one modality (e.g., Albe-Fessard *et al.*, 1960). Moreover, the participation of the caudate nucleus in motor conditioned responses has been well documented (e.g., Brust-Carmona and Zarco-Coronado, 1971; Chorover and Gross, 1963). More recently, Grinberg-Zylerbaum *et al.*, (1973) found that gross potentials in the caudate nucleus produced by a CS increased during conditioning trials and decreased during extinction. These findings suggest that sensory impulses reaching the extrapyramidal system may be importantly involved in the development of motor CRs. On the basis of the findings of our extracellular recording experiment, it would be of interest to locate the sensory units in the caudate nucleus that show changes during conditioning and to determine whether they are also involved in the response selection stage of cardiovascular URs and CRs within the hypothalamus. Thus, the studies examining sensory influences upon the extrapyramidal system together with our own findings suggest the existence of possible pathways mediating cardiodecelerative CRs. In the case of a diffuse-light CS, for example, such a conditioning circuit might conduct impulses via a retinal–tectal pathway, through the caudate nucleus and hypothalamus to the cardioinhibitory region of the dorsal motor nucleus. The finding that cardiovascular classical conditioning can occur in the decorticate animal is consistent with the hypothesis that such a subcortical pathway may exist. However, our observation that limbic as well as extrapyramidal structures are involved in cardiovascular response selection suggests that the pathways involved in cardiovascular conditioning are actually more complex than described by our simplified circuit.

7. Relations Between Learned and Unlearned Cardiovascular Responses

In this chapter we have begun to examine the role of the CNS in the regulation of learned and unlearned cardiovascular responses. Our examination has furnished us with a brief outline of the supramedullary mechanisms involved in cardiovascular regulation. This outline, in turn, suggests some hypotheses about the manner in which cardiovascular CRs and URs are related to each other.

Recently, Schneiderman (1974) has proposed that cardiovascular CRs in classical conditioning are adaptive responses that prepare the organism to either augment or cope with the effects of the US. During instances in which the US leads to increased muscular exertion and increased demands upon the cardiovascular system (e.g., Bolme and Novotny, 1969), the heart rate CR is likely to be accelerative. In contrast, during situations in which the US does not lead to muscular exertion, but in which sympathetic activation occurs (e.g., Sideroff et al., 1972; VanDercar et al., 1970) a decelerative heart rate CR would serve to decrease the stress placed upon the cardiovascular system. The hypothesis that heart rate CRs have a compensatory function was originally proposed by Subkov and Zilov (1937). They observed that dogs did not initially reveal heart rate changes when injected with Ringer solution. This initial injection procedure can be conceived of as furnishing a neutral CS. After the initial injection of Ringer solution, the dogs were subsequently given systemic injections of adrenaline. The adrenaline injections were given every 2 or 3 days for several weeks. Each of these injections produced cardioacceleration. After the series of adrenaline injections were given, Subkov and Zilov again injected the dogs with Ringer solution. This time the injection elicited a cardiodeceleration. Pairing of the injection procedure (CS) with the administration of adrenaline (US) apparently elicited a compensatory bradycardia as the CR. Subsequent injection of adrenaline again elicited tachycardia.

Siegel (1972) has also provided evidence that CRs can serve a preparatory, compensatory function. Rats initially injected with saline did not show a change in the level of blood glucose. Subsequently, the animals received insulin injections on alternate days for several sessions. Each injection elicited a decrease in blood glucose (hypoglycemia). After receiving several injections of insulin, the rats were tested with an injection of saline. The saline injection now induced an increase in blood glucose (hyperglycemia) as the CR.

Because it is essential for animals to maintain an adequate glucose level, giving an injection of insulin to a normal animal would be dangerous. Therefore, a hypoglycemic CR would be maladaptive. In contrast, the hyperglycemic CR observed by Siegel could be viewed as a preparatory CR made by the organism in anticipation of a reduction of blood glucose due to the insulin US.

In our own experiments (e.g., Sideroff et al., 1972; VanDercar et al., 1970) in which overt movement did not occur, the primary URs were sympathetic in origin, but the CR consisted of bradycardia. Similarly, in the Adams et al. (1968) experiment, heart rate, cardiac output, total peripheral resistance, and vasodilation in muscle all increased once frightening began. Conversely, in the foreperiod during which it was not clear to the animal whether fighting would be permitted, and apparently in most instances it was not, decreases occurred in heart rate, cardiac output, and total peripheral resistance.

The results of the Adams et al. (1968) experiment suggest that in ambiguous situations some species may respond with decreased motor activity and a compensatory heart rate response. In contrast, during highly predictable situations involving exertion (e.g., Bolme and Novotny, 1969) organisms may be expected to make augmenting rather than coping responses. Brady (1967) and Brady et al. (1969) have observed that ambiguous situations (e.g., early training trials) produced one kind of autonomic–endocrine response pattern; whereas, highly predictable contingencies (e.g., during later training) produced another set of responses. The former situation included a conditioned bradycardia, while the latter included conditioned tachycardia. Our present experiments in which we are examining conditioned and unconditioned cardiovascular changes induced by stimulation of the anterior or posterolateral hypothalamus should furnish us with opportunities to further investigate how compensatory and augmenting cardiovascular CRs are integrated.

8. Concluding Statement

In this chapter we have attempted to describe what is presently known about the CNS integration of learned cardiovascular adjustments. An examination of the literature concerning the CNS control of the circulation, as well as our own experimental findings, has convinced us that the detailed analysis of learned circulatory behavior requires a thorough characterization of the major cardiovascular events occurring during conditioning. The administration of selective autonomic blocking agents has helped us to understand some of the extrinsic sympathetic and parasympathetic interactions occurring during the performance of CRs and URs. More direct examination of the performance of individual components of the cardiovascular system is required to clarify the nature of the dynamic circulatory relationships occurring during conditioning. Thus, for example, a detailed assessment is needed of the relative contributions that changes in cardiac output and peripheral resistance make to the performance of cardiovascular CRs and URs. In addition, our comprehension of the CNS integration of learned cardiovascular behavior requires that we be able to relate such mechanisms as sympathetic vasodilation, shunting of the blood flow, and baroreceptor modulation to the performance of CRs.

Although most of our research has been conducted upon rabbits, we have also spent several years developing a chronic preparation to study the cardiovascular dynamics occurring during learned circulatory adjustments in the rhesus monkey. In this preparation we are chronically measuring heart rate, blood pressure, left ventricular pressure, and blood flow from the ascending aorta. By transferring the intracranial stimulation and extracellular unit recording procedures we have developed in the rabbit to our studies using monkeys, we intend to compare the neural and circulatory adjustments made by the two species during the performance of cardiovascular CRs.

As our research program has developed, it has become increasingly evident to us that an understanding of the CNS integration of learned cardiovascular responses at the neuronal level requires the concomitant recording of cardiovascular acivity and the extracellular discharge patterns of individual neurons. Thus far, we have used the rabbit to develop a conscious, nonparalyzed preparation from which stable unit recordings can be obtained over the course of several experimental sessions. We have also recorded from cardioinhibitory neurons in the dorsal motor nucleus, from higher-order baroreceptor afferents in the nucleus solitarius, and from the anterior and posterolateral hypothalamus.

In our present experiments we are recording unit activity from the anterior and posterolateral hypothalamus during classical conditioning. The USs in these experiments consist of peripheral electric shock or intracranial stimulation. The effects of baroreceptor afferent stimulation upon hypothalamic neurons that may be involved in conditioning are being assessed. This phase of our research program should provide us with information at the neuronal level about the role of baroreceptor modulation during cardiovascular adjustments. It should also help us in our endeavor to trace the neural pathways mediating cardiovascular CRs. By synthesizing information, viewpoints and techniques derived from cardiovascular physiology, neurophysiology and behavior we have thus begun to focus our attention upon the CNS integration of learned cardiovascular adjustments.

ACKNOWLEDGMENTS

We thank Mike Gimpl for his advice and comments and Dr. Harvey Swadlow for his key role in the development of our method for recording unit activity from the conscious, nonparalyzed rabbit.

9. References

Abrahams, V. C., Hilton, S. M., and Zbrozyna, A., 1960, Active vasodilation produced by stimulation of the brain stem: Its significance in the defense reaction, *J. Physiol.* (London) *154:*491–513.
Abrahams, V. C., Hilton, S. M. and Zbrozyna, A. W., 1964, The role of active muscle vasodilation in the alerting of the defense reaction, *J. Physiol. 171:*189–202.
Achari, N. K., Downman, C. B., and Weber, W. V., 1968, A cardio-inhibitory pathway in the brain stem of the cat, *J. Physiol. 197:*35.
Adams, D. B., Baccelli, G., Mancia, G., and Zanchetti, A., 1968, Cardiovascular changes during preparation for fighting behavior in the cat, *Nature 220:*1239–1240.
Albe-Fessard, D., Oswaldo-Cruz, E. and Rocha-Miranda, C., 1960, Activités évoquées dans le noyau caudé du chat en réponse a des types divers d'afférences. II. Étude microphysiologique, *Electroenceph. Clin. Neurophysiol. 12:*405–420.
Antal, J., 1962, Carotid sinus reflexes during locomotion and food intake in dogs, *Inter. Physiol. Congr.* 22nd, Leiden, 1962, abstract, *157:*1963.
Augenstein, J., 1974, Differential classical conditioning of heart rate and blood pressure in the rhesus monkey. Unpublished Master's Thesis, Department of Psychology, University of Miami, 1974.
Baccelli, G., Guazzi, M., Libretti, A., and Zanchetti, A., 1965, Pressoceptive and chemoceptive aortic reflexes in decorticate and decerebrate cats, *Am. J. Physiol. 208:*708–714.
Ban, T., 1966, The septo-preoptico-hypothalamic system and its autonomic function, in *Progress in brain research: Correlative neurosciences. Part A. Fundamental mechanisms,* T. Tokizane & J. P. Schade, eds., Elsevier Publishing Company, Amsterdam.
Ban, T., and Shinoda, H., 1961, Experimental studies on the relation between the hypothalamus and conditioned reflex. III. Conditioned response in the variation of the leukocyte count and the blood sugar level, *Med. J. Osaka Univ. 11:*439–453.
Bernard, C., 1852, De la influence du systéme nerveux grand sympathique sur la chaleur animale, *Compt. Rend. 34:*472.
Berne, R. M., and Levy, M. N., 1972, *Cardiovascular physiology,* (2nd ed.) C. V. Mosby, St. Louis.
Biscoe, T., and Sampson, S., 1970, Responses of cells in the brain stem of the cat by stimulation of the carotid sinus, glossopharyngeal, aortic, and superior laryngeal nerves, *J. Physiol. 209:*341–358.

Bloch-Rojas, S., Toro, A., and Pinto-Hamuy, T., 1964, Cardiac vs. somatic-motor conditioned responses in neodecorticated rats, *J. Comp. Physiol. Psychol. 58:*233–236.
Bolme, P., and Novotny, J., 1969, Conditional reflex activation of the sympathetic cholinergic vasodilator nerves in the dog, *Acta Physiol. Scand. 77:*58–67.
Bolme, P., Novotny, J., Uvnäs, B., and Wright, P. G., 1970, Specie distribution of sympathetic cholinergic vasodilator nerves in skeletal muscle, *Acta Physiol. Scand. 78:*60–64.
Brady, J. V., 1967, Emotion and the sensitivity of psychoendocrine systems, in *Neurophysiology and emotions*, D. C. Glass, ed., Rockefeller University Press, New York.
Brady, J., and Nauta, W., 1953, Subcortical mechanisms in emotional behaviors: Affective changes following septal forebrain lesions in the albino rat, *J. Comp. Physiol. Psychol. 46:*339–346.
Brady, S. V., Kelly, D., and Plumlee, L., 1969, Autonomic and behavioral responses of the rhesus monkey to emotional conditioning, *Ann. N.Y. Acad. Sci. 4:*24–31.
Brodal, A., 1957, *The reticular formation of the brain stem: Anatomical aspects and functional correlations,* Oliver and Boyd, Edinburgh.
Brown, A. M., 1969, Sympathetic ganglionic transmission and the cardiovascular changes in the defense reaction in the cat, *Circulation Res. 24:*843–849.
Brust-Carmona, H., and Zarco-Corondao, I., 1971, Instrumental and inhibitory conditioning in cats. II. Effects of paleocortical and caudate nucleus lesion, *Boletin del Instituto de Estudies Medicos y Biologicos* (National University, Mexico), *27:*61–70.
Bülbring, E., and Burn, J. H., 1935, The sympathetic vasodilator fibres in the muscles of the cat and dog, *J. Physiol. 83:*483–501.
Bunzl-Federn, E., 1899, Der centrale Ursprung des Nervus Vagus, *Monat. Psychiat. Neurol. 5:*1–22.
Carlton, P. L., 1962, Some behavioral effects of atropine and methylatropine. *Psychol. Rep. 10:*579–582.
Chai, C. Y., and Wang, S. C., 1962, Localization of central cardiovascular control mechanism in lower brain stem of the cat, *Am. J. Physiol. 202:*25–30.
Chorover, S. L., and Gross, C. G., 1963 Caudate nucleus lesions: Behavioral effects in the rat, *Science 141:*826–827.
Cottle, M. K., 1964, Degeneration studies of primary afferents of IXth and Xth cranial nerves in the cat, *J. Comp. Neurol. 122:*329–343.
Crill, W. E. and Reis, D. J., 1968, Distribution of carotid sinus and depressor nerves in the cat brain stem, *Am. J. Physiol. 214:*269–276.
Dell, P., 1952, Corelations entre le systeme vegetatif et le systeme de la vie de relation. Mesencephale, diecephale et cortex cerebral, *J. Physiol.* (Paris) *44:*471–557.
DiCara, L. V., Braun, J. J., and Pappas, B. A., 1970, Classical conditioning and instrumental learning of cardiac and gastrointestinal responses following removal of neocortex in the rat, *J. Comp. Physiol. Psychol. 73:*208–216.
Dittmar, C., 1873, Ueber dei Lage des sogennanter Gefässzentrums in der Medulla oblongata, *Ber Sachs. Ges. Wiss. Mat. Phys. Kl., 25:*449.
Djojosugito, A. M., Folkow, B., Kylstra, P., Lisander, B., and Tuttle, R. S., 1970, Differentiated interaction between the hypothalamic defense reaction and baroreceptor reflexes. I. Effects on heart rate and regional flow resistance. *Acta Physiol. Scand. 78:*376–383.
Doty, R. W., 1969 Electrical stimulation of the brain in behavioral context, in, P. H. Mussen and M. R. Rosenzweig (eds.), *Ann. Rev. Psychol. 20:*289–321.
Downs, D., Cardozo, C., Schneiderman, N., Yehle, A. L., VanDercar, D. H., and Zwilling, G., 1972, Central effects of atropine upon aversive classical conditioning in rabbits, *Psychopharmacol. 23:*318–333.

Dreifuss, J. J., and Murphy, J. T., 1968, Convergence of impulses upon single hypothalamic neurons, *Brain Res. 8:*167–176.

Durkovic, R. G., and Cohen, D. H., 1969, Effects of caudal midbrain lesions and conditioning of heart and respiratory rate responses in the pigeon, *J. Comp. Physiol. Psychol. 69:*329–338.

Eliasson, S., Folkow, B., Lindgren, P., and Uvnäs, B., 1951, Activation of sympathetic vasodilator nerves to the skeletal muscle in the cat by hypothalamic stimulation, *Acta Physiol. Scand. 23:*333–351.

Eliasson, S., Lingren, P., and Uvnäs, B., 1952, Representation in the hypothalamus and the motor cortex in the dog of the sympathetic vasodilator outflow to the skeletal muscle, *Acta Physiol. Scand. 27:*18–37.

Ellen, P., and Powell, E., 1962, Effects of septal lesions on behavior generated by positive reinforcement, *Exptl. Neurol. 6:*1–11.

Elster, A. J., VanDercar, D. H., and Schneiderman, N., 1970, Classical conditioning of heart rate discriminations using subcortical electrical stimulations as conditioned and unconditioned stimuli, *Physiol. Behav. 5:*503–508.

Enoch, D. M., and Kerr, F. W. L., 1967a, Hypothalamic vasodepressor and vesicopressor pathways I. Functional studies, *Arch. Neurol. 16:*290–306.

Enoch, D. M., and Kerr, F. W. L., 1967b, Vasopressor and vesicopressor pathways II. Anatomic study of their course and connections, *Arch. Neurol. 16:*307–320.

Euler, U. S. von and Folkow, B., 1958, The effect of stimulation of autonomic areas in the cerebral cortex upon adrenaline and noradrenaline secretion from the adrenal gland of the cat, *Acta Physiol. Scand. 42:*313–320.

Fang, H. S., and Wang, S. C., 1962, Cardioaccelerator and cardioaugmentor points in the hypothalamus of the dog, *Am. J. Physiol. 203:*147–150.

Folkow, B., and Uvnäs, B., 1950, Do adrenergic vasodilator nerves exist? *Acta Physiol. Scand. 20:*329–337.

Folkow, B., Langston, J., Oberg, B., and Prerovsky, I., 1964, Reactions of the different series-coupled vascular sections upon stimulation of the hypothalamic sympatho-inhibitory area, *Acta Physiol. Scand. 61:*476–483.

Folkow, B., Heymans, C., and Neil, E., 1965, Integrated aspects of cardiovascular regulation, *Handbook of Physiology. Circulation,* Section 2, Vol. 1, 1787–1824.

Francis, J., Sampson, L., Gerace, T., and Schneiderman, N., 1973, Cardiovascular responses of rabbits to ESB: Effects of anesthetization, stimulus frequency and pulse train duration, *Physiol. Behav. 11:*195–203.

Fredericks, A., Moore, J. W., Metcalf, F. U. Schwaber, J. S., and Schneiderman, N., 1974, Selective autonomic blockade of conditioned and unconditioned heart rate changes in rabbits, *Pharmacol. Biochem. Behav. 2:*in press.

Gebber, G. L., and Snyder, D. W., 1970, Hypothalamic control of baroreceptor reflexes. *Am. J. Physiol. 218*(1):124–131.

Gellhorn, E., 1957, *Autonomic Imbalance and the Hypothalamus,* University of Minnesota Press, Minnesota.

Gellhorn, E., 1964, Motion and emotion: The role of proprioception in the physiology and pathology of the emotions, *Psychol. Rev. 71:*457–472.

Giarman, H. J., and Pepeu, G., 1964, The influence of centrally acting cholinolytic drugs on brain acetylcholine levels, *Brit. J. Pharmacol. 23:*123–130.

Goldfein, A., and Ganong, W. F., 1962, Adrenal medullary and adrenal cortical responses to stimulation of the diencephalon, *Am. J. Physiol. 202:*205–211.

Green, J. H., 1967, Physiology of baroreceptor function: Mechanism of receptor stimulation, in *Baroreceptors and Hypertension,* P. Kezall, ed., Pergamon, Oxford.

Green, H. D., and Hoff, E. C., 1937, Effects of faradic stimulation of the cerebral cortex on limb and renal volumes in the cat and monkey, *Am. J. Physiol. 118:*641.

Grinberg-Zylerbaum, J., Prado-Alcala, R., and Brust-Carmona, H., 1973, Correlation of evoked potentials in the caudate nucleus and conditioned motor responses, *Physiol. Behav. 10:*1005-1009.

Hardy, J. D., 1961, Physiology of temperature regulation, *Physiol. Rev. 41:*521-606.

Hess, W., 1957, *Functional organization of the diencephalon,* Grune and Stratton, New York.

Hess, W. R., and Brügger, M., 1943, Das subkorticale zentrum der affektiven abwehr-reaktion, *Helv. Physiol. Acta 1:*33-52.

Heymans, L., and Neil, E., 1958, *Reflexogenic areas of the cardiovascular system,* J. A. Churchill, London.

Hilton, S. M., 1963, Inhibition of baroreceptor reflex on hypothalamic stimulation, *J. Physiol.* (London) *165:*56.

Hilton, S. M., and Spyer, K. M., 1969, The hypothalamic depressor area and the baro-receptor reflex, *J. Physiol. 200:*107-108.

Hilton, S. M., and Spyer, K. M., 1971, Participation of the anterior hypothalamus in the baroreceptor reflex, *J. Physiol. 218:*271-293.

Hilton, S. M., and Zbrozyna, A. W., 1963, Amygdaloid region for defense reactions and its efficient pathway to the brain stem, *J. Physiol.* (London) *165:*160-173.

Hirata, Y., 1965, Subcortical projections from the orbital surface of the cat's brain, *Acta Med. Biol.* (Miigata), *13:*123-142.

Hockman, H., and Talesnik, J., 1971, Central nervous system modulation of baroreceptor input, *Am. J. Physiol. 221*(2):515-519.

Hoff, E. C., and Green, H. D., 1936, Cardiovascular reactions induced by electrical stimulation of the cerebral cortex, *Am. J. Physiol. 117:*411-422.

Honig, C. R., and Myers, H. A., 1968, Evaluation of possible adrenergic and cholinergic mechanisms in sympathetic vasodilation, *Fed. Proc. 27:*1379-1383.

Humphreys, P. W., Joels, N., and McAllen, R. M., 1971, Modification of the reflex response to stimulation of carotid sinus baroreceptors during and following stimulation of the hypothalamic defense area in the cat, *J. Physiol. 216:*461-482.

Kaada, B. R., 1960, Cingulate, posterior orbital, anterior insular, and temporal pole cortex, in *Handbook of Physiology,* Vol. II, J. Field, H. W. Magoun, and V. E. Hall, eds., Williams and Wilkins, Baltimore.

Kaada, B. R., Pribram, K. H., and Epstein, J. A., 1949, Respiratory and vascular responses in monkeys from temporal pole, insula, orbital surface and cingulate gyrus, *J. Neurophysiol. 12:*347-356.

Klevans, L. R., and Gebber, G. L., 1970, Faciliatory forebrain influence on cardiac component of baroreceptor reflexes, *Am. J. Physiol. 219:*1235-1241.

Klose, K. J., 1974, Adrenergic and cholinergic blockade of cardiovascular classical condi-tioning in the rhesus monkey. Unpublished Master's Thesis, Department of Psychology, University of Miami.

Koch, E., 1931, *Die Reflextorische Selbsteurung des Kreislaufes,* Steinkopf, Leipzig.

Kohnstamm, O., 1901, Zur anatomie und physiologie der vagus kerne, *Neurol. Zbl. 16:*767-793.

Korner, P. I., 1971, Integrative neural cardiovascular control, *Physiol. Rev. 51:*312-367.

Korner, P. I., Uther, J. B., and White, S. W., 1969, Central nervous integration of the respira-tory responses to arterial hypoxia in the rabbit, *Circulation Res. 24:*757-776.

Kylstra, P. H., and Lisander, B., 1970, Differential interaction between the hypothaalmic defense area and baroreceptor reflexes. II. Effects on aortic blood flow as related to work load on the left ventricle, *Acta Physiol. Scand. 78:*386-392.

Lico, M. C., Hoffman, A., and Covian, M. R., 1968, Autonomic conditioning in the anesthetized rabbit, *Physiol. Behav., 3:*673–675.

Lindgren, P., and Uvnäs, B., 1953, Vasodilator responses in the skeletal muscles of the dog to electrical stimulation in the oblongata medulla, *Acta Physiol. Scand. 29* (Suppl. 137):105–108.

Lindgren, P., and Uvnäs, B., 1954, Postulated vasodilator center in the medulla oblongata, *Am. J. Physiol. 6:*68–76.

Lindgren, P., Rosen, A., Strandberg, P., and Uvnäs, B., 1956, The sympathetic vasodilator and vasoconstrictor outflow—a cortico-spinal autonomic pathway, *J. Comp. Neurol. 105:*95–104.

Löfving, B., 1961, Cardiovascular adjustments induced from the rostral cingulate gyrus, *Acta Physiol. Scand. 53:* (Suppl. 84):1–82.

Magoun, H. W., 1938, Excitability of the hypothalamus after degeneration of corticofugal connections from the frontal lobe, *Am. J. Physiol. 112:*530–532.

Magnitskii, A. M., 1953, Attempt to apply the "dominant" concept to the analyses of blood pressure changes in hypertension, "Problemy eksperimental 'noi gipert. onicheskoi bolezni", *Trudy Akad. Med. Nauk. 3:*22. Cited by E. Simonson and J. Brojek, 1959, Russian research on arterial hypertension, *Ann. Int. Med.* pp. 129–193.

Malmo, R. B., 1965, Classical and instrumental conditioning with septal stimulation as reinforcement, *J. Comp. Physiol. Psychol. 60:*1–8.

Miller, F., and Bowman, J., 1916, The cardioinhibitory center, *Am. J. Physiol. 39:*149–153.

Obrist, P. A., 1965, Heart rate during conditioning in dogs: Relationship to respiration and gross bodily movements. *Proceedings of 73rd Annual Convention of the American Psychological Association*, pp. 165–166.

Obrist, P. A., and Webb, R. A., 1967, Heart rate during conditioning in dogs. Relationship to somatic-motor activity, *Psychophysiol. 4:*7–34.

Obrist, P. A., Sutterer, J. R., and Howard, J. L., 1972, Preparatory cardiac changes: A psychobiological approach, in *Classical Conditioning. II. Current Theory and Research*, A. H. Black & W. F. Prokasy, eds., Appleton-Century-Crofts, New York, pp. 312–340.

Owsjannikow, P., 1871, Die tonischen und reflectorischen centern der gefässnerven, *Ber. Sachs. Ges. Wiss. Mat-Phys. Kl. 23:*135.

Powell, D. A., Goldberg, S. R., Dauth, G. W., Schneiderman, E., and Schneiderman, N., 1972, Adrenergic and cholinergic blockade of cardiovascular responses to subcortical electrical stimulation in unanesthesized rabbits, *Physiol. Behav. 8:*927–936.

Ramon y Cajal, 1909, *Histologie du systeme nerveux de l'homme et des vertebres*, A. Maloine, Paris.

Ranson, S. W. and Billingsley, P. R., 1916, Vasomotor reactions from stimulation of the floor of the fourth ventricle, *Am. J. Physiol. 41:*85.

Reis, D., and Cuenod, N., 1965, Central neural regulation of carotid baroreceptor reflexes in the cat, *Am. J. Physiol. 209:*1267–1279.

Reis, D. J., and Oliphant, M. C., 1964, Bradycardia and tachycardia following electrical stimulation of the amygdaloid region in the monkey, *J. Neurophysiol. 27:*893–912.

Rushmer, R. F., 1959, Constancy of stroke volume in ventricular responses to exertion, *Am. J. Physiol. 196:*745–750.

Rushmer, R. F., 1962, Effects of nerve stimulation and hormones on the heart: The role of the heart in general circulatory regulation, in *Handbook of physiology: Circulation*, W. F. Hamilton, section ed., Section 2, Volume 1, *American Physiology Society* Washington, pp. 533–550.

Rushmer, R. F., and Smith, O. A., 1959, Cardiac control, *Physiol. Rev.* 39:41–68.

Schneiderman, N., 1974, The relationship between learned and unlearned cardiovascular responses, in *Cardiovascular psychophysiology: Current issues in response mechanisms, biofeedback and methodology,* P. A. Obrist, A. H. Black, J. Brenner, and L. V. DiCara, eds., Aldine-Atherton Press.

Schneiderman, N., Schwaber, J. S., and Gimpl, M., 1974, 'Cardiovascular Units' in anterior and posterolateral hypothalamus, *Fed. Proc. 33:*430.

Schneiderman, N., VanDercar, D. H., Yehle, A. L., Manning, A. A., Golden, T. and Schneiderman, E., 1969, Vagal compensatory adjustment: Relationship to heart rate classical conditioning in rabbits, *J. Comp. Physiol. Psychol. 68:*175-183.

Schramm, P., and Bignall, K. E., 1971, Central neural pathways mediating active sympathetic muscle vasodilation in cats, *Am. J. Physiol. 223:*754-767.

Schramm, L. P., Honig, C. R. and Bignall, K. E., 1971 Active muscle vasodilation in primates homologous with sympathetic vasodilation in carnivores, *Am. J. Physiol. 221:*768-777.

Schwaber, J. S., 1973, Cardioinhibitory units in dorsal motor nucleus and cardiovascular units in hypothalamus and nucleus solitarius of the conscious rabbit. Unpublished doctoral dissertation, Department of Psychology, University of Miami, 1973.

Schwaber, J. S., and Schneiderman, N., 1974, Cardiac units in dorsal motor nucleus and nucleus solitarius of the rabbit, *Fed. Proc. 33:*429.

Sideroff, S., Elster, A. J., and Schneiderman, N., 1972, Cardiovascular classical conditioning in rabbits (Oryctolagus cuniculus) using appetitive or aversive hypothalamic stimulation as the US, *J. Comp. Physiol. Psychol. 81:*501-508.

Siegel, S., 1972, Conditioning of insulin-induced glycemia, *J. Comp. Physiol. Psychol. 78:*233-241.

Smith, O. A., Nathan, M. A., and Clarke, N. P., 1968, Central nervous system pathways mediating blood pressure changes, *Hypertension 16:*9-22.

Subkov, A. A., and Zilov, G. N., 1937, The role of conditioned reflex adaptation in the origin of hyperergic reactions, *Bull. Biol. Med. Exptl. 4:*294-296.

Uvnäs, B., 1967, Cholinergic vasodilator innervation to skeletal muscles, *Circulation Res.* 20 (Suppl. 1):83-90.

VanDercar, D. H., Elster, A. S., and Schneiderman, N., 1970, Heart rate classical conditioning in rabbits to hypothalamic or septal US stimulation, *J. Comp. Physiol. Psychol. 72:*145-152.

Wall, P. D., and Davis, G. D., 1951, Three cortical systems affecting autonomic functions, *J. Neurophysiol. 14:*507-517.

Weber, E. F. W., and Weber, E. H., 1845, Experimenta quibus probatus nervos vagos rotatione machinae galvano-magneticae irritatos, motum cordi retardare et adeo intercipare, *Ann. Univ. Med. Milano 20:*227-228.

Wilson, M. F., Clarke, N. P., Smith, O. A., and Rushmer, R. F., 1961, Interrelation between central and peripheral mechanisms regulating blood pressure, *Circulation Res.* 9:491-496.

Yehle, A., Dauth, G., and Schneiderman, N., 1967, Correlates of heart-rate classical conditioning in curarized rabbits, *J. Comp. Physiol. Psychol. 64:*98-104.

CHAPTER 9

A Psychobiological Perspective on the Cardiovascular System *

Paul A. Obrist, James E. Lawler, and Claude J. Gaebelein

Department of Psychiatry, Medical School
University of North Carolina
Chapel Hill, North Carolina

1. Introduction

Our research concerns the interaction between cardiovascular and behavioral processes. It primarily involves two parameters of the activities of the heart, rate and contractile force, and deals with two interrelated questions. First, can cardiovascular activity tell us anything about behavioral processes? This is the traditional approach of using a biological event as an index of some behavioral state or process. Second, can behavioral processes influence the cardiovascular system, particularly in regard to the etiology of pathological conditions of the cardiovascular system? This is the question of psychosomatics.

Over the past decade, cardiovascular activity, particularly heart rate (HR), has drawn considerable interest in psychophysiological endeavors for several reasons. For one thing, there is likely no parameter of biological function that is as easily and as reliably measured as is HR. Second, HR is consistently modified by behavioral interventions. Third, some interesting and at times paradoxical results have emerged. For example, contrary to motivational concepts, e.g., activation theory, HR has been observed in some species and with some paradigms to decrease either in anticipation of or in the presence of motivating events. Such effects have in turn resulted in

* This chapter is based on research supported by grant MH 07995, National Institute of Mental Health, USPHS, and institutional grant HD 03110 from the National Institute of Child Health and Human Development, USPHS, to the Biological Research Center of Child Development Institute, University of North Carolina, Chapel Hill.

a conceptual reorientation such as is illustrated by the work of the Laceys (1970; 1974). Fourth, HR has been shown to be subject to modification by operant or biofeedback techniques, sometimes quite dramatically.

The purpose of this chapter is to provide a perspective as to how HR, and to a lesser extent cardiac contractility and blood pressure, might interact with behavioral processes. In doing so, we will rely particularly on our own research. Certain issues and problems will be highlighted, and an argument will be made for the necessity of a biological strategy in the study of the cardiovascular–behavioral interaction.

One implication which consistently emerges from contemporary research is that HR does not provide the simple, unidimensional index of behavioral processes, such as motivational and affective states, which many of us had either believed or hoped it would (see Lacey, 1967; Rescorla and Solomon, 1967; Elliott, 1974; Roberts, 1974). Although the recent evidence that HR is subject to modification by operant procedures has acted to sustain if not revitalize interest in this biological event, there remains both conceptual controversy as to the significance of the data as well as methodological issues over replicability (see Black, 1974; Brener, 1974; Brener et al., 1974; DiCara, 1974; Hahn, 1974; Miller and Dworkin, 1974; Obrist et al., 1974; Roberts et al., 1974). On the other hand, some consensus is evolving that HR reflects what our behavioral paradigms have done to modify striate muscular or somatic activity, among other things. This would come as no great surprise to the exercise physiologist except that we are not usually talking about an exercising organism, but rather about quite subtle activity which in order to be observed commonly requires the recording of bioelectric potentials. This has been bothersome because it has reawakened the artifact issue (Smith, 1967) and leaves us in the position of questioning the significance of HR to behavior.

It is important that we do not ignore the relationship HR can have to somatic activity because it provides us with a perspective as to what HR might tell us about behavioral processes, information which at least in one context has proven useful (see next section). However, we believe that heart rate, as well as other cardiovascular parameters, will relate to or be influenced by behavioral processes independently of what they tell us about the state of the striate musculature, but not in the abiological–unidimensional manner we have traditionally believed. The basis of this faith is that cardiovascular processes are likely more continually atuned to the organism's interaction with its environment than other visceral process. On the other hand, it is a system commonly subject to pathological influences. Thus, something must intervene between this highly functional, adaptable system, as seen in the normal individual and pathological states. Furthermore, it is not too far fetched to believe that this intervention must, among other things, involve the way the system has been influenced by the organism's interactions with its environment. Our further belief is that we shall not understand the relevance of this system to behavior or pathology unless we resort to a biological strategy, an approach more typical of current research. By a biological strategy we refer to any approach that is concerned with how different parameters of cardiovascular function relate to one another or to other visceral and somatic events within the confines of behavioral paradigms, and how in turn the central nervous system modulates and controls these events. The remainder of this chapter will illustrate more concretely the application of a biololgical strategy and hopefully demonstrate its validity in behavioral research.

2. Cardiac–Somatic Coupling

It is only recently that any effort has been made to evaluate the relationship between HR and somatic activity within the more commonly used behavioral paradigms. A fair degree of consensus is developing that there is a pronounced relationship between each type of event (see Black and DeToledo, 1972; Brener, 1974; Elliott, 1974; Obrist *et al.*, 1974; Roberts, 1974). Our own efforts in evaluating this relationship stem from studies concerning the anticipatory deceleration of HR during classical aversive conditioning in humans. This anticipatory deceleratory effect was perplexing since it was in the opposite direction than the acceleratory unconditioned response and was contrary to our expectation that under such conditions sympathetic acceleratory effects should be seen. We had little success in understanding this effect by more traditional explanations involving stimulus parameters like UCS intensity (Obrist, *et al.*, 1965), the CS–UCS interval (interstimulus interval or ISI) (Hastings and Obrist, 1967), and the type of UCS (Wood and Obrist, 1968). Similarly, when we first looked at the deceleration biologically we found no evidence that it was secondary to the conditioning of still other peripheral events like blood pressure (Obrist *et al.*, 1965) or respiration (Wood and Obrist, 1964; Obrist *et al.*, 1969). The only evidence that evolved from these latter studies was that the deceleratory effect involved an increase in vagal (i.e., parasympathetic), restraint on the heart that masked a weak sympathetic excitatory effect on the heart (Obrist *et al.*, 1965; Obrist *et al.*, 1970b). That is, once the vagal innervation was blocked pharmacologically, a small sympathetic acceleratory effect was observed. This was of some interest since sympathetic effects could be observed galvanically, and in the vasomotor response at the same time they were masked on heart rate by vagal effects.

That there might be a relationship between HR and somatic activity in behavioral studies was first suggested when we subjected dogs to classical aversive conditioning, and found a relationship between anticipatory increases in HR and increased somatic activity (Obrist and Webb, 1967). On the basis of this finding as well as some less direct evidence, it was hypothesized that if increases in HR were concomitant with increases in somatic activity, then perhaps anticipatory decreases in HR would be related to anticipatory decreases in somatic activity. This was verified in both the classical conditioning and the reaction time (RT) paradigms where the decrease in both effects anticipate the UCS or the execution of the motor response (Obrist, 1968; Obrist et al., 1969; 1970; Webb and Obrist, 1970).

2.1. Overview of Data

Several aspects of these results deserve emphasis. First, the phasic changes in HR and somatic activity are directionally related, either both increasing or decreasing, and are frequently related in magnitude. Only the latency of the effects differs, with HR usually lagging somatic changes by about a second, an effect which seems accountable by intrinsic latency differences (Smith, 1945; Lofving, 1961). Second, except in dogs, where the increases in activity can be very pronounced, both the cardiac and somatic changes usually are of small amplitude and a short duration. For example, HR changes are in the range of 2–6 beats per minute (bpm) with a duration of 2–6 seconds. The types of somatic activity measured involve events ranging from postural adjustments to such subtle activities as eye movements, and activities in and around the mouth, e.g., swallowing. Figure 1 illustrates the concomitance between two somatic measures and HR averaged over 240 nonreinforced test trials during classical aversive conditioning in 20 adult humans. Depicted are the second-by-second changes from CS onset with regard to base level, for HR, chin EMG, and eye movements. Third, the alterations in somatic activity involve task irrelevant background activity. That is, activities a subject indulges in while sitting in a chair waiting for the next trial. The phasic decreases in somatic activity can be likened to a momentary state of suspended animation.

Our evidence quite consistently indicates that the cardiac–somatic effects we are dealing with are a biologically substantive phenomenon, i.e., events that have a common mediating mechanism. For example, we have up until recently been unable to demonstrate changes in HR unaccompanied by reliable and directionally related changes in somatic activity, although a fair effort has been made to do so. In dogs, for example, cardiac

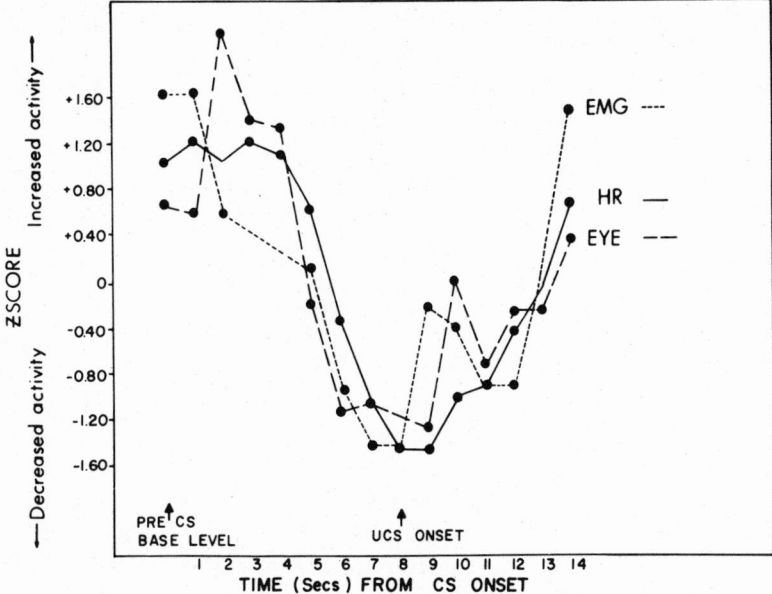

FIG. 1. Second-by-second changes from base level in heart rate, chin EMG, and eye movements and blinks on nonreinforced test trials during classical aversive conditioning in humans. Note: based on 12 trials on each of 20 subjects.

and somatic activity were related during an experimental conflict procedure (Obrist and Webb, 1967), in an appetitive task where reinforcement was contingent on first an increase and then a decrease in somatic activity (Webb and Obrist, 1967), and when a classical aversive conditioning procedure was superimposed on a appetitive variable interval operant baseline (Sutterer and Obrist, 1972). It was believed at the time that with these procedures an influence of affective–motivational processes on HR would be disentangled from influences associated solely with somatic activity for two reasons. First, with a conflict procedure, the motivational impact of the situation should be far greater than with aversive procedures alone (Masserman, 1943). Second, in two of the studies, somatic activity was experimentally controlled; this should allow any nonsomatic influences on HR associated with behavioral processes to be manifested.

In humans, several lines of evidence indicate the significance of the cardiac–somatic relationship. In several experiments, the consistency was evaluated between phasic alterations in somatic activity and HR. It was found, for example, that EMG activity from chin muscles was associated with an accelerated HR during the base period of an aversive classical con-

ditioning study. In turn, this elevated base level resulted in a larger anticipatory decrease in HR on trials where anticipatory EMG activity was observed to decrease during the interstimulus interval (ISI) (Obrist, 1968). In
a RT task, trials on which HR is slowest during the preparatory interval
were associated with less somatic activity than trials where HR was more
accelerated (Obrist et al., 1970b). Experimental manipulation of either the
duration and certainty of the preparatory interval (PI) of a RT task (Webb
and Obrist 1970) or the ISI during classical aversive conditioning (Obrist,
1968) influenced HR and somatic activity in a similar manner. The phasic
HR and somatic decreases associated with the executive of the motor
response in a RT task have not only been observed with adults, but in four
age groups of children ranging from 4 to 10 years of age (Obrist et al.,
1973). This was an important observation since it was believed that particularly in the younger age groups, the cardiac or somatic changes might not
be consistently related if they were not in fact integrated events. Within the
aversive conditioning paradigm manipulation of one somatic parameter,
respiration, had a similar influence on HR and two other somatic measures
(Obrist et al., 1969). Using an operant paradigm in which HR increases or
decreases were shaped to avoid shock, somatic activity was influenced in a
similar manner. When recourse was made to control somatic activity, the
HR changes were appreciably reduced with little evidence that the contingency had any influence on HR independent of somatic activity (Obrist et
al., 1974b). Finally, within the aversive conditioning paradigm, the anticipatory HR deceleration observed in cats has been found to be concomitant with decreases in the electrical activity of the pyramidal tract
(Howard et al., 1974).

2.2. Biological and Behavioral Significance

This relationship between HR and somatic activity raises two fundamental issues. First, how can this effect be understood biologically? The
neurophysiological evidence indicating that cardiovascular and somatic
activity have common integrating mechanisms within the central nervous
system (Obrist et al., 1970a) has led us to conclude that HR and somatic
effects may be different aspects of the same response process. This conclusion is not contraindicated by the demonstration of HR changes in the
curarized   preparation,   since   curare   only   blocks   the   peripheral
manifestation of somatic activity and the resulting afferent processes, not
the central mechanisms that could initiate each effect. We have further
viewed the HR changes as tied to the metabolic function of the heart. That
is, in the exercising organism HR tends to be directly related to both

cardiac output and O_2 consumption (Wang *et al.*, 1960). That we can still observe a relationship between HR and somatic activity even when metabolic requirements and cardiac output are virtually unaltered indicates to us that HR can be very intimately integrated with somatic activity. Thus, we propose, that even these subtle HR effects involve CNS processes which are similar to those involved when an appreciable metabolic load, such as exercise, is placed on the organism. We know of no alternative mechanism that could account for the effects observed.

The second issue concerns the significance of these somatically coupled HR changes to behavioral processes. In this regard one can conclude that HR, to the extent that it provides a more or less global estimate of the state of the striate musculature, will be relevant to behavioral events if the state of the striate musculature is of some significance. As such, a case can be made that such information is useful in both the aversive conditioning and RT paradigm. In the former situation one possibility is that the decreases in both HR and somatic activity reflect the response of an organism when shock is unavoidable and inescapable—one might liken it to conditioned helplessness (Seleigman *et al.* 1971). It is even possible that such changes are functional, acting to attenuate the aversiveness of the stimuli since recourse to flight or fight is not possible. There is only clinical and anecdotal evidence which bears on this possibility (Obrist *et al.*, 1969). However, there is experimental evidence that in the nonaversive RT paradigm the phasic decreases in HR and somatic activity are biological manifestations of attentional processes. For example, the magnitude of the HR deceleration has been found to be directly related to performance as assessed both intra- and interindividually (Lacey and Lacey, 1970). A similar direct relationship has been observed between speed of performance and the magnitude of the phasic decreases in both somatic activity and HR (Obrist *et al.*, 1969; 1970b; Webb and Obrist, 1970). It is, of course, not very parsimonious for similar biological events to have a different significance to behavioral processes in the two types of situations, i.e., aversive and nonaversive. A unitary hypothesis would be to consider the HR and somatic effects which anticipate aversive stimuli as a hightened attentional state occurring when some environmental danger is imminent (see Hastings and Obrist, 1967; Lacey and Lacey, 1974).

The relationship between phasic somatic and HR changes and the relationship of each to attentional processes in the RT paradigm illustrates the advantage of a biological strategy. Such an approach establishes the biological mechanism by which HR is decelerated (i.e., cessation of irrelevant somatic activity), which in turn suggests the basis of the covariation between the HR deceleration and performance (i.e., cessation of irrelevant somatic activity enhances performance). A question that remains unanswered is whether the phasic HR effects are particularly sensitive to alterations in attentional states. This is a particularly important problem since HR, in contrast to the somatic measures, is simpler to measure, more reliable, and may provide in one muscle the best single estimate of what the total striate musculature is doing; this would have significant methodological advantages.

The evidence on this problem is equivocal. Several studies using a RT paradigm primarily with adults and assessing only HR have manipulated attentional states in several manners, and all have found that HR is more decelerated with heightened attention (Lacey and Lacey, 1970; Higgins, 1971; Jennings et al., 1971; Sroufe, 1971). On the other hand, we have found in two separate studies in children that manipulating attention by using different age groups (Obrist et al., 1973), or within an age group by the use of incentives (Meyers and Obrist, 1972), did not influence the magnitude of the phasic HR deceleration. Similarly, two somatic measures, general activity and chin EMG, were not influenced by these manipulations except on one occasion when the influence of age related differences in base levels was corrected by covariance. Elliott (1974) also reports that a manipulation of incentive in the RT paradigm influenced neither cardiac nor somatic effects in 7-year-olds. This failure to find an influence of attentional manipulation in the developing human suggests that in the immature organism that HR may lack the necessary sensitivity to be very useful.

There can be no question in our own studies that the manipulation of attention by either age or incentive was successful, since in both studies performance time and one measure of task-irrelevant somatic activity, namely, occular activity, were both influenced by the attentional manipulation. Somatic activity has been observed to have greater sensitivity and certainty than HR to the manipulation of foreperiod duration in adults (Obrist et al., 1970b; Webb and Obrist, 1970). Therefore, as things stand, the phasic HR deceleration coincident with responding in an RT task appears to be sensitive inconsistently to the manipulation of attentional states, and either no more sensitive or even less sensitive than the phasic decrease in one or more measures of task-irrelevant somatic activity. There appear to be no studies which have evaluated the sensitivity of HR and somatic effects in tasks involving more sustained periods of attention.

In summary, a considerable amount of evidence indicates that the vagally mediated phasic HR effects observed in several simple behavioral paradigms primarily reflect the state of the striate musculature. Within the RT paradigm, a case can be made that the phasic HR deceleration reflects momentary shifts in attentional states and to varying degrees of sensitivity. The consistency with which somatic activity has been observed to relate to HR should not be misconstrued to indicate that nonsomatic influences associated with behavioral processes do not influence HR. It is our judgment that such nonsomatic influences have not been convincingly demonstrated to influence the vagally mediated phasic changes observed in the RT, and the operant and the classical conditioning paradigms.

In the next section, data will be presented demonstrating such nonsomatic influences, but involving sympathetic influences on the heart and in more stressful experimental paradigms. Also, the recent work of the Laceys (Lacey and Lacey, 1974), indicating that events within the cardiac cycle influence sensory–motor processes via afferent processes, does not directly involve somatic coupling. It is, of course, desirable to demonstrate that HR can tell us more about behavioral processes than the state of the striate musculature since it makes HR more significant to behavioral processes, as Elliott (1974) has suggested. However, we do not feel that we should continue to delude ourselves that these vagally mediated, phasic HR changes have unique qualities regarding attentional, motivational, or emotional states of the organism which do not concern the state of the musculature, until it can be shown that in fact this is the case.

3. Cardiac–Somatic Uncoupling

It has been our contention, and apparently that of many other investigators, that the heart can be influenced by behavioral processes independently of somatic activity. However, this contention was not based on particularly definitive experimental evidence. It is suggested by observations in humans with hyperkinetic beta-adrenergic circulatory states (Frohlich *et al.,* 1969), as well as in both normals and hypertensives (Brod, 1963), of stress-induced alterations in cardiac output which appear excessive relative to the metabolic requirements of the situation. In these studies, somatic activity or metabolic requirements have not been systematically assessed although Brod (1963) did evaluate O_2 consumption in the forearm muscles and observed no significant change. Brod did not assess total oxygen consumption.

The observation that was particularly intriguing was our failure to observe appreciable sympathetic influences on HR, particularly in the classical conditioning paradigm. The fact that sympathetic influences could be seen in vasomotor and sudomotor responses indicated that sympathetic activation had been elicited. The hypothesis was then made based on still other evidence (see Obrist *et al.,* 1970a) that sympathetic influences on HR were not observed because they are more clearly manifested on the force of the cardiac contraction rather than HR. It was further hypothesized that any nonsomatic behavioral influence would be mediated via sympathetic activity. This was suggested by the observation that somatic activity decreased (Obrist, 1968) under conditions in which a weak sympathetic influence on HR was observable once vagal influences were pharmacologically blocked. If sympathetic influences were metabolically relevant or somatically coupled, they should be directly, not inversely, related to somatic activity such as in exercise (Robinson et al., 1966).

3.1. An Evaluation of Sympathetic Effects

Our first effort was to determine in a chronic dog preparation using classical aversive conditioning procedures whether contractile force depicted sympathetic influences more clearly than HR. This necessitated developing a measure of contractile force. Based on a suggestion by Rushmer (1964) an indirect technique was used which involved rate of change measures in one of three manifestations of left ventricular performance: the rate at which blood is accelerated in the aorta, the rate at which the left ventricle contracts, and the rate at which aortic blood pressure climbs from diastole to systole. All measures were found to have an acceptable degree of reliability and validity. Measurement of the rate of change in pressure, however, seemed to be the best technique, particularly since it can be used in humans. It is not possible to measure contractile force more directly, such as by assessing the rate at which individual muscle units contract and the synchrony in which the units contract (see Lawler and Obrist, 1974, for a discussion of the problem). It should be emphasized that we are dealing with a rate of change measure, and not a volumetric or magnitude measure.

This first work in the chronic dog preparation did in fact indicate that contractile force more clearly depicted sympathetic influences than HR (Obrist et al., 1972b). The next study involved human subjects; contractile force was measured noninvasively by assessing the rate of change or slope of the ascending limb of the carotid pulse wave (Obrist et al., 1974c). This study verified the results obtained in the dog, but also demonstrated for the first time that the sympathetic effects were independent of somatic activity. The study involved a RT task in which subjects were instructed that they would be shocked sometimes if their performance on any one trial was not fast enough. On each trial changes in the two cardiovascular parameters, rate and force of contraction, and in three measures of somatic activity were evaluated relative to baseline in each of 30 seconds commencing with the ready signal. The PI was 8 seconds and shock, if administered, occurred 8 seconds after the execution of the motor response. In 11 of the 33 subjects, the sympathetic innervation of the heart was blocked pharmacologically so

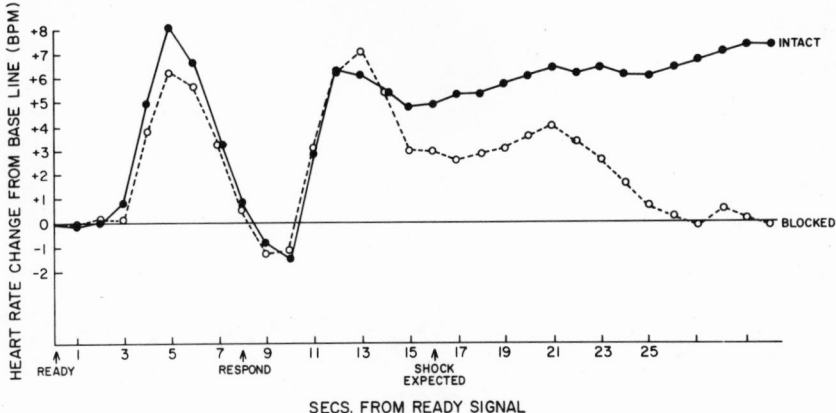

FIG. 2a.   Second-by-second changes from base level in heart rate on nonshock trials during a stressful reaction time task in humans with (N = 483 trials) and without (N = 253 trials) an intact sympathetic innervation.

as to determine the contribution of sympathetic influences to any observed changes in either HR or contractile force.

Figures 2a,b,c depict the second-by-second changes in HR, contractile force and one of the somatic measures, general activity, for each experimental group excluding trials when shock was administrated. During the 8-second PI and over the course of the next 4–5 seconds, HR showed a

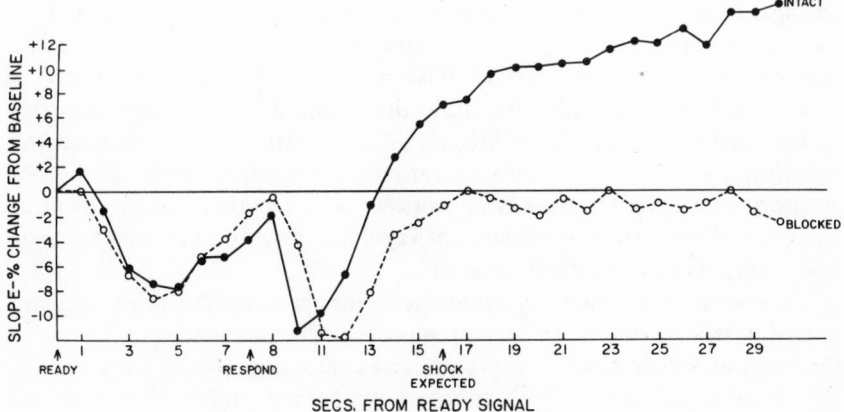

FIG. 2b.   Second-by-second changes from base level in cardiac contractility, i.e., slope of the carotid pulse wave, on nonshock trials during a stressful reaction time task in humans with (N = 483 trials) and without (N = 253 trials) an intact sympathetic innervation.

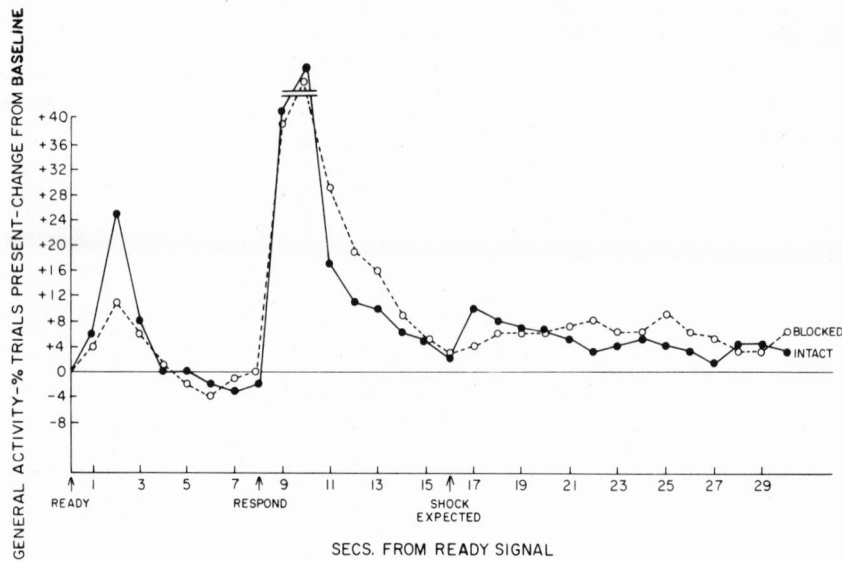

FIG. 2c.   Second-by-second changes from base level in general activity on nonshock trials during a
stressful reaction time task in humans with (N = 483 trials) and without (N = 253 trials) an intact
sympathetic innervation.

triphasic response, first increasing, then decreasing as the subject
responded, and then increasing again. This effect was seen with and without
an intact sympathetic innervation, indicating that it was due to variations
in vagal tone. A concomitant triphasic effect was also seen with each of the
somatic measures. Contractility during this interval did not increase.
Rather, the slope of the carotid pulse wave extended below base level in
both experimental groups, indicating that some influence other than that
contributed by sympathetic effects on contractile force modified this
manifestation of left ventricular performance. Therefore, in this part of the
measurement period there was no evidence of sympathetic involvement on
the heart. There was only evidence of vagal influences on HR which was directionally related to somatic activity.

However, a pronounced sympathetic influence on the heart that appeared unrelated to somatic activity was observed commencing just prior to
the point at which shock is expected, and continuing for the remainder of
the measurement period. With an intact sympathetic innervation there was
an increase in the slope of the carotid pulse wave above baseline and a
further acceleration of HR, both of which continually increased through
the remainder of the measurement period. These effects represent sym-

pathetic influences on both HR and contractile force since, with the sympathetic innervation blocked, the slope of the carotid pulse wave did not increase above baseline and HR decreased toward baseline. Therefore, it appeared that heart rate as well as contractility can be influenced by sympathetic activity, once it is evoked. However, sympathetic influences were more clearly manifested on the contractile measure. That is, when the slope of the carotid pulse wave first became elevated above baseline, synergistic vagal and sympathetic influences on HR were evident.

Two aspects of the data indicate that these sympathetic effects are independent of somatic activity. First, with an intact innervation the cardiac and somatic changes are in the opposite direction. Second, with a blocked innervation, the HR changes parallel the somatic effects throughout the measurement period. We have one other study in which HR was also observed to be independent of somatic activity, although the influence of the sympathetic innervation has not yet been evaluated. In the study attempting to modify HR by operant techniques using shock avoidance (Obrist *et al.*, 1974b) seven groups of between 12–15 subjects each have been run. The groups varied with respect to whether increases or decreases in HR were reinforced, to the extent to which somatic activity was experimentally controlled, and to whether reinforcement was contingent upon HR changes. Regardless of the experimental condition, on the first block of three trials, and particularly on the first trial, an acceleration of HR of approximately the same magnitude was observed in all groups while there was no consistent somatic effect. Such an independence of HR and somatic activity was of short duration, however, since on later trials and where the reinforcement contingency was found to be effective as defined by acquistion effects, HR and somatic activity were then found to be significantly related.

3.2. Possible Significance of Sympathetic Effects

We have now found in two paradigms that HR, and in one pardigm contractile force, can be independent of somatic activity, i.e., an increase in HR and contractile force was observed either in the absence of reliable changes in somatic activity, or when somatic activity was decreasing. The cardiac effects appeared to involve the sympathetic innervation in the one study where they were evaluated. These data raise several questions which at the present cannot be definitely answered. However, enough data is available from various sources to warrant some educated guessing.

One question concerns why these effects have been observed in the more recent studies and not in the previous ones. There are at least two possible reasons. First, the recent studies were intended to be more stressful by recourse to several procedural changes. These changes involved procedures such as not giving the subjects experience with the aversive stimulus prior to its first administration for a less than criterion response. With the pervious aversive conditioning procedures, subjects had experienced the shock prior to conditioning since they set their own shock levels. Also, feedback on the adequacy of performance was both delayed and not consistently given, and in the case of the operant paradigm, it was difficult for subjects to determine on any one trial whether the criterion was being met. With the operant procedure, subjects were also never instructed in what they specifically must do to avoid shock. In all, these procedural changes might be thought to result in a more stressful situation than those used in the previous aversive conditioning studies because of the greater uncertainty they create about several aspects of the experiment.

Second, the more recent tasks differ from the earlier ones using aversive conditioning procedures by making it possible for subjects to avoid the aversive events rather than just sitting there and taking it with no possibility of escape or avoidance. On the face of it, the opportunity to avoid might be considered a procedural change which would act to weaken the effectiveness of the other procedural changes instituted to elevate the stressful quality of the situation. We do not yet have evidence on this. However, we believe that the opportunity to avoid or cope is a necessary dimension of the situation in order for sympathetic effects to be evoked. That is, the evocation of sympathetic effects on the heart is a function of both stress intensity and the opportunity to cope with the stress. There are several lines of evidence which bear on this latter possibility. For example, in a follow-up study using the shock-avoidance reaction-time task, direct recordings of arterial blood pressure were made which involved a puncture of the radial artery. There can be no question that a radial puncture is a stressful procedure in which the subjects passively accept the circumstances. Yet invariably associated with the puncture is a rather pronouced vagal inhibition of HR and hypotensive effect. In one subject, who actually fainted, a very pronouced sympathetic effect was observed 20 minutes later on the avoidance task which was associated with a hypertensive episode. Such data clearly argue that there is not a simple direct relationship between sympathetic activity and stress intensity. However, the situations do differ with regard to the opportunity to avoid or cope. There is still other evidence suggesting the relevance of what might be best referred to as a passive–active parameter to sympathetic effects (see Obrist et al., 1974a,c; Elliott, 1974; Brod, 1963).

In a sense, the possibility that active coping is a relevant stimulus condition suggests that a somatic component might be still relevant with regard to sympathetic effects, but in this case the cardiovascular effect is likely greatly exaggerated or excessive relative to metabolic requirements. It may be, as Brod (1963) has suggested, that these sympathetic effects are anticipatory to exercise such as flight or fight. Brod (1963) observed very appeciable increases in cardiac output and muscle blood flow during a stressful mental arithmetic task. He likened the effects to exercise, but considered them anticipatory since the subject clearly was not exercising, nor did it appear that elevated output was required metabolically. If these anticipatory effects are considered in the light of the vagally mediated HR changes seen in the nonstressful RT paradigm, the aversive conditioning paradigm, and in exercise itself, where they seem very closely coupled to somatic activity, it appears that when the sympathetic component is evoked, there is clearly a short-circuiting of the integrating mechanisms concerned with metabolic function.

A second question raised by our observation of an independence of sympathetic effects on the heart and somatic activity concerns the significance of sympathetic influences with respect to the effects of stress on cardiovascular function. We are particularly fascinated by several aspects of the data which suggest that we are dealing with a very substantive biological phenomena. For one thing, these sympathetically mediated effects are larger than any we have seen using classical aversive conditioning and the nonstressful RT task. For example, in the recent RT stress study some subjects were observed to go from a resting base level HR of 75 bpm to a base level of 120 bpm during the RT task, with further phasic increases in HR following execution of the motor tasks reaching 140 bpm which were sustained for as much as 20–30 seconds. Figure 3 shows an example of such an effect during one of the early RT trials.

A second aspect of the data concerns pronounced individual differences with regard to the size of these effects. Some subjects show very small cardiovascular changes even though they indicate that the task is very stressful. For example, in the follow-up RT stress study in which blood pressure was directly recorded, several subjects showed virtually no cardiovascular changes except for a small 5–6-mm-Hg pressor response during the PI, and the triphasic vagally mediated HR effect during the first 12–14 seconds of a trial. The basis for these individual differences is not clear. The observation that some nonresponsive subjects clearly judged the task as very stressful suggests that hypo- or hyperresponsiveness is an inherent characteristic of the organism and is relevant to what the Laceys (Lacey and Lacey 1958) have called response stereotypy.

Also, in the study where blood pressure was directly recorded, there are several aspects of the blood pressure data worth noting. First, all subjects, regardless of how responsive they are, demonstrate the small pressor

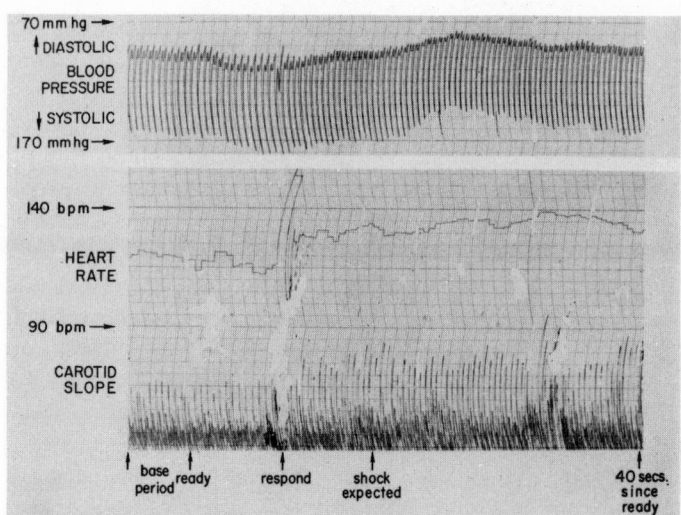

FIG. 3.   An example of a single trial during a stressful reaction time task in a
human subject demonstrating heart rate, contractility as measured by the
slope of the carotid pulse wave, and blood pressure changes. Note: Blood
pressure recorded so that diastolic blood pressure is on the upper part of the
tracing and systolic blood pressure on the lower part of the tracing.

response during PI, where in the previous study (see Fig. 2a,b) no sympathetic influence on the heart was seen. This quite clearly demonstrates
the presence of sympathetic influences which is specific to vasomotor
activity.

A second, and perhaps most perplexing observation, was that in the
most reactive subjects a depressor response was observed which commenced 5–6 seconds after sympathetic influences on HR and contractility
were manifested, and which terminated while HR and contractility were
still elevated. This depressor response was particularly pronounced on trials
where HR and contractility increases were greatest. It is also illustrated in
Fig. 3. On a couple of occasions, it peaked at 60-mm Hg below the elevated
base level. One possible explanation for this depressor effect is that it
reflects a massive sympathetic discharge which involves not only the heart,
but an appreciable vasodilation of the musculature, such as Kelly *et al.,*
(1970) and Mathews and Lader (1971) have reported with a stressful
arithmetic task. The vasodilation results in a drop in pressure because of a
decrease in total peripheral resistance (TPR), which is momentarily greater
than the increase in cardiac output associated with the elevated HR and
contractility. If this is so, it suggests, in the light of other aspects of our
data from past as well as present experiments, that we might have to con-

ceptualize sympathetic activity as involving two subsystems. One involves sympathetic influences on the sudomotor and vasomotor–constrictor responses which are evoked by novel stimuli which are not necessarily very stressful. A second system is evoked by more intense stress, when the subject attempts to cope, and involves not only sudomotor and vasomotor activity, but the heart and vasodilatory processes as well. This latter subsystem is more in line with the emergency function sympathetic influence has been viewed as having (Cannon and Rosenblueth, 1937).

A third aspect of the blood pressure data is that base levels of blood pressure in sympathetically responsive subjects were higher than with the nonresponsive subjects. Also, base levels of HR were elevated, and there appeared at times to be a direct relationship between base levels of HR, contractility, and blood pressure. For example, one of these subjects had a resting HR prior to the start of the RT task of 60 bpm and a resting blood pressure of 110/55. During the RT task his base level HR was 93 bpm and his blood pressure was 143/72. The phasic depressor effect and the further acceleration of HR and contractility following the execution of the motor response were superimposed on these higher base levels. These various aspects of the blood pressure data and how they relate to HR and contractility are not simple and warn us that blood pressure, like HR, does not provide a simple unidimensional depiction of what stress does to the organism. Nonetheless, the fact that elevations of tonic levels of blood pressure are associated with elevations of tonic levels of HR and contractility suggests that these effects may be relevant to one current conceptualization regarding the etiology of essential hypertension. This is the model which considers a high cardiac output state as the initial hemodynamic process in the development of hypertension (Frohlich et al., 1970). We do not have data in human subjects directly relevant to this problem. However, a recent animal study by Dr. James E. Lawler (Lawler et al., 1974) in our lab bears on this problem and represents our first systematic effort to evaluate this hemodynamic model.

4. Hypertensive Effects—Chronic Dog Preparation

There are several purposes to this work, among which is to create a hypertensive effect and then to assess the hemodynamic basis of the effect. For this purpose, dogs were chronically implanted with an electromagnetic blood flow probe on the ascending aorta and an aortic catheter. From these we can obtain, among other things, cardiac output, blood pressure, a continuous estimate of TPR, and an indirect estimate of contractility. The dogs were exposed daily to a 1-hour avoidance session using signaled shock to shape them to a Sidman avoidance schedule. In three dogs on which data are collected and reasonably completely quantified, a very pronounced hypertensive effect has been seen in one, while modest and small effects have been seen in the other two. The effects were most pronounced during the initial training period, and became attenuated over the 10 or more sessions on which the dogs are on the Sidman schedule.

Figure 4 presents the average systolic and diastolic blood pressure, cardiac output, and TPR during 17 consecutive daily sessions in the most reactive dog. The data are presented separately for the initial seven training sessions; during the first and last five sessions the dog was on the Sidman schedule. Also presented are the average values during a 1-hour rest period just prior to each avoidance session (preavoidance) and a 15-minute rest just following avoidance (post-avoidance). The preavoidance hour just prior to the first training session was used as a reference point or baseline to compare the effects of the aversive procedures on each cardiovascular parameter. These values appear as the first single bar graph and are labeled rest; they are henceforth referred to as the resting baseline. Blood pressure during the pre-, post-, and avoidance periods was elevated over the resting baseline by approximately 70 mm Hg during training and by 40 mm Hg

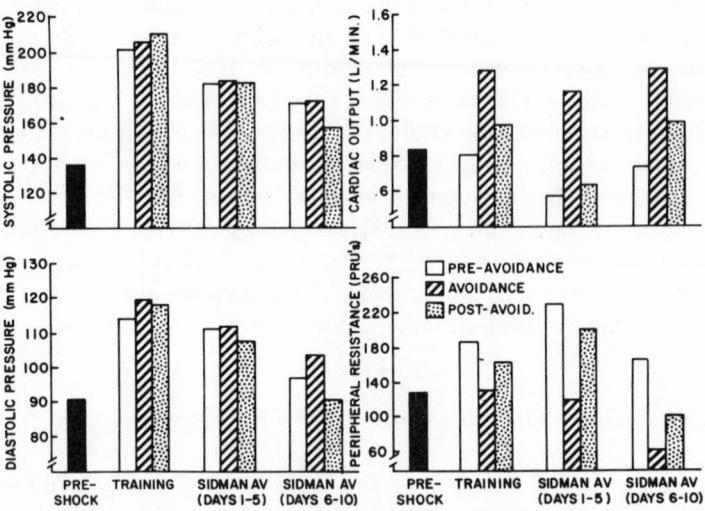

FIG. 4. Systolic and diastolic blood pressure, cardiac output and total peripheral resistance averaged over a 1-hour pre-avoidance period, a 1-hour avoidance period and a 15-minute post-avoidance period in a dog using a Sidman avoidance procedure. Data broken down into a rest or baseline values prior to the first avoidance session, during training, and the first and last half of the days the dog was on the Sidman schedule.

once the dog was on the Sidman schedule. The hemodynamic basis of this pressure elevation, however, varied between the pre–post periods and the avoidance hours. During the pre- and post- avoidance periods, it was primarily attributable to an elevation of peripheral resistance, but during avoidance primarily to an elevation of cardiac output. The latter was due to an elevation of HR and a large increase in contractility which maintained stroke volume. Although the magnitude of the blood pressure rise became attenuated once the dog was on the Sidman schedule, the hemodynamic processes maintained the same pattern. Similar but less pronounced effects were seen in the other two dogs whose blood pressure elevations on the training days peaked at approximately 50 mm Hg above the resting baseline in one and 10 mm Hg in the other dog.

In all dogs, the influence of cardiac output on pressure was most pronounced during the first minutes of each avoidance session. For example, in the most reactive dog, cardiac output was at its maximum while pressure peaked at approximately 150 mm Hg above the resting baseline. It is not clear why these large pressure changes were not sustained within sessions. A similar time effect is seen in humans for whom heart rate and carotid slope increases were most pronounced on the first trials.

The effects observed during the avoidance sessions are consistent with the hypothesis concerning the influence of an elevated cardiac output in the etiology of hypertension. Another facet of this model stipulates that an increased TPR occurs secondary to cardiac output increases due to excessive tissue perfusion which initiates autoregulatory processes (Coleman et al., 1971). The data are not definitive with respect to this possibility. Total peripheral resistance is elevated, particularly during the pre- and post-avoidance hour in the most reactive dog, whereas in the least reactive dog it is elevated only during training. However, there is no way to evaluate autoregulatory influences more definitively in the present data since tissue perfusion was not evaluated.

Overall, these first data from the chronic dog preparation serve several purposes. First, they establish the feasibility of a relatively long-term chronic preparation which provides up to seven parameters of cardiovascular function. The only significant parameter not known is the distribution of blood. Second, the data establish that an appreciable hypertensive effect can be found in some dogs, and that such effects can have a different hemodynamic basis. Third, the approach is promising in that it is relevant to evaluating models of the etiological basis of an experimental hypertension and lends some credence to one model. However, this work is preliminary and asks more questions than it answers. Perhaps one of the more significant unknowns is the extent to which the cardiovascular effects are relevant to metabolic requirements. We believe that this is the cornerstone on which to evaluate the influence of behavioral stress on cardiovascular function. Put another way, this is the problem of cardiac–somatic coupling and uncoupling. If a given behavioral stressor results in a cardiovascular adjustment which is metabolically relevant, i.e., somatically coupled, then it can be argued that the stress has not had any unique influence on cardiovascular activity. That is, it acts like any metabolic load such as exercise to result in an appropriate adjustment of the system. On the other hand, to the extent behavioral stress results in a cardiovascular adjustment which is excessive to metabolic requirements, then the stress assumes unique significance and added importance and may well be relevant to pathological conditions.*

5. Summary

This chapter may be summarized by proposing several hypotheses which seek to depict the means by which the functioning of the heart and behavioral processes interact. In reasonably non- or mildly stressful behavioral paradigms, which are likely characteristic of most paradigms used with normal human subjects, there is no significant influence of the sympathetic innervation on the heart. The changes in HR observed under these conditions, to the extent that they are controlled by extrinsic, i.e., neural–humoral processes, are due either to increases or to decreases in vagal (i.e., parasympathetic) restraining influences. In turn, the available data indicate that these variations in vagal activity are somatically coupled. Thus, these HR changes are only relevant to behavioral processes to the extent to which they reflect the activity of the striate musculature. This does not deny that nonsomatic behavioral processes may influence the vagal innervation, but rather, that under the conditions studied, available data do not convincingly indicate such an influence, nor the means by which it is mediated. Should such a nonsomatic influence be demonstrated, new vistas concerning the possible behavioral significance of HR changes may emerge. At present, a case can be made that these vagally mediated HR effects are related under certain circumstances to attentional processes because of their relationship to task-irrelevant somatic activity. Similarly, if somatic activity is related to other aspects of behavioral processes, e.g., immobility of freezing associated with affective states, then HR might serve to depict these states.

* The problem of assessing metabolic relevance is not insurmountable since one can obtain both O_2 consumption (if cardiac output is known) and tissue perfusion from the measurement of arterio-venous oxygen differences.

Although sympathetic influences on the heart, as manifested by both rate and force of contraction, are normally very minimal, it is proposed that they can be evoked by reasonably intense stress and situations in which the organism actively engages in preparing or executing activities that will cope with the stress. This is in contrast to helplessness or passivity. It may also be that sympathetic effects under such conditions are only evoked in certain individuals, and as such might be considered as an inherent characteristic. The cardiovascular response observed when sympathetic influences are evoked appears to be an excercise response, yet the organism is not exercising, but only engaging in less extensive somatic acts or anticipating activity. Thus, the cardiovascular response is metabolically maladaptive. In this context, somatic activity is critical only in the sense that it is one way an organism can actively involve itself in coping. It is this sympathetic effect which we believe now has the most significance to behavior, since it may be the means by which behavioral stressors uniquely influence the heart and may be relevant in the etiology of pathological conditions of the cardiovascular system, particularly some types of essential hypertension.

This scheme regarding the significance of sympathetic influences is not new. It differs from more traditional views only in that it suggests the conditions under which sympathetic effects are significant, and attempts to correct the assumption that sympathetic influences on the heart are constantly involved in behavioral processes.

6. References

Black, A. H., 1974, Operant autonomic conditioning: The analysis of response mechanisms, in *Cardiovascular Psychophysiology*, P. A. Obrist, A. H., Black, J. Brener, and L. V. DiCara, eds., Aldine, Chicago, p. 229.

Black, A. H., and DeToledo, L., 1972, The relationship among classically conditioned responses: Heart rate and skeletal behavior, in, *Classical Conditioning II: Current Theory and Research*. A. H. Black and W. F. Prokasy, ed., Appleton-Century, Crofts, New York, pp. 290–311.

Brener, J., 1974, A general model of voluntary control applied to the phenomena of learned cardiovascular change, in *Cardiovascular Psychophysiology*, P. A. Obrist, A. H. Black, J. Brener, and L. V. DiCara, eds., Aldine, Chicago, p. 365.

Brener, J., Eissenberg, E., and Middaugh, S., 1974, Respiratory and somatomotor factors associated with operant conditioning of cardiovascular responses in curarized rats, in *Cardiovascular Psychophysiology*, P. A. Obrist, A. H. Black, J. Brener, and L. V. DiCara, eds., Aldine, Chicago, p. 251.

Brod, J., 1963, Haemodynamic basis of acute pressor reactions and hypertension, *Brit. Heart J. 25:227*.

Cannon, W. B., and Rosenblueth, A., 1937, *Autonomic Neuro-Effector Systems*, MacMillan, New York.

Coleman, T. G., Granger, H. J., and Guyton, A. C., 1971, Whole body circulatory autoregulation and hypertension, *Circulation Res. 28*(Suppl. II): 76.

DiCara, L. V., 1974, Some critical methodological variables involved in viseral learning, in *Cardiovascular Psychophysiology,* P. A. Obrist, A. H. Black, J. Brener, and L. V. DiCara, eds., Aldine, Chicago, p. 276.

Elliott, R., 1974, The motivational significance of heart rate, in: *Cardiovascular Psychophysiology,* P. A. Obrist, A. H. Black, J. Brener, and L. V. DiCara, eds., Aldine, Chicago, p. 505.

Frohlich, E. D., Tarazi, R. C., and Dustan, H. P., 1969, Hyperdynamic B-adrenergic circulatory state. Increased B-receptor responsiveness, *Arch. Internal Med. 123:*1.

Frohlich, E. D., Kozul, V. J., Tarazi, R. C., and Dustan, H. P., 1970, Physiological comparison of labile and essential hypertension, *Circulation Res. 27:*(Suppl.): 6.

Hahn, W. W., 1974, The learning of autonomic responses by curarized animals, in *Cardiovascular Psychophysiology,* P. A. Obrist, A. H. Black, J. Brener, and L. V. DiCara, eds., Aldine, Chicago, p. 295.

Hastings, S. E., and Obrist, P. A., 1967, Heart rate during conditioning in humans: Effect of varying the interstimulus (CS–UCS) interval, *J. Exptl. Psychol. 74:*431.

Higgins, J. D., 1971, Set and Uncertainty as factors influencing anticipatory cardiovascular responding in humans, *J. Comp. Physiol. Psychol. 74:*272.

Howard, J. L., Obrist, P. A. Gaebelein, C., and Galosy, R. A., 1974, Multiple somatic measures and heart rate during classical aversive conditioning in the cat, *J. Comp. Physiol. Psychol.* (in press).

Jennings, J. R., Averill, J. R., Opten, E. M., and Lazarus, R. S., 1971, Some parameters of heart rate change: Perceptual versus motor task requirements, noxiousness, and uncertainty, *Psychophysiol. 7:*194.

Kelly, D. H. W., Brown, C. C., and Shaffer, J. W., 1970, A comparison of physiological measurements on anxious patients and normal controls, *Psychophysiol. 6:*429.

Lacey, J. I., 1967, Somatic response patterning and stress: Some revisions of activation theory, in *Psychological Stress: Issues in Research,* M. H. Appley and R. Trumbull, eds., Appleton-Century-Crofts, New York, pp. 14–42.

Lacey, J. I., and Lacey, B. C., 1958, Verification and extension of the principle of autonomic response sterotypy, *Am. J. Psychol. 71:*50.

Lacey, J. I., and Lacey, B. C., 1970, Some autonomic-central nervous system interrelationships, in *Physiological Correlated of Emotion,* P. Black, ed., Academic Press, New York, pp. 205–227.

Lacey, B. C., and Lacey, J. I., 1974, Studies of heart rate and other bodily processes in sensorimotor behavior, in *Cardiovascular Psychophysiology,* P. A. Obrist, A. H. Black, J. Brener, and L. V. DiCara, eds., Aldine, Chicago, p. 538.

Lawler, J. E., and Obrist, P. A., 1974, Indirect indices of cardiac contractility and sympathetic innervation: Their utility for cardiovascular psychophysiologists. Submitted for publication.

Lawler, J. E., Obrist, P. A., and Lawler, K. A., 1974, Cardiovascular function during pre-avoidance, avoidance, and post-avoidance in dogs, *Psychophysiol.* (in press).

Lofving, B., 1961, Cardiovascular adjustments induced from rostral cingulate gyrus, *Acta Physiol. Scand. 53* (Suppl. 181).

Masserman, J. H., 1943, *Behavior and Neurosis,* University of Chicago Press, Chicago.

Mathews, A. M., and Lader, M. H., 1971, An evaluation of forearm blood flow as a psychophysiological measure, *Psycholphysiol. 8:*509.

Meyers, K. A., and Obrist, P. A., 1972, Psychophysiological correlates of attention in children. Paper presented at the Annual Meeting of Society for Psychophysiological Research, Boston, Mass.

Miller, N. E., and Dworkin, B. R., 1974, Visceral learning: Recent difficulties with curarized rats and significant problems for human research in *Cardiovascular Psychophysiology,* P. A. Obrist, A. H. Black, J. Brener, and L. V. DiCara, eds., Aldine, Chicago, p. 312.

Obrist, P. A., 1968, Heart rate and somatic motor coupling during classical aversive conditioning in humans, *J. Expl. Psychol. 77:*180.

Obrist, P. A., and Webb, R. A., 1967, Heart rate during conditioning in dogs: Relationship of somatic-motor activity, *Psychophysiol. 4:*7.

Obrist, P. A., Wood, D. M., and Perez-Reyes, M., 1965, Heart rate during conditioning in humans: Effects of UCS intensity, vagal blockade and adrenergic block of vasomotor activity, *J. Expl. Psychol. 70:*32.

Obrist, P. A., Webb, R. A., and Sutterer, J. R., 1969, Heart rate and somatic changes during aversive conditioning and a simple reaction time task, *Psychophysiol. 5:*696.

Obrist, P. A., Webb, R. A., Sutterer, J. R., and Howard, J. L., 1970a, The cardiac-somatic relationship: Some reformulations, *Psychophysiol. 6:*569.

Obrist, P. A., Webb, R. A., Sutterer, J. R., and Howard, J. L., 1970b, Cardiac deceleration and reaction time: An evaluation of two hypotheses, *Psychophysiol. 6:*695.

Obrist, P. A., Howard, J. L., Lawler, J. E., Sutterer, J. R., Smithson, K. W., and Martin, P. L., 1972b, Alterations in cardiac contractility during classical aversive conditioning in dogs: Methodological and theoretical implications, *Psychophysiol. 9:*246.

Obrist, P. A., Sutterer, J. R., Hennis, H. S., Murrell, D. J., 1973, Cardiac-somatic changes during a simple reaction time task: A developmental study, *J. Exptl. Child Psychol. 16:*346.

Obrist, P. A., Howard, J. L., Lawler, J. E., Galosy, R. A., Meyers, K. A., and Gaebelein, C. J., 1974a, The cardiac-somatic interaction, in *Cardiovascular Psychophysiology,* P. A. Obrist, A. H. Black, J. Brener, and L. V. DiCara, eds., Aldine, Chicago, p. 136.

Obrist, P. A., Galosy, R. A., Lawler, J. E., and Gaebelein, C. J., Howard, J. L., and Shanks, E. M., 1974b, Operant conditioning of heart rate: Somatic correlates. *Psychophysiology,* in press.

Obrist, P. A., Lawler, J. E., Howard, J. L., Smithson, K. W., Martin, P. L., and Manning, J., 1974c, Sympathetic influences on cardiac rate and contractility during acute stress in humans, *Psychophysiol. 11:*405.

Rescorla, R. A., and Soloman, R. L., 1967, Two-process learning theory: Relationships between Pavlovian condition and instrumental learning, *Psychol. Rev. 74:*151.

Roberts, L. E., 1974, Comparative psychophysiology of the electrodermal and cardiac control systems, in *Cardiovascular Psychophysiology,* P. A. Obrist, A. H. Black, J. Brener, and L. V. DiCara, eds., Aldine, Chicago, p. 163.

Roberts, L. E., Lacroix, J. M., Wright, M., 1974, Comparative studies of operant electrodermal and heart rate conditioning in curarized rats, in *Cardiovascular Psychophysiology,* P. A. Obrist, A. H. Black, J. Brener, and L. V. DiCara, eds., Aldine, Chicago, p. 332.

Robinson, B. F., Epstein, S. E., Beiser, G. D., and Braunwold, E., 1966, Control of heart rate by the autonomic nervous system: Studies in man on the interrelationship between baroreceptor mechanisms and exercise, *Circulation Res. 19:*400.

Rushmer, R. F., 1964, Initial ventricular impulse: A potential key to cardiac evaluation, *Circulation, 29:*268.

Seligman, M. E. P., Maier, S. F., and Soloman, R. L., 1971, Unpredictable and uncontrollable aversive events, in *Aversive Conditioning and Learning,* F. R. Brush, ed., Academic Press, New York, pp. 347–400.

Smith, K., 1967, Conditioning as an artifact, in *Foundation of Conditioning and Learning,* G. A. Kimble, ed., Appleton-Century-Crofts, New York, pp. 100–111.

Smith, W. K., 1945, The functional significance of the rostral singular cortex as revealed by its responses to electrical excitation, *J. Neurophysiol. 8:*241.

Sroufe, L. A., 1971, Age changes in cardiac deceleration within a fixed fore-period reaction time task: An index of attention, *Develop. Psychol. 5:*338.

Sutterer, J. R., and Obrist, P. A., 1972, Heart rate and general activity alterations in dogs during several aversive conditioning procedures, *J. Comp. Physiol. Psychol. 80:*314.

Wang, Y., Marshall, R. J., and Sheppard, J. T., 1960, The effect of changes in posture and of graded exercise on stroke volume in man, *J. Clin. Inves. 39:*1051.

Webb, R. A., and Obrist, P. A., 1967, Heart rate change during complex operant performance in the dog, *Proc. Am. Psychol. Assoc. 3:*137.

Webb, R. A., and Obrist, P. A., 1970, The physiological concomitants of reaction time performance as a function of preparatory interval and preparatory interval series, *Psychophysiol. 6:*389.

Wood, D. M., and Obrist, P. A., 1964, Effects of controlled and uncontrolled respiration on the conditioned heart rate response in humans, *J. Exptl. Psychol. 68:*221.

Wood, D. M., and Obrist, P. A., 1968, Minimal and maximal sensory intake and exercise as unconditioned stimuli in human heart rate conditioning, *J. Exptl. Psychol. 76:*254.

CHAPTER 10

Factors Influencing the Specificity of Voluntary Cardiovascular Control*

Jasper Brener
Department of Psychology
University of Hull
Yorkshire, England

1. Introduction

The recent prolific growth in the literature relating to learned control of cardiovascular and other internal activities has not been paralleled by an equivalent growth in the theoretical or conceptual superstructure relating to these phenomena. Although the phenomena reported in this literature may be described by existing theories of learned control, the resultant assimilation leaves much to be desired. This is true in terms of a conceptual clarification of the processes of learned control in general, and specifically with respect to the processes involved in learned modification of what have hitherto been considered to be reflexively organized vegetative functions. The primary intent of this chapter is to describe a theoretical appreciation of the processes of voluntary cardiovascular activity with special reference to the role of feedback in the development of differentiated control.

2. Operant and Voluntary Control

That the highest levels of the nervous system exert a systematic effect on cardiovascular performance is not in question. As Figar (1965) points out, acknowledgment of the systematic relationship between higher mental processes and cardiovascular activity (blushing, heart rate changes, and penile erection) preceded the inception of the scientific method by several

* This research was supported by NIMH Grant #17061.

millenia. Furthermore, laboratory studies of classical cardiovascular conditioning may be traced to the work of Tsitovich (1918), thereby empirically implicating the intersensory mechanisms of learned control in the modification of cardiovascular activities. The observation that individuals may display voluntary control of cardiovascular activities also precedes the new literature on operant and voluntary cardiovascular modification by a considerable period of time. Wenger *et al.* (1961) point out that systematic observations of such voluntary cardiovascular activities among practitioners of Yoga were reported by Rele in 1927. In view of these well-established phenomena relating to learned cardiovascular control, we are led to inquire into the precise nature of the theoretical contributions implicit in the new experimental literature on operant and voluntary cardiovascular control.

Psychology and physiology alike have drawn a distinction between learned and unlearned behavioral control. In all of its subdivisions, biology acknowledges that the response repertoires of organisms are unconditionally bounded by genetically determined anatomical constraints. In this sense it may be said that no response which an organism displays is learned. Intrinsic structural factors are also acknowledged to underly those forms of response control which we call unlearned. Thus, reflexive behavior is attributed to fixed structural connections between the relevant receptor and effector aparatus. The energy transformation that is implicit in the reflexive mechanism, from environmental energy to motor energy, represents not only an empirical element of the behavior control process, but also a fundamental conceptual element: the concept of transduction. In the light of this fundamental concept, the problem of learned response control becomes one of accounting for the processes by which environmental energy comes to be transformed into motor energy where innate structural pathways subserving this transduction are not in evidence. In other words, the problem of learned control lies in accounting for how stimuli that do not exhibit an intrinsic ability to elicit particular responses acquire this ability.

Just as the reflex defines one fundamental concept in the theoretical description of the behavior control process—that of energy transduction—so does classical conditioning define another fundamental concept—that of association. When two stimuli reliably occur in close temporal contiguity, each acquires some of the response-controlling properties of the other. The precise mechanisms that underlie this process, although not immediately specifiable, appear to be well within the immediate descriptive repertoire of neurophysiology. By and large, theorists have favored Pavlov's proposition that the neural connections which mediate such learned control develop between the sensory or afferent elements of the control mechanism.

In other words, plastic changes in behavioral control are attributed largely to the process of sensory interpenetration rather than to the formation of new connections between sensory and motor elements.

Although the paradigmatic aspects of operant control have been meticulously examined (Ferster and Skinner, 1957), the mechanisms (what becomes connected to what) underlying this process have been sorely neglected. Kendler (1952) has in fact suggested that the question of "what is learned" in operant conditioning is a theoretical blind alley. Since this view pervades much of this area of research, it is not surprising that the theoretical implications of operant and voluntary cardiovascular control remain obscure.

In general, an operant is defined as a response which is systematically influenced by its programmed consequences (reinforcing stimuli). The heuristic device which is employed to explain the acquisition of operant control is the Law of Effect. The use of this *law* as a primary explanatory principle has continued to foster the assumption of behavior as being subject to a *vis a fronte*. Despite the vociferous denial of teleology in the writings of biological researchers from Darwin to Skinner, the *purposiveness* of operant behavior (its goal-directedness) has maintained its colloquial meaning. Organisms are seen as acting *in order to* achieve goals. Because the goal or reinforcing stimulus is the most identifiable and manipulable stimulus determinant of the operant control process, its importance has been successively emphasized while the antecedent preconditions to operant behavior have gradually receded from consideration. We may note for example that Skinner relegates the stimulus antecedents of operant behavior to obscurity by virtue of the difficulty of their identification. Holt (1915) acknowledged the same point in observing that as the number of antagonistic and synergic reflexes composing an act increases, the stimulus antecedents of that act recede further and further from view. The difficulties of specifying the stimulus antecedents of operant behavior do not, however, justify their neglect when attempting to define a theoretical analog of the operant control process. Within the traditional framework of scientific explanation, the concept of events being the effects of their future consequences is totally alien. Blanshard (1958) raises this point with respect to our appreciation of the concept of *choice*. He points out that "you are too much preoccupied with the ends to which the choice would be a means to give any attention of the causes of which your choice may be an effect." The traditional approach to operant behavior which invokes the Law of Effect as a final explanatory concept is responsible for perpetuating precisely this theoretical tendency in behavioral theorists. For these reasons, to assert that cardiovascular behavior is subject to the Law of Effect is of marginal theoretical significance. Certainly it does violate the traditional notion that visceral responses are not amenable to the influence of response-contingent reinforcement, but because the mechanisms of operant control are unspecified, the conceptual reorganization regarding the nature of plastic changes in visceral control is obscured rather than being facilitated.

Much of what has been said concerning the use of the concept of *operant* applies equally if not more vigorously to the concept of a *voluntary response*. Like an operant, a voluntary response is one that is not defined with respect to its external antecedents. The covert process of conscious intentionality is the essential characteristic of volition, and it is this process which identifies the fundamental cause of the voluntary as opposed to the nonvoluntary act. Not only are operants and voluntary responses identical with respect to this definitional criterion (that they occur in the absence of an objectively identifiable antecedent stimulus), but in addition, they parallel one another closely with respect to their empirical properties. Most notably, the development of both operant and voluntary control depends upon the availability of response-contingent stimulation.

James (1890) was among the first behaviorists to recognize the theoretical impasse implied by explaining behaviors in terms of their consequences. He also provided an extremely plausible hypothesis to account for the processes by which the programmed consequences of an act (reinforcing or feedback stimuli) might acquire antecedent eliciting properties for that act. Stated in its most colloquial form, James's ideo-motor theory of voluntary action states that the necessary and sufficient condition for the occurrence of an act is the focussing of attention on the "image" or "memory" of the stimulus consequences of that act. Since this hypothesis as it applies to the phenomena of learned cardiovascular change has been elaborated elsewhere (Brener, 1974a, 1974b), it will suffice for the present to summarize its basic assumptions and predictions.

1. It is assumed that prior to the establishment of voluntary control over any act, that act must be elicited in an involuntary reflexive fashion.

2. The afferent feedback stimuli that are consequent upon the response impinge upon the sensory areas of the brain to produce a specific pattern of excitation. This pattern of excitation was termed by James the response "image" and represents a precise specification of the intensive and topographical dimensions of the motor actions comprising the response. In the present context the afferent feedback stimuli whioh give rise to the response image are assumed to be interoceptive in origin. No distinction is drawn between interoception and proprioception.

3. If an exteroceptive stimulus is made to consistently follow a particular response, it will by the process of association with the interoceptive consequences of the response come to elicit the central representation or image of the response. This associative process is termed *calibration,* and the interoceptive consequences of the response are said to be calibrated in terms of the exteroceptive consequences.

4. Following calibration, an exteroceptive stimulus will activate the neural circuits which store the central representation or image of the response that the stimulus was previously consequent upon.

5. Activation of the response image will lead to the occurrence of motor activity resulting in the pattern of interoceptive feedback specified by the image.

To grant the validity of this hypothesis is also to acknowledge the mechanism by which the prior consequences of an act acquire eliciting properties for that act. The mechanism does not postulate that voluntary behavior is subject to a *vis a fronte,* but rather that by virtue of certain associative processes, the previous stimulus consequences of an act acquire the properties of a *vis a tergo.* This point of view is readily assimilable with existing neurophysiological and anatomical evidences. Recently Guyton (1972) has described the development of voluntary motor control as follows:

> "A person performs a motor movement mainly to achieve a purpose. It is primarily in the sensory and sensory association areas that he experiences effects of motor movements and records memories of the different patterns of motor movements. These are called sensory engrams of the motor movements. When he wishes to achieve some puposeful act, he presumably calls forth one of these engrams and then sets the motor system of the brain into action to reproduce the sensory pattern that is laid down in the engram." (p. 200)

Thus, a sensory activity that has previously been consequent upon a motor act becomes a prerequisite to the voluntary control of that act. Given the biological utility of plastic motor change, it is difficult to imagine a more efficient means of delineating *effective or instrumental* motor programs than in terms of their consequences.

An illustrative example of the operation of this mechanism is described by Razran (1961). Patients with urinary bladder fistulas were permitted to observe manometers indicating the distension of their bladders. They were provided with a means of signalling the time and intensity of their urinary urges. Following the consistent association of manometer readings with varying degrees of bladder distension, it was noted that when the manometer dial was made to read high although the bladder distension was minimal, the patients reported a strong urge to urinate. Conversely, when the manometer was made to read low, although the bladder was considerably distended, no urge to urinate was reported. In terms of the ideomotor theory, it would be said that manometer dial readings had acquired the ability to elicit the response images previously consequent upon interoceptive feedback from stimulation of the stretch receptors of the urinary bladder.

In the case of verbal instructions, the procedure of calibration involves the systematic pairing of verbal labels with the occurrence of the motor acts to which they refer. Thus, before an instruction to "increase the heart rate" will lead to a compliant response, it is necessary that the subject has learned to label the internal sensations consequent upon increasing the heart rate with the words "heart-rate increase."

3.   Nonspecific Voluntary Control of Cardiovascular Activities

Over the past several years it has been well established that instructional control may be developed over a wide variety of cardiovascular responses in humans. These include increases and decreases in mean heart rate (Brener, 1966; Brener and Hothersall, 1966; Engel and Chism, 1967a; Engel and Hansen, 1966), decreases in heart-rate variability (Hnatiow and Lang, 1965; Lang, Sroufe and Hastings, 1967), increases and decreases in both systolic and diastolic blood pressures (Brener and Kleinman, 1970; Shanks, 1973; Shapiro et al., 1969; Shapiro et al., 1972), and control of vasomotor activity (Snyder and Noble, 1968). Almost without exception these effects have been observed under conditions of exteroceptive feedback of the activity in question. Entrenched prejudices against the possibility of a native form of voluntary cardiovascular control have led to an almost universal neglect of systematic and controlled observations of these phenomena. For example, on the basis of the extant literature, it is presently impossible to determine whether or not augmented sensory feedback (biofeedback) is a prerequisite to voluntary cardiovascular control. The necessity of this form of feedback to the development of instructional cardiovascular control has been accepted on a priori grounds. In the light of evidence to be presented below, this assumption appears to be unwarranted.

For example, Brener et al. (1969) demonstrated that in the absence of exteroceptive feedback, when naive subjects were instructed to increase their heart rates in the presence of one visual stimulus and to decrease their heart rates in the presence of another, 9 of 10 subjects complied. Although the mean heart-rate differences were small (about 3 beats per minute, bpm), they were statistically reliable. In a second experiment, a group of five subjects displayed similar instructionally produced heart-rate changes in the absence of any special conditions. Subsequent experiments in our laboratory (Brener, 1974) have established the reliability of this phenomenon. The results of 7 independent experiments including two by Bergman and Johnson (1971, 1972) indicate that when humans are instructed to increase their heart rates in the absence of any special conditions, they display mean heart rates that are between 3 and 8 bpm higher than when they are instructed to decrease their heart rates. Furthermore, the magnitude of this instructionally produced heart-rate response is observed to be inversely related to the extent of somatomotor restraint imposed upon the subjects. The smallest heart-rate differences are observed when subjects are instructed not to move or alter their respiratory activity during the procedure and the largest heart-rate differences are observed when no constraints on somatomotor activity are explicitly imposed. A similar effect has been reported by Obrist et al., (1974).

From these observations, we may draw two conclusions: Heart rate is amenable to instructional control in the absence of any special conditions and therefore meets the criterion for classification of a voluntary response. Since somatomotor restraint negatively influences the magnitude of such instructionally produced heart-rate changes in the absence of any special conditions, it may be concluded that the processes underlying this control are *not* independent of somatomotor activity.

The role of somatomotor involvement in learned cardiovascular change has been the focus of considerable debate. In terms of the proposals made by Katkin and Murray (1968), evidence of somatomotor involvement in learned cardiovascular change disqualifies the observed cardiovascular changes from classification as voluntary or operant responses. However, from the point of view developed in the introduction to this chapter, the occurrence of such correlated activities are irrelevant to the classification of cardiovascular responses as voluntary or not. Such activities are, however, definitely germane to an assessment of the processes involved in the observed cardiovascular effects. Before delving into this issue, certain other related observations made in our laboratory require consideration.

It has been reported that naive human subjects comply with instructions to increase and decrease their heart rates by exhibiting a mean heart-rate difference between the increase and decrease conditions of 3 to 8 bpm. It has also been observed, however, that in the absence of any special conditions, instructions to increase and decrease respiratory activity and instructions to increase and decrease blood pressure result in heart-rate changes of approximately the same magnitude. The heart-rate changes in these experiments were likewise observed to be inversely related to the degree of somatomotor restraint imposed upon the subjects. It would appear, therefore, that the heart-rate response to instructions is not specific to the activity referenced in the instruction, but appears rather to be a component of a general motoric adjustment produced by the "increase" and "decrease" elements of the verbal instructions.

Since equivalent heart-rate changes may be produced by instructions to modify either heart rate, blood pressure, or respiration, it may be considered that the conclusion presented above, namely, that heart rate is a voluntary response, requires modification. In terms of the present frame of reference, however, these observations are not germane to the voluntary–nonvoluntary classification of the response, but rather to a dimension of voluntary activity that is sometimes referred to as *specificity of control.* For example, consider that if every time the subject complied with the instruction to press a key with his index finger, he also reliably engaged in other unnecessary actions such as moving other fingers, his arm, his torso, his head, etc. These correlative behaviors would be considered to be components of a general behavioral adjustment of which the instructionally referenced activity was also a component. It would not disqualify the key press as a voluntary act any more than it would disqualify reliable correlative behaviors as components of the instructionally produced behavioral adjustment or voluntary response. Nevertheless, we are forced to admit that there is a significant difference between a behavioral adjustment which is nondifferentiated with respect to the activity referenced in the instruction, and one that is specific to the activity referenced in the instruction. Increased specificity of responding is a characteristic property of the development of motor control. During the initial stages of training, the motoric adjustment is of a gross nature involving numerous components that are irrelevant to the *purpose* of the act in question. As training progresses, these superfluous activities tend to drop out eventuating ideally in a nonredundant or maximally efficient motor act. Clearly the mechanism underlying this process of response differentiation is of fundamental importance to the understanding of learned motor control.

As has been pointed out, the motoric adjustment induced by instructions to increase and decrease various visceral activities such as heart rate, blood pressure, and respiration in the absence of special feedback conditions is of a gross nondifferentiated nature. In particular, instructions to increase some visceral activity result in a general motoric activation, and instructions to decrease the activity result in a general motoric quiescence. The two basic responses are of the sort previously described by Hess (1954) as ergotropic and trophotropic responses. Gellhorn (1957) described the ergotropic syndrome as consisting of sympathetico-adrenal events, increased somatomotor activity, and a desynchronization of the EEG. Trophotropic responses are characterized by reverse changes. Given these two basic response modes, it is clear that subjects may meet the stipulated requirements of instructions to increase almost any activity by displaying the erogtropic response syndrome, and may meet the requirements stipulated by a decrease instruction by engaging in the trophotropic response mode. In a recent experiment by Shanks (1973), it was observed that of 60 subjects submitted to procedures involving various combinations of instructions and feedback conditions, 51 displayed higher heart rates, 47 higher respiratory activity, 42 more EMG, and 40 higher diastolic blood pressures during increase than during decrease trials, regardless of the activity referenced in the instructions or the feedback conditions obtaining during the tests. Similarly, Brackin (1973) has observed that subjects displayed significantly lower levels of alpha activity when instructed to "speed up" their brain waves than when instructed to "slow down" their brain waves in the absence of special feedback conditions. Furthermore, the magnitude of alpha rhythm control evidenced under conditions of instructions-only was found not to be different from the magnitude of such control produced by instruction plus feedback of alpha performance. Further evidence in support of the power of the increase and decrease components of verbal instructions comes from a study by Brener and Goesling (1968). Increases in heart rate may be produced by compliance with instructions to either "increase the production of short inter-heartbeat-intervals (IBI's)" or to "decrease the production of long IBI's." Similarly, low heart rates may be produced by compliance with the instruction to "decrease the production of short IBI's" or to "increase the production of long IBI's." In this experiment subjects were provided with exteroceptive feedback of heart rate in the form of a low-pitched tone following each long IBI and a high-pitched tone following each short IBI. Four groups of ten subjects each were instructed respectively to "produce high-pitched tones," "inhibit the occurrence of high-pitched tones," "produce low-pitched tones," and "inhibit the occurrence of low-pitched tones." It was observed that the group instructed to produce high-pitched tones displayed significantly greater increases in heart rate than the group instructed to inhibit low-pitched tones, whereas the group instructed to inhibit high-pitched tones displayed significantly greater heart-rate decrements than the group instructed to produce low-pitched tones. These results again support the notion that the instruction to produce something (like the instruction to increase something) produces an ergotropic response set in human subjects that facilitates the production of heart-rate increments. Similarly, the instruction to inhibit something (like the instruction to decrease something) produces a trophotropic response set which facilitates the production of heart-rate decrements.

In view of these findings, it must be recognized that instructions *per se* are an important systematic source of influence over cardiovascular activity. Neglect of the pretreatment influence of instructions on the activity under study has led to a confounding of the effects produced by this variable with the effects of exteroceptive feedback provided during training. As a consequence of this confounding, it is difficult on the basis of the extant literature to partial out the influence of exteroceptive feedback on the development of learned cardiovascular control.

4. Criteria Employed in Assessing Specificity of Control

Since we have traditionally tended to confuse the concept of voluntary control with the concept of specificity of control, experimenters in the area of learned cardiovascular control have gone to considerable lengths to establish that the voluntary and operant cardiovascular effects observed in their experiments were independent of other activities, particularly activities of the somatomotor system. Despite these efforts, however, the evidence in support of specific cardiovascular effects is not at all compelling.

Two approaches are to be distinguished in the various attempts to establish a case for the independence of learned cardiovascular change from learned changes in, particularly, somatomotor activity. These two approaches may be termed *interventional* and *correlational* methods. In the interventional approach, an attempt is made to independently control likely or potential behavioral correlates of cardiovascular change during procedures directed toward the modification of cardiovascular activity. In the correlational approach, no attempt is made to control potential correlates of cardiovascular change, and the case for specificity of learned cardiovascular control is made on the basis of *post hoc* correlational procedures. Thus, in assessing the relationship of respiratory activity to learned cardiovascular control, Brener and Hothersall (1967) employed an interventional procedure in which the respiratory activity of subjects was paced during the training of heart-rate control. The results of this procedure tended to support the conclusion that changes in respiratory activity were not prerequisite to learned heart-rate control. A similar conclusion was reached by Engel and Chism (1967) on the basis of correlational data where no attempt was made to control respiratory activity. In neither case, however, does the conclusion that learned heart-rate changes may occur independently of correlated respiratory activity seem to be fully justified by the data presented. Neither procedure obviates the possibility that unmeasured aspects of respiratory activity covaried systematically with the observed heart-rate changes. A similar criticism may be applied to any attempt to demonstrate response-specific effects in the intact organism. Regardless of the number of specific activities recorded, a larger number of unrecorded activities might potentially covary with the activity under study.

When interest in this area of research became dominated by the apparent need to demonstrate response-specific effects, the interventional method of choice was curarization. In view of historical prejudices against the operant or voluntary status of cardiovascular phenomena, it was thought necessary to demonstrate that such phenomena were not the reflexive after-effects of learned changes in somatomotor and respiratory activities. By immobilizing the striate musculature with the peripheral myoneural blocking agent, curare, and maintaining the subjects on artificial respiration, it was possible to eliminate the potential influence of peripheral somatomotor activity on cardiovascular activity. Under these very stringent control conditions, the strongest evidence of operant cardiovascular conditioning was obtained. Although recent difficulties in replication (Brener *et al*; 1974, Hahn, 1974, Miller and Dworkin, 1974) somwehat detract from the force of these demonstrations, the basic phenomena reported remain worthy of careful consideration.

Under the conditions of total quiescence of the striate musculature induced by curare, substantial alterations in heart rate, vasomotor activity, and blood pressure have been conditioned by the use of reward and punishment precedures (Miller, 1969, DiCara, 1970). Although one might be tempted to conclude from these demonstrations that cardiovascular activity is modifiable independently of somatomotor activity, careful examination of the relevant data indicates that such a general conclusion is unwarranted. For example, DiCara and Miller (1969), employing a shock-avoidance procedure, conditioned increases in heart rate in one group of curarized rats and decreases in a second group. Subsequent tests in the non-curarized state indicated that rats previously reinforced for heart-rate increases displayed substantially higher levels of general activity and respiratory rates than animals previously reinforced for decreases in heart rate. Since during the curare conditioning sessions, fortuitous reinforcement of activity and respiratory changes was impossible, it must be concluded that what had been modified in this procedure was not a cardiovascular-specific response, but rather the activity of some neural center responsible for the parallel efferent control of the functionally related responses of heart rate, respiration, and somatomotor activity. These activity constellations fit well with the ergotropic–trophotropic distinction made earlier. Curare established only that the observed cardiovascular changes were not dependent upon afferentation from the striate musculature. Since such a mechanism of cardiovascular change finds few modern proponents, the use of this extreme interventional procedure is of dubious theoretical utility. The most profound effect of curarization seems to be that it prevents the experimenter from observing the naturally occurring covariates of cardiovascular change, thereby serving to further entrench the erroneous notion of response-specific operant modification.

Evidence opposed to the notion of learned response independence derives from a variety of sources. A large body of neurophysiological literature (Germana, 1969) indicates that somatomotor and visceral responses are coupled at a central level with the two effector systems being influenced in parallel by the same central processes. Behavioral data likewise (Obrist *et al.*, 1974) indicate an extremely close parallel between cardiovascular and somatomotor effects. Goesling and Brener (1972) have demonstrated that training of somatomotor activity and immobility prior to curarization has a more profound influence on cardiovascular change under curare than do heart-rate reinforcement contingencies imposed under the latter procedure. This result clearly reinforces the view that curarization does not eliminate the possibility that somatomotor processes proximal to the myoneural junction may retain a profound influence over cardiovascular activity. All in all, it must be concluded that learned cardiovascular control is not generally manifested in specific activity changes in specific components of this effector system.

Although specificity of learned cardiovascular control is difficult to justify in this sense, as has already been mentioned, increases in the relative specificity of response control as a function of training are commonly observed. This process of increasing specificity of control is characterized by the successive differentiation of an initially gross behavioral adjustment. In a recent appraisal of the literature on learned motor control, Clemens (1972) points out that at the inception of training two classes of behavior are differentiated: those containing instances of the desired behavior and those not containing instances of the desired behavior. Since a given response, particularly of the cardiovascular system, is likely to be embedded within a great variety of behavioral contexts, these classes will necessarily be very broad. If we are dealing with increases and decreases in cardiovascular activity, the classes will in fact be those referred to previously as the ergotropic and trophotropic response modes. Unfortunately the available literature on learned cardiovascular control does not satisfactorily establish whether or not a further differentiation of cardiovascular control occurs. There is, however, certain evidence that favors this bility.

The strongest claims for learned specificity of cardiovascular control derive from the curare literature. An example of what is generally implied by specific control is contained in the report by DiCara and Miller (1968) of differential control of vasomotor responding in the two ears of a curarized rat. Although these data appear to establish that the vasomotor activity in one ear of a rat may be controlled independently of the vasomotor activity in the other ear, they do not establish whether, for example, these vasomotor responses are independent of the somatomotor activities they accompany in the normal state. Independent motor control of the ears may be observed to accompany auditory localization in this species of animal—we might therefore legitimately expect such differential motor activity to be accompanied by associated vascular changes. The point made here is that specificity of control is remarkable only where this process involves the differentiation of normally integrated behavioral constellations. For example, to demonstrate that movement of the second toe occurs independently of hand movements is of doubtful significance whereas to demonstrate that movement of the second toe occurs independently of movements of the third toe would be of considerable interest. The procedural conditions defining this demonstration would serve to identify factors involved in the refinement of motor control. For these reasons, the various demonstrations that blood pressure may be modified independently of heart rate (e.g., Brener and Kleinman, 1970; Shapiro *et al.*, 1969) or that heart rate may be modified independently of gastrointestinal activity (Miller and Banuazizi, 1968) are of marginal significance in evaluating the processes involved in the development of response-specific control. Such differentiations of activity are to be expected in terms of functional organization of the activity elements concerned.

More germane to the present notion of what is important in the process of specificity of control are data derived from the experiment by DiCara and Miller (1969) described above. As was mentioned, following heart-rate training under curare, when subjects were tested in the noncurarized state, rats previously reinforced for heart-rate increments displayed substantially higher activity levels and respiration rates than animals previously reinforced for heart-rate decrements. However, with further testing and training in the noncurarized state, the somatomotor correlates of the learned heart-rate changes tended to recede while the heart-rate responses became accentuated. This change in the magnitude of the cardiovascular effect relative to other components of the behavioral complex in which this effect was initially embedded is a characteristic example of the general process of response differentiation. This process which may be described as an increase in the efficiency of a behavioral adjustment to the specific demands of the environment as a function of training is commonly acknowledged. Although this increase in specificity of control is generally attributed to the procedural factor of continued training, the mechanisms mediating this effect have not been generally agreed upon. Inhibitory processes of the sort referred to by Hull (1943) provide a useful explanatory base, but because they are implied by the concept of behavioral efficiency (which they purportedly explain), their use necessarily involves a tautology. In other words, to say that redundant acts fall out because they involve an unnecessary and maladaptive expenditure of energy is nothing more than to define what is meant by "redundant" in the biological sense. Although the assumption of a *principle of least effort* is by no means extraneous to the approach to response differentiation adopted here, a need is seen for a more molecular specification of the mechanism underlying this important behavioral process.

5.   Feedback and the Discriminability of Responses

The provision of response-contingent exteroceptive feedback is generally conceded to provide a powerful technique in the development of specific or differential motor control. A compelling illustration of the power of this technique is contained in an experiment by Basmajian (1963) on the development of instructional control over the rate of firing in single motor units. This investigator observed that when subjects are provided with auditory feedback, they rapidly learn to produce specific patterns of firing in single motor nerve cells. Not only was such control observed to be specific to a single motor neuron, but it was also observed that the control was maintained following withdrawal of the exteroceptive feedback. In no case could subjects report how they were effecting the observed control. A similar effect has been reported by Hefferline *et al.* (1959). These investigators developed control over a virtually imperceptible muscle twitch in human subjects by making avoidance of an aversive stimulus complex dependent upon the occurrence of criterion EMG responses. A criterion response was defined as one that fell within a narrow amplitude band, thereby disqualifying responses which were components of a general motor activation (ergotropic) response. Again subjects demonstrated an inability to describe how they achieved criterion performance. For example, one subject "professed to have discovered an effective response sequence, which consisted of subtle rowing motions with both hands, infinitesimal wriggles of both ankles, a slight displacement of the jaw to the left, breathing out—and then waiting." The inference to be drawn from this example is that what subjects say they are doing often has little relevance to what they are in fact doing. Verplanck (1962) has demonstrated that the verbal descriptions humans apply to their behavior may be manipulated independently of the behavior itself. The significance of such verbal reports in the assessment of factors underlying voluntary motor control is, therefore, very questionable. Basmajian reports that "To this day I cannot put into words how I was able to call three different motorneurons unerringly into activity in the total absence of artificial aids." As Sherrington among many others has indicated, the mind is not apprised of how we execute even the most primitive voluntary acts—it knows but the consequences of having executed the act. This point is raised here to emphasize that consciousness is not a necessary prerequisite to voluntary control and may more legitimately be considered an aftereffect of voluntary behavior.

Nevertheless, the ability of humans to apply different verbal labels to the various acts that comprise their voluntary repertoire is considered here to be an essential prerequisite to the instructional control of those acts. In terms of the model of voluntary control described earlier, the fact that we are able to describe, for example, the position of our arms relative to our bodies implies that the interoceptive feedback consequent upon the various positions the arms may assume has been previously calibrated in terms of the verbal labels employed in the description. This calibration process is prerequisite to the ability of such verbal labels to evoke appropriate motor adjustments when later employed in an instructional context. In other words, it is unlikely that an individual who was unable to accurately describe the position of his arm when it was extended at right angles to his body would respond appropriately to the instruction to "extend the arm so that it makes a right angle with the body."

The precision with which an instruction might produce a specific motor effect may be assumed, therefore, to depend upon the precision with which the interoceptive feedback from the effector has been calibrated. Thus, the finer the discriminations an individual can make between variations in the activity of an effector apparatus, the finer will be the demonstrable control of that effector. Stated in the form of an hypothesis, it is suggested that the potential specificity of voluntary motor control is a direct function of the discriminability of variations in the activity of the effector in question. Although the ability of humans to discriminate responses may be substantially enhanced by the procedure of calibration via exteroceptive feedback, it is clear that structural anatomical factors as well as psychophysical functions impose constraints on the potential fineness of such discriminations, and therefore on the potential specificity of control.

It seems reasonable to assume that the most cogent anatomical determinants of response discriminability are the density of the afferent innervation of the effector apparatus and the relative size of the cortical projection area receiving these afferent fibers. Thus, the cortical projections of the buccal effectors are proportionately much greater in animals such as dogs, which employ these effectors for fine-grain technical activities, than they are for, say, the marmoset, which employs its hands in the accomplishment of such activities (Woolsey, 1953). It may furthermore be assumed that the psychophysical processes which determine such constants as absolute and difference thresholds in the exteroceptive senses are operative in the determination of interoceptive sensory abilities. An important factor to be considered in relation to this issue is the signal-to-noise

ratio of the interoceptive stimuli consequent upon an act. This idea, that
the motor adjustments demanded by the environment will be met by acts
which provide the most discriminable interoceptive feedback, is supported
by research on deafferentation with monkeys. Although Mott and Sherrington (1895) concluded that unilateral deafferentation results in the loss
of voluntary movement of the affected limb, it has been shown (Taub and
Berman, 1968) that the extent of this impairment is lessened by bilateral
deafferentation. In other words, in meeting environmental demands,
organisms tend to employ those effectors whose activities are most discriminable. Following unilateral deafferentation, movements of the
contralateral limb may be more effectively regulated in meeting environmental demands than movements of the deafferented limb. However, where
this advantage in discriminability is eliminated by bilateral deafferentation,
voluntary activities in both limbs may be observed.

In summary, then, it might reasonably be suggested that the discriminability of, and hence, the potential specificity of voluntary control over,
the activities of an effector are determined by (1) the channel capacity of
the afferent system serving that effector, (2) the absolute sensory threshold
and Weber fraction defining the psychophysical properties of that afferent
channel, and (3) the immediate sensory context (interoceptive and exteroceptive) in which activity in that afferent channel occurs.

Considering these issues in relation to voluntary control of cardiovascular activities, our long commitment to the nonvoluntary status of such
activities is scarcely surprising. Not only is the afferent innervation of the
cardiovascular effector system less prolific than that of the striate muscle
system, but in addition, the cortical projections of the viscera in general are
inconspicuous. Visceral sensations are poorly defined and are frequently
referred to loci other than their points of origin (Kuntz, 1953). For these
reasons, the ability of humans to provide verbal descriptions of visceral
activities is very limited as is the specificity with which they respond to
instructions to modify visceral activity.

Despite these apparent limitations in the visceral afferent system, it
will be recognized that visceral afferent stimuli are not only capable of
eliciting profound behavioral adjustments as in the operation of primary
drives, but they are also capable of acquiring motor effects via the associative processes of classical conditioning (Bykov, 1957; Razran, 1961). On
the basis of the Russian literature on interoceptive conditioning, it may be
concluded that the visceral afferent system participates fully in the
intersensory mechanisms of learned motor control. Because current
knowledge of the psychophysical properties of the cardiovascular afferent
system is virtually nonexistent, the potential discriminability of cardiovascular activity must remain for the present a moot point. However, it

would seem reasonable to assume that the cardiovascular afferent system is capable of providing discriminable information to the same degree as has been demonstrated for other visceral afferent systems. Armed with this assumption, and because the demonstration that interoceptive feedback from the cardiovascular system is crucial to the proposed theory of voluntary cardiovascular control, we undertook a series of experiments in our laboratory to investigate the ability of humans to discriminate cardiovascular action.

Although the interoceptive conditioning procedures employed by the Russians have provided a substantial body of useful evidence relating to the discriminability of visceral afferent signals, these procedures are not readily adaptable to the study of interoceptive discrimination in intact humans. The problems associated with an adequate demonstration of this phenomenon are considerable. For example, it must be adequately demonstrated that the subject is employing stimuli derived from cardiovascular action as the basis of his discrimination, rather than stimuli derived from other related activities. The reason for this is that the ability of an instruction to produce specific cardiovascular changes (e.g., exclusive of the somatomotor contexts in which they are normally embedded) is assumed to rest upon the ability of the subject to discriminate cardiovascular feedback from feedback contingent upon other activities that might normally provide the behavioral context of the specific response.

Thus, if a subject was required to press one button whenever his heart rate was high and another button whenever his heart rate was low, successful compliance might result from the discrimination of somatomotor afferentation accompanying these responses. For this reason, it was decided to investigate discrimination of the heart beat, a response which occurs regardless of somatomotor activity. Our initial attempts proved that even so mundane an ambition as this is fraught with measurement difficulties. If the subject is instructed to press a button every time his heart beats, his discriminative performance may be assessed by recording the relative frequencies of different sequences of heart beats and button presses. Perfect discrimination would be evidenced in a performance in which every heart beat was followed by a button press. The relative frequency with which heart beats were followed by heart beats without an interpolated button press would provide an index of the subject's failure to detect the signal. Finally, the relative frequency with which button presses were followed by button presses without an interpolated heart beat would provide an index of the subject's tendency to confuse some other signal with the signal to be detected. This measurement procedure, while plausible, failed to differentiate those subjects who were responding to the afferent consequences of heart beats from those subjects who learned to press the button at a frequency approximating their heart rates. Improvement in either of these aspects of performance leads to a systematic increase in the relative frequency of heart-beat–button-press sequences.

The procedure that we have finally adopted to demonstrate that humans may learn to discriminate their pulses involves a successive discrimination procedure in which the subject is required to discriminate between signals that are contingent upon his heart action and signals which display similar intensive, qualitative, and temporal properties, but which are not contingent on the heart beat. This procedure is broken into successive 10-second trials. On each trial, a sequence of vibratory stimuli is delivered to the subject's left wrist. On half the trials, the onset of each brief vibratory stimulus is determined by the occurrence of an R-wave in the EKG. On the other half, the onset of the vibratory stimulus is determined by the firing of a multivibrator which is set to develop a pulse frequency equal to the subject's pulse rate. These two types of trials are presented in a random order. Following the sequence of stimuli on each trial, a red light comes on. Subjects are instructed that on the presentation of the red light, they are to indicate whether the preceding sequence of vibratory stimuli was correlated with their heart beats (by pressing a button in their right hands) or not (by pressing a button in their left hands.). Following the occurrence of each discriminative (button-press) response, the next trial commences. Because the qualitative and temporal (duration and mean frequency) characteristics of the two stimulus sources are identical, the ability of individuals to discriminate those sequences that are heart-contingent from those that are not, must rely upon the ability of the individuals to associate the heart-contingent vibratory stimuli with the interoceptive stimulus consequences of cardiac action. The only other basis for discriminating between the two stimulus sequences in this procedure is in terms of the temporal distributions of vibratory stimuli that are heart-contingent and those that are dependent on the output of the multivibrator. In the former case, the interstimulus intervals are normally distributed about the mean IBI whereas in the latter case, the interstimulus intervals are invariant. To control for the possibility that subjects may be learning to discriminate between regular and irregular pulse trains, a second group of subjects was run.

Experimental and control subjects (10 per group) each received 20 pretraining trials. During these trials, subjects were not provided with knowledge of results (KOR). Thereafter, experimental subjects received discrimination training with KOR (a brief tone following each correct discrimination) until they reached a criterion of at least 80% correct on two successive blocks of 10 trials. When this criterion had been achieved, KOR was withdrawn and subjects given a further 20 post-training discrimination trials. The experimental and control procedures differed only with respect to the treatment given during the training phase of the experiment. The sequences of heart-contingent and multivibrator-contingent vibratory stimuli that control subjects received during the initial 20 pretraining trials were recorded as discrete events on magnetic tape and replayed to them during the subsequent training trials. These stimulus sequences were replayed on successive training trials with KOR until control subjects reached an 80% discrimination criterion or until they had received 200 training trials. Following this phase of the experiment, control subjects received an identical post-training discrimination test to that administered to experimental subjects. Since control subjects were trained to discriminate heart-contingent vibratory stimuli (variable interpulse time) from multivibrator (invariant interpulse time) stimuli, they provided a control for the possibility that subjects may learn to discriminate a variable from an invariant pulse train. The median pretraining and post-training discrimination performances for these two groups of subjects are presented in Fig. 1. As will be seen, experimental subjects display an increase in correct discrimination from 50% (chance level) during the pretraining to 77.5% during the post-training test. Control subjects, on the other hand, display a median pretraining performance of 57.7% correct and a post-training performance of 51.6% correct. Nine of the ten subjects in the experimental group displayed an improvement in discriminative performance from pre- to post-training, whereas only one of the ten control subjects did. This difference is significant at beyond the .01 level.

It is proposed that these data provide strong, if not conclusive, evidence that humans may be trained to discriminate the consequences of cardiac action. It is also suggested that variants of this basic procedure may be employed effectively to examine the psychophysical properties of the interoceptive sensory system. Acceptance of the conclusion that these data provide evidence that humans may be trained to discriminate the interoceptive consequences of cardiac action establishes, within the framework of the proposed model, the possibility of establishing specific control of such activity.

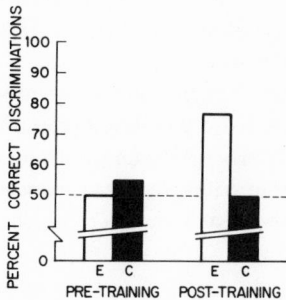

FIG. 1. The effects of training on discrimination of the pulse.

6. Development of Specific Motor Control

It has been argued that the development of specific control over a response which is normally embedded within the context of other functionally related activities will depend upon the extent to which the unique sensory consequences of that response are discriminable from the sensory consequences of the activities which form its normal behavioral context. Data have been offered to provide an empirical basis for the assumption that cardiovascular-specific afferentation is discriminable to humans following certain training procedures. Such training procedures have been termed "calibrating" procedures and are characterized by the programming of exteroceptive stimuli to coincide in a systematic manner with the naturally occurring internal sensory consequences of the act in question.

In the absence of any joint contingencies, when an exteroceptive stimulus is made to consistently follow a particular act, the precise origin and nature of the interoceptive stimuli thereby calibrated is not easily identified. Nevertheless, in terms of the hypotheses proposed here, the behavioral adjustment that is observed to follow a particular instruction does provide a basis for inferring the sources of the interoceptive stimuli previously calibrated by the instructional labels employed. Thus, if an instruction to increase the heart rate does, as has been reported, lead to a general state of motor activation with a pronounced somatomotor component, it is reasonable to assume that the heart-rate response is identified by feedback from the more discriminable somatomotor components of the motor response rather than by cardiovascular feedback per se. Smith (1967) has suggested the operation of such a mechanism in the joint regulation of somatomotor–autonomic response constellations. This author has proposed that somatomotor activity is primary in that feedback from the striate muscles provides the fundamental regulatory basis of learned behavioral adjustments involving the viscera. To amplify this point further attention is drawn to the observation by Davis (1943) that children exhibit much more EMG in response to instructions to perform unfamiliar motor acts than do adults, who have had previous experience in executing these acts. In terms of the proposed model, this result is explicable by recourse to the hypothesis that the interoceptive consequences of the acts referenced in these instructions are calibrated during a development stage not yet reached by the young subjects in this experiment. It would also be expected that these children would display a relatively poor ability to distinguish the interoceptive consequences of the act specified in the instruction from the interoceptive consequences of general adjustment displayed in response to the instructions. The efficiency (specificity) of a motor adjustment to environmental demands is therefore assumed to depend primarily upon the discriminability of the effective component of the act specified in the demand.*

If an exteroceptive stimulus is made to consistently follow a specific act, say movement of the middle finger, and subjects are instructed to produce this tone, it will be observed that as a function of the number of response-feedback couplings, the instructionally-produced act will become more specific. This will be evidenced in an increase in the movement of the middle finger relative to the movements of the other fingers. Presumably this increase in specificity is accounted for by the fact that the exteroceptive stimulus follows movements of the middle finger more reliably than it does movements of the other fingers, thereby differentially calibrating the intrinsic consequences of this act. However, a similar experiment in which an exteroceptive stimulus was made to consistently follow movements of the middle toe will indicate that differentiation of this response will be far more protracted. Movements of the other toes, for anatomical as well as experiential reasons, form a stable behavioral context for the movement of the middle toe. The development of specific control over cardiovascular activities is assumed here to present problems similar to those illustrated by this latter example. Not only is cardiovascular afferentation relatively indiscriminable when compared to afferentation from the somatomotor responses it normally accompanies, but in addition, variations in cardiovascular activity are highly correlated with functionally associated somatomotor activities. Both of these factors militate against the rapid acquisition of response-specific cardiovascular control.

* It is important to note that in terms of this model, the more information that is transmitted by an instruction, the more efficient *in terms of energy expenditure* will be the motor adjustment induced by that instruction. Thus, motor output efficiency as measured by energy expenditure increases at the cost of an increase in the complexity of the mechanism required for the translation of instructional input. A system with a very limited instructional processing capability (e.g., the ability to respectively translate increase and decrease instructions into ergotropic and trophotropic responses) would be capable of complying systematically with instructions to increase or decrease any activity. The instructionally-produced behavioral adjustments exhibited by such a system would, however, be of a very undifferentiated and gross nature and would be relatively inefficient in terms of energy expenditure. As the instructional processing capability of the system increases, the behavioral consequences of instructions become more specific and efficient in terms of energy expenditure. In terms of the ideas presented here, the rate at which a maximally efficient instructionally-produced motor effect will be acquired depends upon the capacity of the system to distinguish the unique sensory consequences of the act referenced by the instruction from the sensory consequences of the other acts which might form its normal behavioral context, and the availability of environmental contingencies which serve to apply a unique verbal label to these intrinsic and discriminable sensory consequences. In terms of this approach the ontogenetic development of the comprehension of verbal instructions and the development of motor control are viewed as two aspects of the same developmental process.

Before I go on to describe some recent experiments that are aimed at the investigation of this process, attention must be directed to a further inference which derives from the hypotheses described above. During protracted training of motor control under conditions of exteroceptive feedback, it may be observed that redundant components of the initially general motor adjustment drop out at a differential rate. Thus, in the toe-movement example described above, we might expect movements of the middle toe to be differentiated from movements of the great toe before they are differentiated from movements of the second and fourth toes. On the basis of such an observation, we might legitimately infer that interoceptive consequences of movements in the great toe are less reliably correlated with movements of the middle toe than are movements of the second and fourth toes, and hence, are less reliably calibrated by the exteroceptive stimulus. Thus, the rate at which initially correlated activities recede from an effective behavioral adjustment during training provides an indication of the organizational properties of the behavioral Gestalt in which the effective response is embedded. Those activities which recede first are most indirectly tied to the effective response, whereas those that are intransigent correlates of the effective act may be considered to represent peripheral consequences of the same central processes responsible for the effective act.

7. The Development of Response-Specific Cardiovascular Control

It has been mentioned that instructions to increase and decrease visceral activities in the absence of any specific conditions result, respectively, in subjects displaying ergotopic and trophotropic responses. These general motoric adjustments tend to occur regardless of the specific activities referenced in the instructions. However, it is possible to discern, superimposed on such generalized responses, certain differences between the behavioral effects of instructions that reference different activities.

Recently, Brener and Shanks (1974) reported an experiment in which 60 naive subjects were submitted to procedures which were distinguished by different combinations of instructions and feedback conditions.* The two instructional conditions required subjects to either successively increase and decrease their heart rates *or* their blood pressures. These instructions were delivered to different groups of subjects who received exteroceptive feedback of changes in either heart rate *or* blood pressure *or* who were given no feedback. Table I describes the instruction/feedback conditions for each of

---

* These data were collected by E. M. Shanks as part of her doctoral dissertation, University of Tennessee.

TABLE 1

Feedback conditions	Instructions	
	Heart rate	Blood pressure
None	HRI/NFB	BPI/NFB
Heart rate	HRI/HRFB	BPI/HRFB
Diastolic blood pressure	HRI/DPFB	BPI/DPFB

the 6 groups of subjects. Throughout the procedure recordings were made of heart rate, diastolic blood pressure, chin EMG, and respiratory volume. Control was assessed by subtracting the mean activity levels for each reponse recorded during decrease trials from the equivalent measures recorded during increase trials. This yielded a set of four difference measures for each subject, with positive differences indicating higher levels of activity during increase than decrease trials.

The median difference scores for all conditions and combinations of conditions are presented in Fig. 2. The top left-hand diagram in this figure illustrates the median increase–decrease difference scores for the four measures of activity for all 60 subjects in the experiment. As will be seen, the scales for each measure were adjusted so as to make bars representing these grand medians approximately equal in height. It should be noted that this diagram indicates that the grand median diastolic blood pressure difference was 1.44 mm Hg., the heart-rate difference, 7.21 bpm, and the EMG and respiration differences (measured in arbitrary units), 64 and 11.5 units, respectively. These measures are representative of the difference between the ergotropic and trophotropic response tendencies previously described to be associated with "increase" and "decrease" instructions in similar experimental situations.

The two diagrams labeled BPI and HRI, respectively, illustrate the influence of the blood pressure and heart-rate instructions across all feedback (FB) conditions. It will be seen that under equivalent FB conditions, the behavioral adjustment produced by instructions to control heart rate exhibits a significantly more pronounced EMG component than does the behavioral adjustment produced by blood pressure instructions. In terms of the approach adopted here, this finding suggests that the labels "heart-rate increase" and "heart-rate decrease" are generally employed to identify the interoceptive consequence of increases and decreases in somatomotor activity. Associated with this pronounced difference between the two

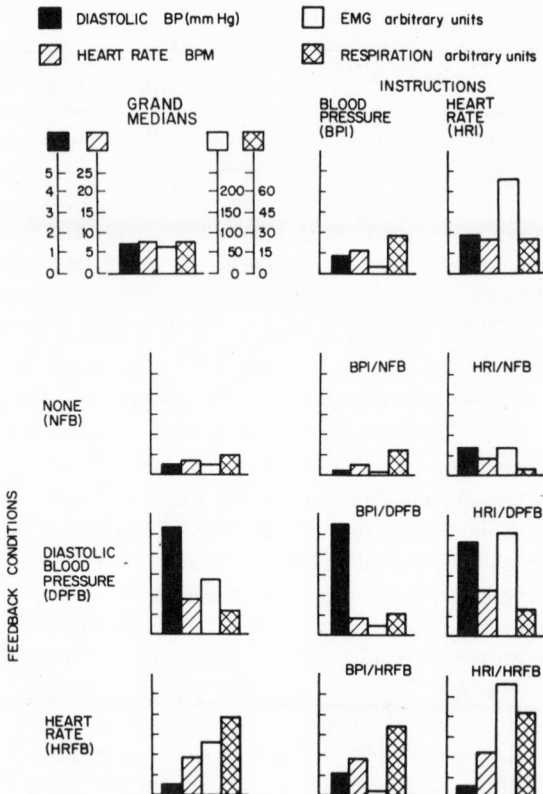

FIG. 2.   The effects of various combinations of instructions and
feedback on four measures of activity.

instructional effects are smaller cardiovascular effects. Comparison of the
diagrams in the HRI column with the corresponding diagrams in the BPI
column reveals that under equivalent feedback conditions the EMG
component associated with heart-rate instructions is consistently and significantly higher than that associated with blood pressure instructions.
These data support the conclusion that when subjects are instructed to
increase and decrease their heart rates they characteristically increase and
decrease their striate muscle tension to a significantly greater degree than
when they are instructed to increase and decrease their blood pressures.
The profile of activity differences associated with blood pressure instructions will be observed to bear a close similarity to the profile illustrated by
the grand medians suggesting that these instructions lead to nondifferentiated ergotropic–trophotropic response constellations of the sort
referred to earlier.

The left-hand diagram in each row illustrates the median activity differences associated with the three feedback conditions across instructions. Several pronounced effects will be observed. First, it will be noted that the response profile associated with the no-feedback (NFB) condition is similar to that described by both the grand medians and the blood pressure instructions (BPI). Not surprisingly, the same nondifferentiated response profile may be observed in response to the combination of blood pressure instructions and the no-feedback condition (BPI/NFB). We may infer from these observations that the label "blood pressure" has not been employed in the history of these naive subjects to systematically describe (calibrate) the intrinsic sensations arising from variations in this cardiovascular parameter or its more discriminable behavioral correlates. Because variations in diastolic blood pressure may occur in a greater variety of behavioral contexts, this is not surprising.

The response profiles associated, respectively, with diastolic blood pressure feedback (DPFB) and heart-rate feedback (HRFB) indicate substantial and specific effects on the activities studied. In particular, it will be observed that blood pressure feedback is associated with a profound elevation of diastolic blood pressure differences and heart-rate feedback with a similarly profound elevation of respiratory differences. Scrutiny of the diagrams illustrating the interaction of these two forms of feedback with the two instructional conditions suggests that these major feedback effects interact in a simple additive fashion with the instructional effects referred to above. In particular, blood pressure feedback tends to facilitate blood pressure differences, heart-rate feedback tends to facilitate respiration differences, and heart-rate instructions tend to facilitate EMG differences. The heart-rate component is relatively ubiquitous and appears to be a primary response to the "increase" and "decrease" components of the different instructions.

The observation that exteroceptive feedback of heart rate serves to identify a respiratory component may be interpreted as evidence that the relationship between respiration and heart-rate control is relatively intransigent. In support of this conclusion is the recent observation by Levenson and Strupp (1972) that under conditions of differential exteroceptive feedback, correlated phasic changes in respiration and heart rate could not be disrupted. Clearly, the functional interrelationship of these activities is not in question any more than is the functional interrelationship between, for example, heart rate and blood pressure. In the latter case, however, differential feedback procedures have proved effective in producing associative and dissociative phasic changes in the two activities (Schwartz, 1972). As was mentioned earlier, the ease with which normally correlated activities may be made to vary independently may provide an empirical basis for inferring the functional organization of the associated neural control centers.

Comparison of the response profiles associated with the BPI/DPFB and HRI/HRFB conditions in Fig. 2 suggests that specific control over cardiovascular activities may be demonstrated under appropriate conditions of exteroceptive feedback. However, these data do not establish whether or not such control will continue to be manifested when the feedback is withdrawn. This point is important both from a theoretical and practical point of view. Theoretically, the ability to demonstrate specific control following the withdrawal of exteroceptive feedback establishes within the terms of the proposed model that response-specific interoceptive feedback has been calibrated by the exteroceptive feedback during training. From a practical point of view, the advantages of establishing control that is not dependent upon the continual availability of technological hardware is obvious. Such advantages have been realized in the results reported by Engel and Bleecker (1974) in the treatment of cardiac arrhythmias by training under conditions of exteroceptive feedback. These investigators gradually weaned their patients from exteroceptive feedback, thereby forcing more reliance on intrinsic cues in the regulation of their cardiac rhythms. That facilitated heart-rate control may be maintained following the withdrawal of exteroceptive feedback has also been established by Brener et al. (1969), who demonstrated that the degree of learned heart-rate control exhibited by subjects in the absence of exteroceptive feedback was a direct function of the amount of feedback they had received during training. Recently Shapiro et al. (1972) have demonstrated that subjects trained to control their diastolic blood pressures under conditions of exteroceptive feedback displayed evidence of blood pressure control when the feedback was withdrawn. These blood pressure differences were, however, closely paralleled by changes in heart rate suggesting the operation of a generalized control process rather than one that was specific to diastolic blood pressure. Little evidence, therefore, exists that subjects are able to exert specific control over diastolic blood pressure in the absence of exteroceptive feedback or, indeed, that such responses have discriminable interoceptive sensory consequences. For this reason, an experiment was undertaken to examine the differentiation of diastolic blood pressure control under conditions of exteroceptive feedback and to explore the transfer of such control to conditions in which exteroceptive feedback was withdrawn (Brener and Shanks, 1974).

Ten naive undergraduate males were submitted to a training procedure consisting of four phases. In the first and last phases of the experiment, no exteroceptive feedback of diastolic blood pressure was provided, whereas in the middle two phases, subjects received auditory feedback whenever their instantaneous diastolic blood pressures exceeded or fell below a criterion value. The criterion was set separately for each subject and adjusted throughout the procedure to approximate his mean diastolic blood pressure. As in the previous experiment, continuous recordings were made of diastolic blood pressure, heart rate, chin EMG, and respiratory volume. Each experimental phase consisted of two blocks of ten training trials, with blocks of three baseline trials preceding each block of training trials, and one block of baseline trials following the final block of training trials. Five subjects were instructed to increase their blood pressures on the first block of training trials in each phase and to decrease on the second block, whereas the other five received "increase" and "decrease" instructions in the reverse order. The rationale of this design was as follows:

1. The first and last phases of the experiment during which no exteroceptive feedback was provided to subjects enabled the determination of the effects of instructions to modify blood pressure prior to and following exteroceptive feedback. Any systematic changes in performance between Phases I and IV could then be attributed to the interpolated feedback experience.

2. Two successive feedback phases were run to permit an assessment of the development of specific control where such differentiation could be assessed by changes in the relative magnitudes of the four responses under study.

3. Baseline levels of activity were measured throughout the procedure in order to provide a valid basis for assessing the degree to which the experimentally induced changes in activity were attributable to increases above or decreases below the baseline. Continuous redetermination of baselines was also thought advisable in order to compensate for unidirectional changes in tonic levels of activity throughout any phase of the procedure.

Mean baseline activities were computed for each subject for each phase of the experiment by averaging the activity levels recorded during the 9 baseline trials of each phase. Average activity levels were then computed for the increase and decrease trial blocks for each phase of the experiment for each subject. Mean increase and decrease scores were then obtained by subtracting the baseline means for each phase from the corresponding increase and decrease means for that phase, thereby yielding an increase and decrease difference score for each measure of activity for each phase of the experiment. The group means for these difference scores are illustrated in Fig. 3. The scales for the different measures of activity have been adjusted so that the total areas under the set of bars representing changes from baseline for each activity are equal.

As in the previous experiment, it will be seen here that the mean levels

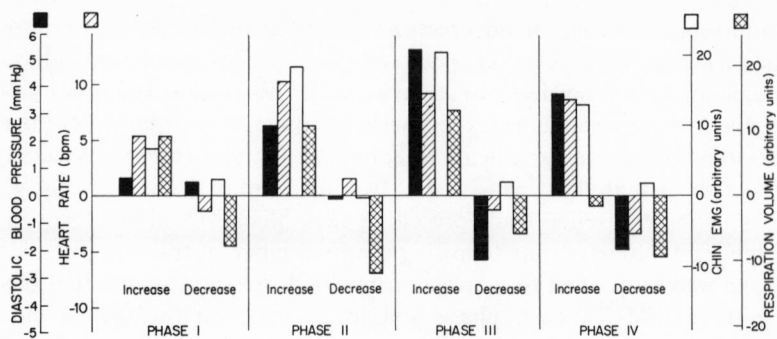

FIG. 3. The effects of training under conditions of diastolic blood pressure feedback on four measures of activity.

of activity recorded during increase trials were consistently greater in all phases of the experiment than the corresponding levels recorded during decrease trials. The absolute increase–decrease differences computed by subtracting the levels of activity recorded during the decrease trials of each phase from the corresponding levels of activity recorded during increase trials are presented below in Table 2. In parentheses beside each absolute difference score is an expression of that difference score as a proportion of the corresponding difference score observed during Phase I of the experiment. Thus, the absolute increase–decrease blood pressure difference recorded during Phase IV of the experiment was 44.9 times greater than that recorded during Phase I. As will be noted from this table, the enhancement of absolute blood pressure differences during Phases II, III, and IV are an order of magnitude greater than the enhancements observed in the other measures of activity. While the Law of Initial Values is clearly operative in determining these proportionate effects, it must nevertheless be conceded that under the conditions imposed by this procedure, diastolic blood pressure control was influenced to a substantially greater degree than any of the other variables monitored. As was mentioned earlier, this relatively greater augmentation of the blood pressure component of the response constellation produced by instructions to modify blood pressure is indicative of the normal process of response differentiation.

The influence of diastolic blood pressure feedback may be observed not only to exert a substantially greater influence on blood pressure than on the other variables, but it will also be observed by reference to Fig. 3 and Table 2 that this influence was more systematically manifested in the blood pressure changes. In particular, it will be noted that when exteroceptive feedback of diastolic blood pressure was provided, blood pressure alone displayed systematic augmentation of both the increase and decrease responses, with greater increases and decreases being displayed during Phase III than Phase II. Although the provision of exteroceptive blood pressure feedback did tend to facilitate the absolute increase–decrease differences for all measures of activity, it will be noted that the heart-rate increment during Phase III was less then that recorded in Phase II, whereas the EMG and respiration decrements during Phase III were smaller than those recorded during Phase II.

The specific effects of providing exteroceptive feedback of diastolic blood pressure on the activities under study were assessed by comparing the activity changes recorded during Phase I with the equivalent changes recorded during Phase III. These analyses revealed that absolute blood pressure differences (increase–decrease) alone were significantly augmented by the provision of blood pressure feedback. Assessment of the increases above and decreases below baseline between Phases I and III indicated that whereas both blood pressure and EMG increases were significantly augmented by feedback, blood pressure decreases alone were significantly augmented.

The effects of training under conditions of exteroceptive diastolic blood pressure feedback on the response-controlling properties of instructions to modify the blood pressure may be assessed by comparing the response profiles associated with Phase I (prior to feedback training) with those associated with Phase IV (following feedback training). Such a comparison reveals that both the absolute (increase–decrease) blood pressure and EMG differences induced by instructions to modify the blood pressure were significantly greater following feedback training than prior to this training. Similar assessments of the changes from baseline indicated that blood pressure increases alone were significantly greater during Phase IV than Phase I. Considerable intersubject variability prevented the augmentation of blood pressure decrements from Phases I to IV from achieving statistical significance. Nevertheless, it will be seen from Fig. 3

TABLE 2. Absolute Increase–Decrease Differences in the Four Measures of Activity as a Function of Experimental Phase

	Blood pressure (mm Hg)	Heart rate (bpm)	Chin EMG (arbitrary units)	Respiration volume (arbitrary units)
Phase I	0.13 (1.00)	6.61 (1.00)	4.2 (1.00)	16.9 (1.00)
Phase II	3.44 (26.5)	8.54 (1.29)	18.5 (4.18)	33.34 (1.32)
Phase III	7.83 (60.2)	10.57 (1.60)	18.27 (4.16)	18.87 (1.12)
Phase IV	5.84 (44.9)	12.19 (1.85)	11.19 (2.53)	8.00 (0.47)

that the blood pressure component represents the only substantial change in the response profile associated with decrease instructions from Phases I to IV.

These results warrant the conclusion that training under conditions of exteroceptive feedback of diastolic blood pressure leads to a specific augmentation of the blood pressure and EMG adjustments induced by instructions to increase blood pressure. Although it is also established that this procedure is effective in producing diastolic blood pressure control that transfers to conditions in which exteroceptive feedback is withdrawn, the conclusion that this control is reliant upon interoceptive feedback that is specific to changes in diastolic blood pressure is unwarranted. Because significant increases in blood pressure control were accompanied by significant increases in EMG control, the possibility remains open that the control process was regulated via interoceptive feedback of somatomotor activity. It should, however, be noted that such EMG changes were associated only with increases in diastolic blood pressure and not with decreases below baseline. This observation suggests the possibility that different mechanisms may have, respectively, been invoked in the production of increases and decreases in diastolic blood pressure.

8. Conclusions

The purpose of this chapter has been to describe a theoretical framework within which the development of voluntary control over specific responses of the cardiovascular system may be analyzed. It has been argued that the specificity of learned cardiovascular control is limited primarily by the discriminability of interoceptive feedback deriving from the specific responses in question. Data have been presented to provide partial validation of this hypothesis, and a method has been described for the experimental investigation of interoceptive discrimination in intact humans.

The functions of exteroceptive feedback in the development of learned cardiovascular control have been examined within a conceptual framework developed from James' *ideo-motor* theory of voluntary action. Exteroceptive feedback stimuli are considered to function primarily as external calibrating referents which serve to identify and label the interoceptive consequences of effective motor adjustments. This calibrating process is seen as a necessary prerequisite to the subsequent environmental (instructional) production of effective motor adjustments.

In terms of this theoretical approach, instructions and exteroceptive feedback are considered to be two sides of the same coin, with instructions embodying the effects of the previous feedback experiences of subjects. An experiment is reported in which the effects of the interaction between instructions and feedback were examined. The results of this experiment indicate that the characteristics of voluntary cardiovascular adjustments may be analyzed in terms of the specific effects of the particular instructions and feedback stimuli employed in the demonstration of that adjustment. This experiment also emphasizes the need for careful asessment of the behavioral influence of instructions per se. It is pointed out that much of the current literature on learned cardiovascular control may be understood in terms of generalized ergotropic and trophotropic responses induced respectively by such common instructional commands as "increase" and "decrease."

Finally, attention is given to the development of response-specific cardiovascular control. The concept of specificity of control is examined and an experiment on the development of diastolic blood pressure control reported. The design of this experiment enabled the determination of changes in the behavioral effects of instructions to modify blood pressure as a function of interpolated feedback training. The results indicated that although diastolic blood pressure control was substantially enhanced by this training procedure, the effect was not specific to this response of the cardiovascular system.

The approach to learned cardiovascular control that is presented in this chapter diverges from the more pragmatic approaches implicit in the conditioning literature. It is argued that the use of feedback (reinforcement) procedures without attention to the functions of such procedures has impaired the understanding of learned cardiovascular phenomena, and inhibited the development of more powerful techniques for the modification of cardiovascular and other visceral activities. A point of major emphasis in the approach adopted here is that closer attention to the sensory and information properties of activity will foster a deeper and more effective understanding of learned motor control in general, and voluntary cardiovascular control in particular. Recently Engel (1972) suggested that the demonstration of operant autonomic phenomena are of no importance to the science of psychology in that they add nothing conceptually to our appreciation of the learning process. In this respect, I find myself in total disagreement with Engel. More than any other recent experimental development, the literature on learned visceral control has served to bring attention to the heuristic inadequacy of prevalent theoretical formulations of the learning process. Of particular significance is the interest that this literature has fostered in the functions of feedback stimuli during the development of motor control. An outgrowth of this theoretical reorientation is manifested in the renewed concern psychophysiologists are displaying in the concept of *voluntary* behavior. By exploring the procedures and mechanisms involved in establishing voluntary characteristics in a traditionally *involuntary* response system, a major conceptual barrier hindering the interaction of psychology and other biological sciences is breached.

9. References

Basmajian, J. V., 1963, Conscious control of single nerve cells, *New Scientist 369:*661–664.
Bergman, J. S., and Johnson, H. J., 1971, The effects of instructional set and autonomic perception on cardiac control, *Psychophysiol. 8:*180–190.
Bergman, J. S., and Johnson, H. J., 1972, Sources of information which affect training and raising of heart rate, *Psychophysiol. 9:*30–39.
Blanshard, B., 1958, The case for determinism, in: *Determinism and Freedom,* (S., Hook, ed.) New York University Press, New York.
Brackin, D., 1973, The effect of visual feedback and instructions on the development of alpha wave control, unpublished doctoral dissertation, University of Tennessee, 1973.
Brener, J., 1966, Heart rate as an avoidance response, *Psychol. Rec. 16:*329–336.
Brener, J., 1974a, Learned control of cardiovascular processes: feedback mechanisms and therapeutic applications, in: *Innovative Treatment Methods in Psychopathology* (K. S. Calhoun, H. E. Adams, and K. M. Mitchell, eds.) John Wiley and Sons, Inc., New York, pp. 245–272.
Brener, J. M., 1974b, A general model of voluntary control applied to the phenomena of learned cardiovascular change, in: *Cardiovascular Psychophysiology,* (P. A. Obrist, A. H. Black, J. Brener, and L. V. DiCara, eds.) Aldine-Atherton, Chicago (in press).
Brener, J., Eissenberg, E., and Middaugh, S., 1974, Respiratory and somatomotor factors associated with operant conditioning of cardiovascular responses in curarized rats, in: *Cardiovascular Psychophysiology* (P. A. Obrist, A. H. Black, J. Brener, and L. V. DiCara, eds.), Aldine-Atherton, Chicago (in press).
Brener, J. M., and Goesling, W. J., 1968, Heart rate and conditioned activity, paper read at Society for Psychophysiology Research meeting, Washington, D.C., October, 1968.
Brener, J., and Hothersall, D., 1966, Heart rate control under conditions of augmented sensory feedback, *Psychophysiol. 3:*23–28.
Brener, J., and Hothersall, D., 1967, Paced respiration and heart rate control, *Psychophysiol. 4:*1–6.
Brener, J., and Kleinman, R. A., 1970, Learned control of decreases in systolic blood pressure, *Nature 226*(170):1063–1064.
Brener, J., Kleinman, R. A., and Goesling, W. J., 1969, The effect of different exposures to augmented sensory feedback on the control of heart rate, *Psychophysiol. 5:*(5):510–516.
Brener, J., and Shanks, E., 1974, The interaction of instructions and feedback in the training of cardiovascular control. Submitted for publication.
Bykov, K. M., 1957, *The Cerebral Cortex and the Internal Organs* (W. H. Gantt, ed.) and Trans., Chemical Publishing Company, New York.
Clemens, W. J., 1972, The role of feedback in the acquisition of a simple skill, unpublished doctoral dissertation, University of Tennessee, 1972.
Davis, R. C., 1943, The genetic development of patterns of voluntary activity, *J. Exptl. Psychol. 33:*471–486.
DiCara, L. V., 1970, Analysis of arterial blood gases in the curarized artificially respirated rat, *Behav. Res. Meth. Instr. 2:*67–69.

DiCara, L. V., and Miller, N. E., 1968a, Instructional learning of vasomotor responses by rats: learning to respond differentially in the two ears, *Science 159:*1485.

DiCara, L. V., and Miller, N. E., 1969a, Transfer of instrumentally learned heart rate changes from curarized to non-curarized state: implications for a mediation hypothesis, *J. Comp. Physiol. Psychol. 68:*159–162.

Engel, B. T., 1972, Operant conditioning of cardiac functioning: a status report, *Psychophysiol. 9:*161–177.

Engel, B. T., and Bleecker, E. R., 1974, Application of operant conditioning techniques to the control of cardiac arrhythmias, in: *Cardiovascular Psychophysiology* (P. A. Obrist, A. H. Black, J. Brener, and L. V. DiCara, eds.), Aldine-Atherton, Chicago, (in press).

Engel, B. T., and Chism, R. A., 1967a, Operant conditioning of heart rate speeding, *Psychophysiol. 3:*418–426.

Engel, B. T., and Hansen, S. P., 1966, Operant conditioning of heart rate slowing, *Psychophysiol. 3:*176–187.

Ferster, C. B., and Skinner, B. F., 1957, *Schedules of Reinforcement,* Appleton-Century Crofts, New York.

Figar, S., 1965, Conditional circulatory responses in men and animals, in: *Handbook of Physiology, Circulation, Am. Physiol. Soc.,* Sect. 2, Vol. III, pp. 1991–2035, Washington, D.C.

Gellhorn, E., 1957, *Principles of Autonomic-Somatic Integration,* University of Minnesota Press, Minneapolis.

Germana, J., 1969, Central efferent processes and autonomic behavioral integration, *Psychophysiol. 6:*78–90.

Goesling, W. J., and Brener, J., 1972, Effects of activity and immobility conditioning upon subsequent heart-rate conditioning in curarized rats, *J. Comp. Physiol. Psychol. 81*(2):311–317.

Guyton, A. C., 1972, *Structure and Function of the Nervous System,* W. B. Saunders Company, Philadelphia.

Hahn, W. W., 1974, The learning of autonomic responses by curarized animals, in: *Cardiovascular Psychophysiology* (P. A. Obrist, A. H. Black, J. Brener, and L. V. DiCara, eds.), Aldine-Atherton, Chicago, (in press).

Hefferline, R. F., Keenan, B., and Harford, R. A., 1959, Escape and avoidance conditioning in human subjects without their observation of the response, *Science 130:*1338–1339.

Hess, W. R., 1954, *Diencephalon: Autonomic and Extrapyramidal Functions,* Grune and Stratton, New York.

Hnatiow, M., and Lang, B. J., 1965, Learned stabilization of cardiac rate, *Psychophysiol. 1:*330–336.

Holt, E. B., 1915, *The Freudian Wish and its Place in Ethics,* Holt, Rinehart and Winston, New York.

Hull, C. L., 1943, *Principles of Behavior,* Appleton-Century Crofts, New York.

James, W., 1890, *Principles of Psychology,* Holt, New York.

Katkin, E. S., and Murray, E. N., 1968, Instrumental conditioning of autonomically mediated behavior: theoretical and methodological issues, *Psychol. Bull. 70*(1):52–68.

Kendler, H. H., 1952, "What is learned?"—A theoretical blind alley, *Psychol. Rev. 59:*269–227.

Kuntz, A., 1953, *The Autonomic Nervous System,* fourth edition, Lea and Febiger, Philadelphia.

Lang, P. J., Sroufe, L. A., and Hastings, J. E., 1967, Effects of feedback and instructional set on the control of cardiac rate variability, *J. Exptl. Psychol. 75:*425–431.

Levenson, R. W. and Strupp, H. H., 1972, Simultaneous feedback and control of heart rate and respiration rate, unpublished manuscript, Vanderbilt University.

Miller, N. E., 1969, Learning of visceral and glandular responses, *Science 163:*434–445.

Miller, N. E., and Banuazizi, A., 1965, Instrumental learning by curarized rats of a specific visceral response, intestinal or cardiac, *J. Comp. Physiol. Psychol. 65:*1–7.

Miller, N. E., and Dworkin, B. R., 1974, Visceral learning: recent difficulties with curarized rats and significant problems for human research, in: *Cardiovascular Psychophysiology* (P. A. Obrist, A. H. Black, J. Brener, and L. V. DiCara, eds.), Aldine-Atherton, Chicago, (in press).

Mott, F. W., and Sherrington, C. S., 1895, Experiments upon the influences of sensory nerves upon movement and nutrition of the limbs, *Proc. Roy. Soc.* (London) *57:*481–488.

Obrist, P. A., Howard, J. L., Lawler, J. G., Galosy, R. A., Meyers, K. A., and Gaebelein, C. J., 1974, The cardiac-somatic interaction, in: *Cardiovascular Psychophysiology.* (P. A. Obrist, A. H., Black, J. Brener, and L. V. DiCara, eds.), Aldine-Atherton, Chicago (in press).

Razran, G., 1961, The observable unconscious and the inferable conscious in current Soviet psychophysiology: Interoceptive conditioning, semantic conditioning, and the orienting reflex, *Psychol. Rev. 68:*81–147.

Schwartz, G., 1972, Voluntary control of human cardiovascular integration and differentiation through feedback and reward, *Science 175:*90–93.

Shanks, E., 1973, The interaction between instructions and augmented sensory feedback in the training of cardiovascular control, unpublished doctoral dissertation, University of Tennessee.

Shapiro, D., Tursky, B., Gershon, E., and Stern, M., 1969, Effects of feedback and reinforcement on the control of human systolic blood pressure, *Science 163:*588–590.

Shapiro, D., Schwartz, G. E., and Tursky, B., 1972, Control of diastolic blood pressure in man by feedback and reinforcement, *Psychophysiol. 9:*296–304.

Smith, K., 1967, Conditioning as an artifact, in *Foundations of Conditioning and Learning* (G. A. Kimble, ed.), pp. 100–111, Appleton-Century Crofts, New York.

Snyder, C., and Nobel, M., 1968, Operant conditioning of vasoconstriction, *J. Exptl. Psychol. 77:*263–268.

Taub, E., and Berman, A. J., 1968, Movement and learning in the absence of sensory feedback, in: *The Neurophysiology of Spatially Oriented Behavior* (S. J. Freedman, ed.), pp. 173–192, Dorsey Press, Homewood, Illinois.

Tsitovich, I. S., 1981, About so-called vasomotor psycho-reflexes, *Russk. Fiziol. Zh.* 1:113.

Verplanck, W. S., 1962, Unaware of where's awareness: Some verbal operants, in: *Behavior and Awareness* (C. W. Eriksen, ed.), pp. 130–158, Duke University Press, Durham, North Carolina.

Wenger, M. A., Bagchi, B. K., and Anand, B. K., 1961, Experiments in India on "voluntary" control of heart and pulse, *Circulation 24:*1319–1326.

Woolsey, C. N., 1953, Patterns of localization in sensory and motor areas of the cerebral cortex, in: *The Biology of Mental Health and Disease* (Milbank Memorial Fund), pp. 193–225, Hoeber, New York.

CHAPTER 11

Cultivated Low Arousal—An Antistress Response? *

Johann Stoyva and Thomas Budzynski
University of Colorado School of Medicine
Denver, Colorado

Assumptions. Our basic working hypothesis, and the unifying principle behind most of our experiments, has been the idea that frequently
stressed individuals will show physiological hyperarousal in one or several
bodily systems. A complementary hypothesis has been that frequently
stressed (or over-reactive individuals) are likely to lose the ability to relax
well; i.e., to shift into a low arousal condition.

When faced by recurring stresses, the individual must repeatedly mobilize his physical and mental resources. Such responding characteristically
involves sympathetic activation and elevated muscle tension, a readiness to
respond to threats and challenges—the *fight-or-flight* response or
defense-alarm reaction. Individuals forced frequently to mobilize
themselves to meet stresses are likely to lose their ability to execute the opposite response, i.e., to shift into the parasympathetic mode in which bodily
recuperation normally occurs. Support for this position can be drawn from
the work and theories of scientists such as Charvat, Folkow, Malmo,
Sternbach, Cannon, Wolff, Lader, and Mathews.

The other major component of our theoretical orientation has been the
assumption that the individual's reaction to psychological stress is capable

* Presented in abridged form as presidential address by the first author at the Fourth Annual
Meeting of the Biofeedback Research Society, November 1972, Boston, Massachusetts.

   This research was supported by the Advanced Research Projects Agency of the Department
of Defense and was monitored by the Office of Naval Research under Contract N00014-70-
C-0350 to the San Diego State College Foundation, by National Institute of Mental Health
Grant Number MH-15596, and Research Scientist Development Award Number K01-MH-
43361-01.

of at least some learned modification. Such learned modification can, we think, be strengthened by means of feedback techniques. Generally, biofeedback techniques employed in our laboratory have been designed to produce low arousal—a condition we assume has physiological effects opposite to those produced by stress.

Although our beginning experimental work focused on alpha feedback, growing evidence for the clinical usefulness of muscle relaxation caused us to shift our efforts to electromyographic (EMG) feedback. Various sources suggested that muscle relaxation would be useful in producing a low arousal condition with certain anti-stress properties. For example, there was Jacobson's (1938) important pioneering work with progressive relaxation, a technique which he employed for a variety of anxiety and stress-related disorders. Also, the German-developed autogenic training (Luthe, 1963; 1969)–essentially a series of exercises designed to produce a shift toward a parasympathetic response pattern—similarly pointed to the clinical usefulness of "cultivated low arousal" and allied techniques. Of more recent origin was the behavior therapy technique of systematic desensitization (Wolpe, 1958), a valuable new approach in reducing anxiety to both real and symbolic situations. In the most commonly used variant of the latter technique, muscle relaxation forms an integral part of the procedure.

A further consideration in favor of muscle relaxation was that since the striate musculature makes up at least 50% of body mass, it would seem likely to have powerful effects on the organism as a whole. Also, there was the obvious fact that muscular activity is an inescapable part of adaptive behavior (and of the response to stress). Without it, there is no behavior. We therefore felt that training in muscle relaxation—and its accompanying low arousal condition—would be an important *first step* in the search to find ways of *moderating the reaction to stress*.

1. Two Clinical Examples of Modifying the Response to Stress

Is there any convincing evidence that the individual's response to stress can be modified? Actually, there are at least two useful clinical examples which may be cited. One is the just-mentioned behavior therapy technique of systematic desensitization. In essence, this technique involves substituting a relaxation response for an anxiety response. When desensitization is complete, the patient is able to think calmly about things which formerly made him extremely anxious.

1.1. Systematic Desensitization

In his development of systematic desensitization, Wolpe (1958) drew on the important pioneering work of Jacobson (1938). Over the years, Jacobson had noted that anxious patients typically show elevated levels of muscle tension. On the basis of clinical observations, he developed the parallel idea that cultivating a condition of thorough muscular relaxation could be useful in reducing a patient's anxiety.

It was for this reason that Wolpe (1958) incorporated the Jacobson technique into the practice of systematic desensitization. Specifically, he postulated that a condition of muscular relaxation is physiologically incompatible with an anxiety response. On the strength of this postulate, muscle relaxation came to play a central role in systematic desensitization.

In Wolpe's desensitization technique, the patient is first taught muscle relaxation by means of an abbreviated Jacobson progressive relaxation technique (usually two to six training sessions). He is next presented with a graded series of anxiety scenes, known as a *"hierarchy."* A given hierarchy is focused around a single theme, such as public-speaking anxiety; and the items are ranked from the one which is the least anxiety-producing to that which is most anxiety-producing. When the actual desensitization is begun, the least-anxiety-evoking scene is used first. The task of the patient is to maintain a condition of thorough relaxation while he imagines the anxiety item. After he masters a given scene, the patient progresses to a more difficult one until finally he becomes able to remain calm even while visualizing the scene which formerly made him the most anxious. Wolpe (1958) reports that transfer from the clinic to everyday life occurs readily, and in the case of specific anxieties, such as phobias, Wolpe and Lazarus (1966) report an impressive successful outcome rate of 80 to 90 percent.

1.2. Tension Headache

In this laboratory, we began working with tension headache. This is a stress-related disorder likely to occur when the patient feels under external pressures (e.g., deadlines, plenty of unfinished work, or mutually conflicting tasks) or feels burdened by emotional conflicts. Since it had been experimentally demonstrated (Wolff, 1963) that the immediate cause of tension headache is the sustained contraction of the head or neck muscles, we hypothesized that systematic training in muscular relaxation might be useful in treating this disorder.

To assist the process of muscular relaxation, we employed an EMG feedback device originally developed by T. H. Budzynski (see Budzynski and Stoyva, 1969). Its essential operation is as follows: surface electrodes detect the EMG activity produced by a particular muscle, such as the frontalis. Through his headphones, the patient hears a train of discrete clicks. If EMG activity is high, the click rate is fast. When EMG activity decreases, the click rate also decreases. The task of the patient is to relax as thoroughly as possible—aided by the information feedback provided by the clicks.

Pilot Work. The EMG feedback technique was applied to several tension headache patients,—the first five individuals available for the study (see Budzynski *et al.*, 1970). With EMG feedback training in muscle relaxation, these patients not only learned to produce lowered EMG activity (frontalis monitored), but showed associated reductions in headache activity. Follow-up results over a 3-month period indicated that for these five patients, headache activity remained at a low level, especially if they continued to practice relaxation for a short time every day. An interesting collateral observation was that many patients, when they felt tension headache beginning to develop in a stress situation, learned to abort the headache by deliberately relaxing their upper body musculature.

Controlled-Outcome Study. In view of our favorable pilot observations, we initiated a controlled-outcome study (Budzynski *et al.*, unpublished observations). The experimental design involved one treatment group and two control groups. The six patients in the experimental group (group A) received accurate information feedback as to their frontalis EMG levels. Over a 9-week period, they received two EMG feedback sessions per week. The six patients in the *pseudo-feedback* group (group B) were given the same number of laboratory sessions of relaxation training, but instead of true feedback they listened to feedback signals which had been tape recorded from the experimental group. To help in applying the relaxation response to everyday life, all patients in both the experimental and pseudo-control groups were told to do the relaxation training at home or work twice a day. The six subjects in the second control group (group C) received no treatment at all.

All persons chosen for the study suffered from frequent tension headaches and had been afflicted for an average of 7 years or more. Patients in all three groups kept daily records of headache activity (a rating scale of intensity recorded on an hour-by-hour basis) during the entire experiment, and for a 3-month follow-up period.

Results. In brief, the results showed that, with training, frontalis EMG levels in the experimental group fell to less than 40 percent of baseline values. In the pseudo-feedback group, levels remained at about 80

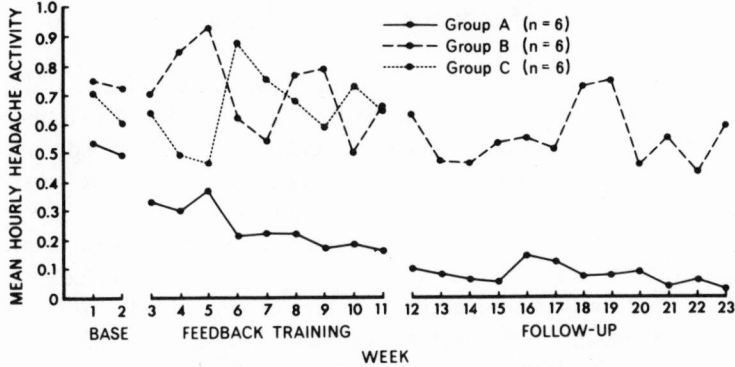

FIG. 1. Headache activity during baseline period, during 2-month feedback training period, and during 3-month follow-up period (A and B only). Group A was experimental group receiving EMG feedback training. Groups B and C were controls.

percent of baseline values. This difference between the two groups was even greater at the end of the 3-month follow-up period (mean frontalis EMG levels for group A = 3.92 mV, and for group B = 8.43 mV; $p < 0.01$).

Figure 1 shows the headache activity over a 23-week period for the three groups. Group A levels of headache activity toward the end of training (weeks 8 and 9) were significantly lower than in groups B and C ($p < 0.001$, Kruskal–Wallis analysis of variance by ranks).

Group A patients also showed a sharply reduced medication usage, when assessed at the end of the 3-month follow-up period. Such a reduction was not characteristically shown by the group B patients.

In summary, then, patients in the treatment group showed diminished headache activity, greatly decreased drug usage, and markedly reduced frontalis EMG levels relative to those of the two control groups. Since the controlled study was completed, a number of additional patients have been run on a case-by-case basis, so that by now over 60 persons have undergone the training. Approximately 75% of them have shown substantial reductions in headache activity. Of the control patients run to date (total of 12), fewer than 25% have shown substantial improvement.

Also, of great interest, from the point of view of modifying the stress response, is that patients typically passed through several stages in terms of their ability to use a *cultivated* relaxation response to reduce headache activity. At first they were able to relax only with deliberate effort. Later, the relaxation response became easier to do, even when the patient felt under some pressure. Finally, with some patients, the relaxation response appeared to have become virtually an automatic reaction, no longer requiring conscious effort.

2. Experiments on Feedback-Induced Muscle Relaxation

The two foregoing clinical examples show that systematic training in muscle relaxation can be useful in treating certain stress-related disorders. It should be noted, however, that in the older techniques of inducing a relaxed, low arousal condition—such as Jacobson's progressive relaxation, systematic desensitization, and autogenic training—the training is generally conducted without continuous physiological monitoring. Such a practice can lead to difficulties. For example, is the subject really relaxed or simply reporting that he is? Or, if he has trouble relaxing—likely to be the case with patients having stress-related disorders—how can he be efficiently and reliably taught to relax?

In view of these problems, and in view of the demonstrated (and potential) clinical value of muscle relaxation, we decided to explore the idea that feedback techniques could be used to improve the learning of muscle relaxation. Therefore, in tandem with our clinical studies (on tension headache and sleep-onset insomnia), we undertook a series of validation and parameter studies addressed to questions such as the following. Is EMG feedback superior to the absence of it in producing muscle relaxation? Does muscle relaxation have effects on other bodily systems, e.g., cortical or autonomic activity? Are some muscles more useful than others for inducing a relaxed, low arousal condition? Can subjects learn to maintain the relaxation response even in the absence of feedback? Described below is a series of interlocking experiments bearing on these questions. Although these studies are chiefly drawn from work in our own laboratory, it should be noted that other investigators have worked with EMG feedback, for example, Green et al. (1970). A strong interest of this group has been the experiential correlates of low arousal conditions.

2.1. Frontalis Feedback

In our first validation study (Budzynski and Stoyva, 1969), we made use of the frontalis, a muscle frequently involved in anxiety and hyperarousal disorders (see Sainsbury and Gibson, 1954; Shagass and Malmo, 1954). If subjects could learn to achieve a high degree of control over this hard-to-relax muscle (see Balshan, 1962), then the feedback procedure should presumably be readily applicable to other less difficult muscle groups.

Three groups of five subjects each were compared with respect to depth of relaxation achieved. The experimental group received accurate feedback of frontalis EMG levels (a tone varying in frequency combined with

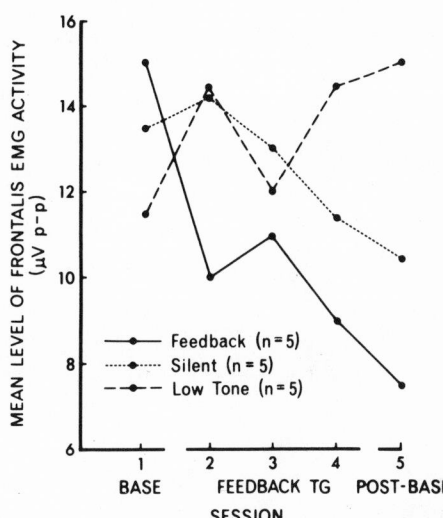

FIG. 2. Mean levels of frontalis EMG activity across sessions.

a shaping procedure). Of the two control groups, one received irrelevant feedback (a steady low tone); the other received no feedback at all (silent condition). Of the approximately 30 subjects who volunteered, the 15 with the highest baseline EMG levels were selected for the experiment.

As indicated in Fig. 2, subjects received one baseline session with no feedback. Next came three training sessions conducted on 3 separate days. Finally, there was a post-baseline day on which there was no feedback of any kind, and subjects were instructed to relax as thoroughly as possible. Additionally, all subjects were given a money reward—the better their performance, the greater the payment for each of the five sessions.

The results clearly showed the superiority of the feedback approach. Following only three training sessions, the feedback subjects had lowered their frontalis EMG levels by 50%; the silent group had decreased by 24%, and the irrelevant feedback group had increased by about 28%.

As Figure 2 shows, although the irrelevant feedback group had the poorest mean performance, the most salient characteristic of this group was its great variability—range of 6.1 to 28.4 mV in Session 5. For the feedback group, the range for Session 5 was 5.3 to 10.8 mV, indicating that correct feedback more reliably produced low levels of EMG activity than did irrelevant feedback.

Further support for the statement that correct feedback more reliably produces thorough relaxation than does irrelevant feedback was demonstrated by comparing one of the subjects from the low tone group

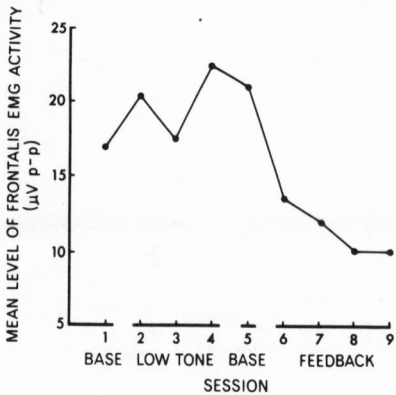

FIG. 3. Mean levels of frontalis EMG activity in same subject under irrelevant (low tone) feedback condition, and under subsequent correct feedback condition.

under both irrelevant feedback and correct feedback conditions. This subject, who had been one of the two poorest performers in the irrelevant feedback group, was provided with correct feedback training over four additional sessions (sessions 6, 7, 8, and 9 in Fig. 3). For this subject, EMG levels had been high throughout the five previous sessions. But, as may be seen in Fig. 3, the mean level dropped sharply with accurate feedback training.

   Cortical Rhythms. An additional observation of interest, especially to electroencephalographers, was that cortical rhythms could be quite clearly distinguished in the forehead EMG after thorough relaxation had been achieved. This phenomenon, although previously noted by Davis (1959), is difficult to observe under ordinary conditions because the dense, high-frequency muscle action potentials from the frontalis mask the cortical rhythms. After feedback training, however, most of the EMG activity drops out of the tracing. Then bursts of cortical frontalis rhythms, in particular alpha (8 to 12 Hertz) and theta (4 to 7 Hertz), are likely to become quite apparent (provided that filter bandpass characteristics are such as to allow the passage of EEG signals).

2.2. Masseter Feedback

   The aim of the second validation study (Budzynski and Stoyva, 1973a) was to see whether the merits of the feedback technique would be apparent even in the course of a single training session. Eighty subjects were told to relax the masseter muscle as deeply as possible. Experimental group 1 consisted of 20 subjects who received accurate auditory feedback (a tone of varying pitch). Experimental group 2 consisted of 20 subjects who received a visual *digital-light* feedback (a small red signal light flashed on or off depending on EMG level). There were two control groups. Twenty control subjects received irrelevant feedback (a steady low tone); and another 20 received no feedback at all. Again the results spoke clearly in favor of the feedback approach.

Mean EMG levels for the *steady low tone* control group ran 70% above those of the two experimental groups. And mean EMG levels for the *silent* control group ran 100% higher than those of the experimental groups (average EMG levels for entire session).

2.3. Frontalis vs. Forearm Feedback

A recent study (Ball *et al.*, unpublished observations) examined whether some muscles are better than others for promoting general bodily relaxation and low arousal. Since work with both patients and normals had suggested that when subjects reached very low EMG levels on the frontalis, that other muscles, especially of the upper body, were also likely to be relaxed, we decided to compare a frontalis feedback group with a forearm (extensor) feedback group. Worth noting in this context is Jacobson's (1970, p. 41) challenging assertion that when EMG activity in the facial and laryngeal muscles falls to very low (close to zero) levels, then the individual is inevitably asleep.

In this study, we ran college age male volunteers under one of three following conditions: (1) Group A received variable rate auditory clicks from frontalis ($n = 7$); (2) Group B received variable rate clicks from forearm extensor ($n = 7$); (3) Group C, the control group, received tape recorded clicks produced by the frontalis subjects.

The three groups were comparable in age ranges, and with respect to means and ranges of EMG levels. Each subject was run for a total of 10 laboratory sessions—including one throwaway adaptation session, two baseline sessions, five training sessions, and two post-baseline sessions (the last without feedback).

TABLE 1. Comparisons Among All Four Groups

Group	Analog-auditory (E)	Digital-visual (L)	Irrelevant (LT)	Silent (S)
Mean EMG (mV)	3.04	3.28	5.33	6.80
S.D.	1.40	1.19	3.47	4.89

Only group A (frontalis feedback) showed a significant decline in frontalis EMG activity when pre-training EMG levels were compared with post-training levels ($p < 0.01$, one-tailed). But perhaps more revealing were pre–post decreases for the three groups expressed as *percentages* (baseline EMG levels minus post-baseline levels).

These results confirmed our hypothesis regarding superiority of the frontalis muscle over the forearm muscle for feedback training purposes. The data showed that only the frontalis feedback subjects decreased on *both* frontalis and forearm EMG levels. In other words, when the frontalis is low, the forearm is also likely to be low. But the reverse relationship does not hold. Subjects receiving forearm feedback decreased 41% on forearm EMG levels, but remained virtually the same on their frontalis EMG levels. Actually, the control subjects showed as much change as did the forearm feedback subjects.

High vs. Low EMG Subjects. Another observation in this experiment—and one likely to be of practical training value—was the differing results for seven high EMG and seven low EMG subjects. (Although 14 frontalis subjects were originally available, it proved possible to match only seven of them with the available forearm and control subjects. However, all 14 received the same frontalis feedback training. For the following comparison, these 14 subjects were divided, on the basis of frontalis EMG, into seven high EMG subjects and seven low ones.)

Figure 4 shows that, in the low frontalis EMG group, pre–post decreases were slight (13%). But, in the high frontalis EMG group, decreases were substantial (46%).

This result is in close agreement with an experiment conducted inde-

TABLE 2

Group A: Frontalis feedback, pre–post declines
$n = 7$
Frontalis decline......31%
Forearm decline.......45%
Group B: Forearm feedback, pre–post declines
$n = 7$
Frontalis decline......2%
Forearm decline.......41%
Group C: Control subjects
$n = 7$
Frontalis decline......9%
Forearm decline.......39%

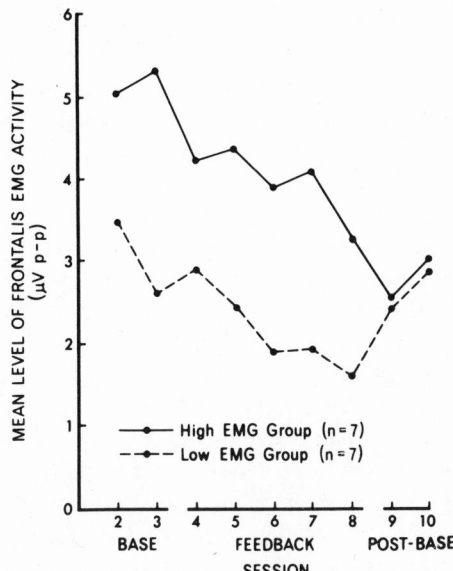

FIG. 4. Frontalis EMB levels across sessions for high and low (baseline) EMG subjects. All subjects trained with frontalis EMG feedback.

pendently at the University of Dusseldorf by Engel and Sittenfeld (personal communication). In their experiment, frontalis EMG's were measured on 200 medical students. Three groups were then chosen for further training— a low frontalis EMG group (n = 12), a medium level frontalis EMG group (n = 12), and a high frontalis EMG group (n = 12). Subjects were given four feedback training sessions on four consecutive days. Control subjects received auditory feedback of their own respiration. High EMG subjects receiving frontalis EMG feedback showed sharp reductions in EMG levels, compared to high EMG subjects receiving only respiratory feedback. However, differences between experimentals and controls were nonexistent in the subjects who had *started* with low frontalis EMG levels.

This finding is valuable in that it helps define the population for whom feedback-induced relaxation is likely to be useful, namely, subjects with high EMG levels. Our impression is that the latter are likely to be older subjects, those with anxiety or stress-linked disorders, people in demanding jobs, or some combination of the foregoing. The observed differences between high and low EMG subjects show that individuals with high muscle tension levels improve considerably in their ability to relax after EMG feedback training. But for subjects who are already quite relaxed, the feedback training produces only minimal changes (a result clearly in keeping with the law of initial values).

2.4.   Effects on Other Bodily Systems

One of the questions raised earlier was whether muscle relaxation would affect other bodily systems. Would it act to dampen autonomic or cortical activity?

Cortical Changes.   A study by Budzynski (1969) demonstrated that the consequences of profound muscle relaxation are not limited to a particular muscle, but are manifested in cortical changes as well. This experiment drew on the work of Venables and Wing (1962), Maley (1967), and Rose (1966) which showed that the fusion threshold for paired flashes of light may be used to determine cortical activation level. In general, individuals who are anxious or hyperalert are usually able to discriminate smaller differences in the time interval between the pairs of successive light flashes than are individuals with more normal activation levels; i.e., the anxious subjects have lower thresholds.

In Budzynski's (1969) experiment, two-flash thresholds were used to assess the cortical effects of profound muscle relaxation. Twelve normal subjects were trained (feedback training on the frontalis, and a neck muscle) to produce thorough muscle relaxation by means of the EMG feedback technique. Each of the 12 subjects showed an increased two-flash threshold (their discrimination interval was longer) in the relaxation condition. Similarly, each subject showed a decreased heart rate and, generally, a decreased respiration rate during profound relaxation (as compared to an isometric, muscle-tensing condition). Thus, when EMG activity diminished, other indicators of activation level such as heart rate and two-flash threshold also changed in the direction of lowered arousal.

Experiential Correlates.   Verbal reports from subjects also indicate that the effects of thorough relaxation are not confined to the particular muscle for which feedback is being provided. Adjective check lists completed after EMG feedback training sessions have shown that sensations of heaviness and tingling of the limbs are common, as are certain body image changes such as experiences of floating, lightness, or turning. Also common are phenomena linked to autonomic changes—sensations of warmth, and increased salivation. Drowsiness and hypnagogic (sleep-onset) imagery are also reported frequently. Subjects generally report the relaxation to be a mildly pleasurable experience, much like waking up from a refreshing nap. These descriptions are in good agreement with those reported in the autogenic training literature (see Luthe, 1965), and although the same pattern of sensations is not reported by every individual, the categories mentioned above occur frequently enough to be of predictive value, when group results are considered.

2.5. The Shaping of Low Arousal

A earlier study (Sittenfield *et al.*, 1972) bears on the question of whether muscle relaxation affects other bodily systems. This experiment supports the concept that muscle, autonomic, and cortical systems (at least in a relaxed, presleep condition) are likely to move in the same direction—although perhaps at different speeds. It further supports the theoretically and practically important idea that muscle relaxation may be an important first step in the biofeedback training of certain autonomic and cortical responses,—particularly those responses associated with a low arousal condition of the organism.

In this experiment we asked whether subjects would acquire some degree of voluntary control over the production of theta. Since we were particularly interested in exploring the use of feedback techniques in cases of sleep-onset insomnia, we sought to determine whether normal subjects could learn to increase theta EEG frequencies above resting baseline levels.

The theta rhythm, 4–7 Hz, is strongly associated with drowsiness, and is recognized as the dominant electroencephalographic (EEG) frequency in Stage 1 of sleep (the sleep-onset stage; see Rechtschaffen and Kales, 1968). It is well known, particularly through the work of Foulkes (1966), that the theta rhythms of sleep-onset are closely associated with hypnagogic or sleep-onset imagery. This materal typically consists of a flow of fleeting, disconnedted visual images, and typically has little or no affect. Recall of specific imagery is reported to occur in over 80% of awakenings (Foulkes, 1966).

Pilot observations soon showed that producing and maintaining a predominantly theta EEG is a very subtle task. Typically, base operant levels of this rhythm are very low—so there is little or nothing to feed back to the subject, a feature which can make learning very frustrating. Also, verbal reports strongly indicate that theta vanishes with the slightest striving on the part of the subject; he must learn to do the opposite, to "let go." Further, when theta is dominant, the subject seems to slip into a dissociated state. And the imagery which occurs is likely to assume a "real" or hallucinatory quality—a feature we were afraid might interfere with learning since attention would probably wander away from the feedback signal.

Because learning to modify theta levels was obviously a demanding and subtle task for most subjects, we hypothesized that a phased training (involving steps of graduated difficulty) might be a more effective approach than using only theta feedback for the entire training period. As Jacobson (1938) had already noted in his extensive work with progressive relaxation—and we had similarly observed—profound muscle relaxation is frequently associated with reports of drowsiness. We therefore decided to test out a two-phase training for the induction of theta. Experimental subjects were first given four sessions of EMG feedback training—to begin the shift toward low arousal. This was followed by four sessions of theta feedback training. Control subjects received theta feedback for each of their eight training sessions.

The ten experimental subjects were divided into five subjects with high baseline EMG levels, and five subjects with low baseline EMG levels. Similarly, the ten control subjects were divided into a high EMG group and a low EMG group. Each of the 20 subjects was run for 13 half-hour sessions—3 baseline sessions, 8 feedback training sessions, and 2 post-baseline sessions (without feedback). In every session the following parameters were continuously measured: theta EEG (filtered output), alpha EEG (filtered output), frontalis EMG, forearm EMG, and heart rate. By means of resetting (Drohocki) integrators, information on each parameter was transformed into a train of digital pulses. These pulses were continuously summed by means of digital counters and totaled on a

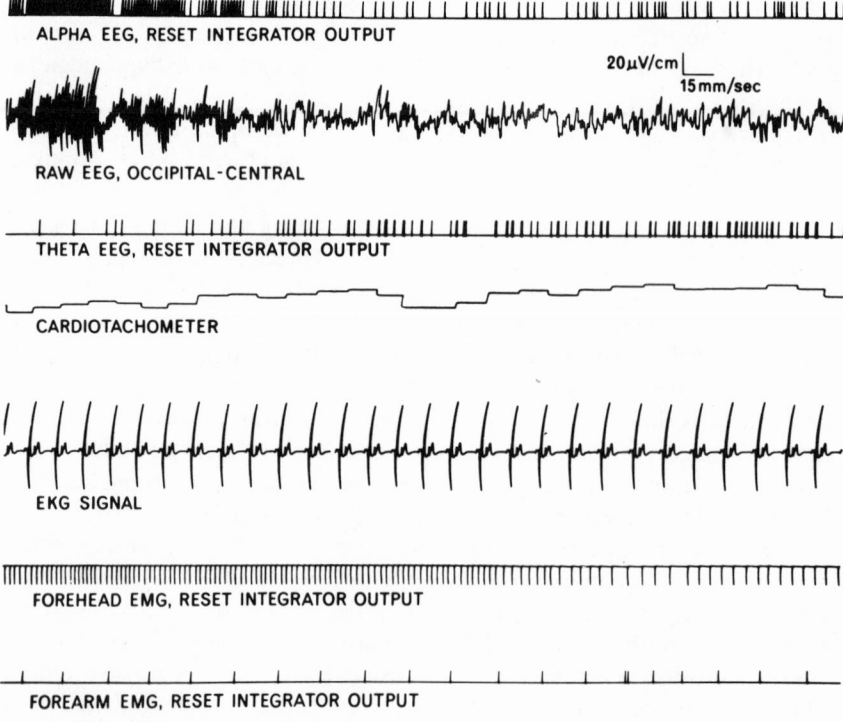

FIG. 5.   Quantification system and digital readout for EMG and EEG.

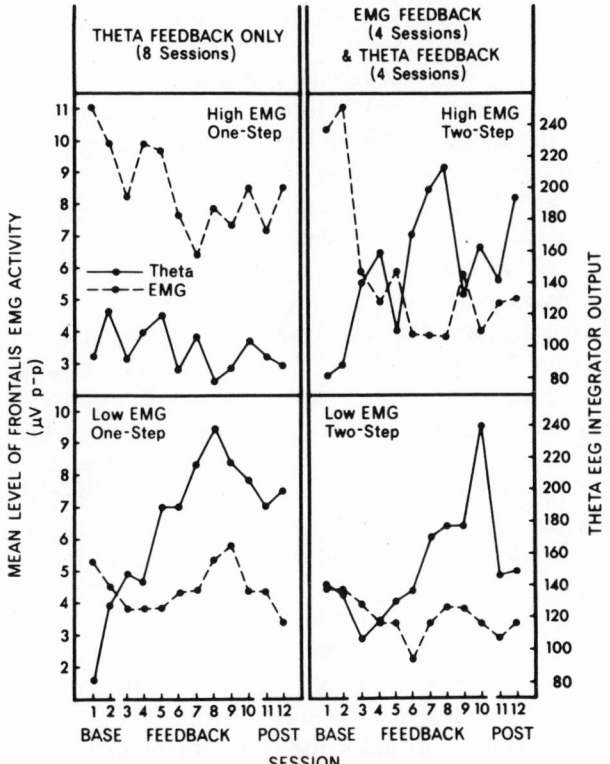

FIG. 6. EMG and theta levels in four different training groups. High
EMG one-step group (n = 5) received eight sessions of theta feedback
only. Low EMG one-step group (n = 5) received eight sessions of theta
feedback only. High EMG two-step group (n = 5) received four sessions
of EMG feedback, followed by four sessions of theta feedback. Low EMG
two-step (n = 5) received four sessions of EMG feedback, followed by
four sessions of theta feedback.

minute-by-minute basis (see Fig. 5 for digital readout and quantification
system).

For the subjects as a whole (n = 20), postbaseline values for theta were
over 50% higher than baseline values, in terms of digital counts produced
by the theta resetting integrator (see Fig. 6). One of the four groups,
however, did *not* succeed in increasing theta levels. This was the high EMG
group in the single-step training condition (eight sessions of strictly theta
feedback). These results indicate that *before high EMG subjects are able to
increase their theta levels, they must first learn to reduce their EMG
activity.* However, in the case of subjects with low baseline EMG values,

either techique (theta feedback for all eight training sessions, or the two-step procedure) can be used for increasing theta level.

Also of interest was that for the group as a whole (n = 20), baseline heart rate and frontalis EMG levels showed a correlation of $+.83$ (rank–order). In the case of the ten high EMG subjects, there was a decline of over 7 beats per minute in heart rate (comparing pre- with postbaseline values). Low EMG subjects showed little or no change. Thus, high EMG subjects showed a combination of decreased EMG activity, decreased heart rate, and increased theta levels—an observation which supports the idea of a shaping technique to produce low arousal.

Another intriguing observation was the evidence of a reciprocal relationship between frontalis EMG levels and abundance of theta. This relationship was particularly strong at sleep onset—where Stage 2 "spindling" sleep begins. At this point, and just prior to it, frontalis EMG regularly showed a sharp drop and theta rhythms displayed a strong increase. Interestingly, this observation is consistent with the previously mentioned statement of Jacobson (1970, p. 41) that, when EMG activity in the facial and laryngeal muscles falls to zero (or close to zero) levels, then the subject is asleep.

An Adaptation Effect? But cannot an objection frequently leveled at the alpha control studies also be raised against this one? Were the increased theta levels merely the result of some nonspecific effect, such as adapting to the laboratory? This interpretation is improbable since, although high EMG subjects given the two-step training showed increased theta levels, high EMG subjects given only the one-step training (theta feedback only) did not, despite 13 sessions in the laboratory. The theta curve for the latter subjects remained flat (see Fig. 6). It should also be noted that alpha levels remained on a plateau for the 13 sessions. This was true for each of the four groups.

These results indicate that, with appropriate feedback training, subjects can learn to increase their levels of theta—an observation in keeping with the commonplace notion that it is difficult to fall asleep if one remains muscularly tense. The study also shows that there is nothing automatic about increasing theta—some techniques work, some do not; the training must be tailored to fit the characteristics of the subject.

Further, the results support the concept of shaping a low arousal condition. In such an approach, subjects would begin their training with the comparatively easy response of learning muscular relaxation—a task which begins a shift toward parasympathetic activity. Subsequently, they would be trained on the more subtle task of changing some specific response such as lowering heart rate or blood pressure, or increasing theta—all associated with low arousal (see last section for further discussion).

2.6. Summary of Validation Studies

In a series of interlocking experiments with EMG feedback we have established the following:

1. Frontalis Study. EMG feedback proved superior to no-feedback and to irrelevant feedback in the production of low frontalis EMG levels (Budzynski and Stoyva, 1969). This superiority was apparent not only during training, but also on a postexperimental session without feedback (see Fig. 2).

2. Masseter Study. In an experiment with masseter relaxation, it was found that the superiority of EMG feedback over the two control conditions was apparent even within a single training session (Budzynski and Stoyva, 1973a; see Table 1).

3. Frontalis vs. Forearm Relaxation. Some muscles are better than others for relaxation training purposes. Thus, subjects who received frontalis feedback training showed substantial decreases on *both* this muscle and on the forearm extensor (which was not receiving feedback). However, the converse relationship was not true. Subjects receiving forearm EMG feedback showed a substantial decline in forearm EMG levels, but little change in frontalis EMG activity. This observation supports the notion that the frontalis is a very useful muscle for relaxation training purposes (see Table 2; Ball *et al.*, unpublished observations).

4. High vs. Low EMG Subjects. The individuals who showed the most dramatic drop in EMG levels were those whose muscle tension levels were comparatively high at the beginning of training. Those whose EMG levels were already low at the beginning of training showed only a moderate decline in EMG activity with feedback training—a result in keeping with the law of initial values (see Fig. 4; Ball *et al.*, unpublished observations).

5. Cortical Changes. Evidence for cortical changes produced by profound muscle relaxation was noted in an experiment by Budzynski (1969). Subjects were less able to detect paired flashes of light in the relaxed condition (i.e., whether a paired flash of lights looked like one light or two). Moreover, verbal reports of thoroughly relaxed subjects indicate that sensations of heaviness, warmth, and drowsiness are common—an observation supporting the idea that muscular relaxation has widespread effects on the organism.

6. Shaping of Theta EEG. Subjects whose baseline EMG levels were high (these are likely to be older subjects, or those in demanding jobs) did better at increasing their theta levels if they were given a two-step feedback training—first, EMG feedback training, then, theta feedback training (Sittenfeld *et al.*, 1972). But subjects with high baseline EMG levels who received only theta feedback training, failed to augment their theta levels (see Fig. 6).

On the other hand, subjects whose starting EMG levels were low did well at increasing theta with either type of training. That is, with low EMG subjects, those who were given simply the one-step training (theta feedback for all training sessions) learned to produce just as much theta as those who were given a two-step training (EMG feedback for first half of training, followed by theta feedback for second half of training).

In addition to increased theta, the (high EMG) subjects showed a decline in heart rate, which appeared to be closely associated with decreasing frontalis EMG levels. Also evident was a clear reciprocal relationship between frontalis EMG activity and theta levels at the moment of sleep-onset. At this point, or shortly prior to it, there was a sharp drop in frontalis EMG activity and a large increase in EEG theta rhythms.

3. Theoretical Background

As already indicated, our basic *working hypothesis* has been that the response to stress can be modified. We regard systematic training in muscle relaxation, and its associated low arousal condition, as a first step in this endeavor.

Our working hypothesis is in turn linked to the idea that in many instances modern man's response to stress is maladaptive—he reacts excessively, or for too long a time. The individual who repeatedly manifests such responding may eventually begin to develop problems, particularly in his most reactive bodily system (e.g., essential hypertensives show large blood pressure increases under stress; see Engel and Bickford, 1961; Wolff, 1968). Fortunately, there is a substantial body of theoretical support which can be marshalled for the foregoing position.

Characteristically, the writers about to be cited point to evidence of hyper-reactivity and sustained arousal in the stress-linked disorders. Coupled with such hyper-reactivity is an inability to return to baseline or resting values after stimulation has occurred.

Charvat, Dell, and Folkow.   For example, Charvat *et al.* (1964) speak of the "defense–alarm" reaction, maintaining that under the conditions of civilized living, the somatomotor component of the defense–alarm reaction is suppressed. However, the visceral and endocrine components of this reaction continue to linger, a phenomenon which may have adverse long-term consequences.

Working under the aegis of the World Health Organization and charged with the task of studying *Mental Factors and Cardiovascular*

Diseases, Charvat, *et al.* (1964, p. 130–131) arrived at the following general conclusions:

> Phylogenetically ancient defense mechanisms—originally intended to meet concrete physical dangers in primitive life—have been gradually transferred to the more subtle threat inherent in complex social relations and competitive situations . . . .
>
> Therefore, it is important to realize that civilized man differs from animals and, from very primitive man, in two respects. Firstly, the situations in which mental stress—and its appropriate efferent expressions—is produced, have become far more complex, subtle and manifold in so far as socio-economic relationships rather than immediate physical danger provide the most commonly occurring afferent stimuli. Secondly, when in civilized man "defense–alarm" reactions are produced, the somatomotor component is usually more or less effectively suppressed; in other words, *the originally well coordinated somatomotor, visceromotor and hormonal discharge pattern becomes dissociated.*
>
> There are, however, good reasons to assume that the visceromotor and hormonal changes, induced in connection with emotional stress and the defense–alarm reaction, will remain essentially the same. This implies that the mobilization of the cardiovascular and metabolic resources, intended to support a violent physical exertion will not be utilized in the natural way. For such reasons the hormonally produced changes of the blood and the chemical environment of the heart and blood-vessels can be expected to be more long-lasting than when a violent muscular exertion ensues.*

Charvat *et al.* are careful to emphasize, however, that the cardiovascular consequences of the dissociation of the originally well-coordinated somatomotor, visceromotor, and hormonal discharge pattern have yet to be thoroughly documented. The critical question which has still to be clearly demonstrated is whether stressful psychological stimuli lasting for long periods contribute substantially to disorders such as the hypertensive states and other cardiovascular disorders.

Cannon. Also pertinent is the well known work of Cannon (1932), who described the *fight-or-flight* or *defense–alarm* reaction. The aroused sympathetic nervous system mobilizes a set of physiological responses marked by increases in blood pressure, heart rate, blood flow to the muscles, and oxygen consumption.

Wallace and Benson (1972, p. 90), writing in the context of the Cannon tradition, have recently voiced sentiments similar to those expressed by Charvat *et al.* (1964). In their view, modern man retains an easily triggered fight-or-flight reaction (well-suited to meet the hazards of Neolithic living).

> During man's early history the defense–alarm reaction may well have had high survival value and thus have become strongly established in his genetic makeup. It continues to be aroused in all its visceral aspects when the individual feels threatened. Yet in the environment of our time the reaction is often an anachronism. Although the

---

* It should be noted that even though modern man may effectively suppress *overt* somatomotor behavior under stress, it is probable that the tension in his skeletal musculature increases.

defense–alarm reaction is generally no longer appropriate, the visceral response is evoked with considerable frequency by the rapid and unsettling changes that are buffeting modern society. There is good reason to believe the changing environment's incessant stimulations of the sympathetic nervous system are largely responsible for the high incidence of hypertension and similar serious diseases that are prevalent in our society.*

Wolff. Again, in the extensive researches of Wolff (1968), ample evidence was found indicating the hyper-reactivity of frequently stressed individuals. Such hyper-reactivity was especially pronounced in the pathologically disturbed organ system; e.g., hypertensives showed large excursions of blood pressure during a stress interview. (The latter was the major experimental manipulation which Wolff employed in his far-ranging series of studies.) This pattern of hyper-reactivity in the affected organ system was noted in a variety of stress-related disorders such as cardiac problems, hypercholesterolemia, vascular headaches, and duodenal ulcers.

Wenger. Another pertinent line of theory is Wenger's (1966) concept of autonomic balance. This refers to whether sympathetic or parasympathetic activity seems to be dominant in an individual. The estimate of autonomic balance ($\bar{A}$) for an individual is a composite of the values obtained by him on each of seven autonomic variables. Low scores reflect sympathetic dominance; high scores indicate parasympathetic dominance.

Wenger (1966) carried out a prospective study on over 1000 healthy aviation cadets. In his follow-up 20 years later, Wenger found that the formerly healthy cadets who had shown lower $\bar{A}$ scores (sympathetic dominance) now displayed a higher incidence of high blood pressure, persistent anxiety, and heart trouble.

Wenger's observation of sympathetic dominance in so many disorders is generally compatible with Charvat's *et al.*'s (1964) theory of the deleterious effects of the *defense–alarm* reaction under the conditions of civilized living, and with Malmo's concept of a deficit in the regulation of the autonomic nervous system.

Malmo. Malmo (1966) hypothesizes that a deficiency of the autonomic nervous system regulatory mechanism may be characteristic of many anxiety and psychotic states. For example, Malmo (1966) noted that in anxiety neurotics, forearm EMG levels in response to a startle stimulus took considerably longer to return to prestimulation values than was the case for normals.

In another experiment, comparing blood pressures in normals against

* Wallace and Benson (1972), who have investigated the physiological effects of regular transcendental meditation, postulate that this practice produces an integrated hypometabolic pattern mediated by the central nervous system. This hypometabolic pattern has effects *opposite* to those seen in the fight-or-flight reaction—decreased oxygen consumption, decreased respiratory and heart rate, diminished blood lactate levels, and increased peripheral blood flow.

those of neurotic patients during a mirror-drawing task, Malmo and Shagass (1952) found that for the neurotics, systolic pressures continued to rise during the task, in contrast to the normal group whose pressures tended to level off.

Observations of this nature led Malmo (1966) to conclude that in anxiety neurotics—and perhaps in acute schizophrenics—there is evidence of defective regulatory mechanisms both of the skeletal musculature and the autonomic nervous system. Malmo speculates that it may be defective inhibitory components of reticular and limbic systems which are involved in the physiological over-reaction to stressful stimulation.

Lader and Mathews. Another theoretical position which postulates defective regulatory mechanisms is that of Lader and Mathews (1968). Lader and Mathews, who suggest that anxiety and physiological arousal are related, developed a model in which they proposed that systematic desensitization can be best thought of as an habituation phenomenon, and that habituation occurs most readily in a low arousal condition. Thus, desensitization works best when the patient maintains as low an arousal level as possible (while at the same time clearly visualizing the anxiety stimulus).

Lader and Mathews further postulate a critical level of arousal beyond which repeated presentation of an anxiety stimulus is not accompanied by any habituation. Instead, the level of arousal becomes higher with each successive stimulus, thus producing a *positive feedback loop*—leading to undamped oscillations experienced as a panic attack of anxiety.*

Sternbach. A formulation combining many of the previously noted ideas is that of Sternbach (1966, p. 156), who envisages stress-linked disorders as involving a sequence of interlocked events.

> We begin with a person who has response-stereotypy to the extent that whatever the nature of the activating stimulus, one response system always or usually shows the greatest magnitudes of change as compared to his other response systems. This person also has a *deficiency in feedback control* so that either in initial responsiveness, or in rebound, some limit is exceeded by this maximally reactive system which results in some tissue damage or symptom appearance. This event will occur either when a stressful situation arises which is specifically stimulating to the responsive system in which the individual is also maximally reactive, or when any stressful situation occurs which is of sufficient intensity and/or frequency to result in maximum and/or frequent

---

* Lader and Mathews (1968) have presented evidence that patients with generalized or pervasive anxiety are at higher arousal levels than patients with specific phobias—their pervasive anxiety patients produced a larger number of spontaneous GSR fluctuations than did their normals, or patients with specific phobias. Pervasive anxiety patients are also much more difficult to desensitize than are persons with circumscribed phobias. For example, in our work with several dozen cases over the past 5 years, we have noted that pervasive anxiety patients typically required over twice as many relaxation training sessions as patients with specific phobias (21 vs. 9). They also required twice as many desensitization sessions (10 vs. 5).

reactivity. In the absence of objective real-life stressors, this condition may be met by the individual whose set is such that he perceives ordinary events as if they were those stressors . . . (italics ours).

3.1.   Some Difficulties with the Working Hypothesis

To many readers, the gap between the experimental data so far presented, and the theoretical objective of modifying the response to stress, may seem rather large. In the hopes of diminishing this gap, and of rendering our argument more plausible, several related questions will now be examined.

Response Specificity. An issue likely to be raised by psychophsyiologists concerns response specificity. Are the physiological response patterns of particular subjects stable enough over time to warrant the assumption that excessive activation of some bodily system leads to a stress-related disorder?

Within psychophysiology, the question of response specificity has been a leading area of investigation for the past two decades. In part, this research has been a justifiable reaction against an oversimplified interpretation of Cannon's conceptualization of the fight-or-flight response—in particular, the idea that there is a *uniform* physiological reaction pattern to stress. As a result of psychophysiological research (see Sternbach, 1966), evidence mounted that the individual's profile of activation under stress was no no means identical with every stressor (response specificity). However, Sternbach (1966, p. 144) notes that though normal subjects show a low degree of response stereotypy, psychosomatic patients, on the other hand, display a high degree of response stereotypy—i.e., a great variety of stress situations trigger the "favored" response. For instance, it has been documented that hypertensives, in a variety of stress situations, show strong pressor episodes (Engel and Bickford, 1961; Wolff, 1968).

Transfer to Everyday Life. Another important issue is whether a cultivated low arousal response, acquired in the laboratory, will later transfer to those everyday life situations in which the individual feels tense, anxious, or under pressure. In other words, can the patient maintain the low arousal response outside the laboratory? Though this transfer question has been insufficiently explored by feedback researchers, the older self-regulation disciplines of progressive relaxation and autogenic training offer some valuable leads.

Probably the most important factor is the need for frequent practice. The autogenic exercises, for example, are carried out several times each day for several months. Finally, the low arousal shift becomes a highly over-learned response, and the individual's excessive reactivity to stress situations is said to diminish (see Luthe, 1969, Vol. IV). Some other promising maneuvers could probably be drawn from autogenic training. (1) The use of brief training episodes. With extended practice the trainee is said to become proficient at producing a low arousal condition quickly (Luthe, 1969, Vol. I). (2) Practicing in several different bodily postures. (3) The use of training phrases (e.g., "My arms and legs are heavy and warm."). These phrases are repeated silently during the exercises and serve not only to help the patient recapture the sensations appropriate to low arousal, but assist in the dampening of conceptual activity—reports from subjects indicate that active, goal-directed thinking acts to prevent a shift into a relaxed, low arousal condition (as, for example, when one is trying to fall asleep).

Other techniques to assist in the transfer problem are presently being explored in this laboratory on a case-by-case basis: (1) The use of a portable home EMG feedback units; (2) Cassette tape-recorded relaxation instructions for home use; (3) The use of fading procedures in the laboratory in which the subject learns to perform the response even as information feedback is gradually withdrawn.

It may also be noted that both progressive relaxation and autogenic training were mainly developed prior to World War II. Advances since that time—in electronics, cybernetics, psychophysiology, the principles of learning, and stress research—should permit the evolution of more powerful versions of these pioneering self-regulation techniques.

Autogenic training and progressive relaxation are both valuable in pointing to clinical applications of systematic training in cultivated low arousal. Both of these independently developed techniques have been applied to a variety of stress-related disorders—sleep-onset insomnia, tachycardia, anxiety neuroses, gastrointestinal disturbances, and essential hypertension (all of which are frequently associated with hyperarousal or hyper-reactivity).

The clinical approach we are beginning to explore in this laboratory is to employ the technique of shaping low arousal to certain stress disorders frequently associated with hyperactivation. Patients are first taught the comparatively easy (whole-body) response of muscle relaxation. Subsequent training depends on the physiological *stress profile* of the individual. Thus, a trainee who shows large heart rate increases under stress receives mainly heart rate feedback for his later phase of training. Insomniacs are later trained in producing theta rhythms.

In a subsequent phase it may be possible for a trainee to learn to control two or three bodily systems simultaneously through multiple feedback. After he proves able to control these systems, even under laboratory stress conditions, systematic desensitization could be added. The trainee could be asked to imagine real-life stressful situations while he maintains a low arousal condition. In this fashion, transfer to *in vivo* situations could be aided. The latter technique has already been used with a number of generalized anxiety patients (Budzynski and Stoyva, 1973b).

3.2. Potential Application to Essential Hypertension

Various sources of evidence suggest that the technique of cultivated low arousal may sometimes be useful in the treatment of essential hypertension. Though the precise causes of this disorder are still a matter of controversy, the reaction to stress is generally thought to play a prominent part in its etiology. Thus, two leading cardiovascular physiologists, Folkow and Neil (1971), maintain that essential hypertension results when the *defense–alarm* reaction is too frequently activated. If the individual, under threats of one kind and another, is *constantly mobilizing* his defense–alarm reaction (and its attendant elevated blood pressure) for extended periods, then blood pressures finally become reset at permanently higher levels. What begins as an adaptive, normal reaction designed to meet stresses of short duration, becomes a pathological one in its consequences when the hypertensive response is extended for too long.

But perhaps the hypertensive's defense–alarm reaction can be modified. A combination of techniques might be attempted, proceeding from a general response to a more specific one—in keeping with the concept of systematically shaping a low arousal condition. If practiced often enough, the low arousal response may become part of the individual's new, and more moderate, reaction to a variety of stressors.

Particularly if the disorder were in its early, labile phase—prior to any permanent renal or vascular changes—the following combination of techniques might be attempted. First, systematic training in general muscle relaxation could be used in training patients to lower their arousal levels. Sources in the autogenic training literature report that the autogenic exercises often produce a reduction in blood pressure levels. For example, Klumbies and Eberhardt, at the University of Jena, applied autogenic training to 26 young adult hypertensives (see Luthe, 1969, Vol. II, pp. 70–72). It should be emphasized that frequent home practice was involved—brief episodes eight to ten times per day. After 4 months of training, systolic pressures showed an average decrease of 35 mm Hg; diastolic pressures showed an average decrease of 18 mm Hg—most of which took place during the first month. It may be noted that Jacobson (1938, p. 423) also has reported pressure decreases when progressive relaxation was applied in cases of moderate essential hypertension.

In a feedback training program, patients could first be trained in readily attaining muscular relaxation. Next, patients could be trained with specific feedback of blood pressure to help them to produce lower pressures, as in the work of Shapiro *et al.* (1969). Finally, if these patients are afflicted by various anxieties, which aggravate their disorders, then systematic desensitization could be used to help them moderate their anxieties.

If the biofeedback techniques are able to prove their mettle in stress-related disorders, then the practical consequences are considerable. These techniques may evolve into a means of modifying man's defense–alarm reaction. Methods of modifying the reaction to stress, such as those suggested by biofeedback techniques, could have widespread applications.

4. References

Balshan, I. D., 1962, Muscle tension and personality in women, *Arch. Gen. Psychiat. 7:*436.

Budzynski, T. H., 1969, Feedback-induced muscle relaxation and activation level, unpublished doctoral dissertation, University of Colorado.

Budzynski, T. H., and Stoyva, J. M., 1969, An instrument for producing deep muscle relaxation by means of analog information feedback, *J. Appl. Behav. Anal. 2:*231.

Budzynski, T. H., and Stoyva, J. M., 1973a, A biofeedback technique for teaching voluntary relaxation of the masseter, *J. Dental Res. 52:*116.

Budzynski, T. H., and Stoyva, J. M., 1973b, Biofeedback techniques in behavior therapy, in *Neuropsychologie der Angst,* (N. Birbaumer, ed.), "Reihe Fortschritte der Klinischen Psychologie," Bd. 3, München, Wien: Verlag Urban and Schwarzenberg, pp. 248–270.

Budzynski, T. H., Stoyva, J. M., and Adler, C. S., 1970, Feedback-induced relaxation: Application to tension headache, *J. Behav. Ther. Exptl. Psychiat. 1:*205.

Cannon, J., 1932, *The Wisdom of the Body*, Norton, New York.

Charvat, J., Dell, P., and Folkow, B., 1964, Mental factors and cardiovascular disorders, *Cardiologia, 44:*124.

Davis, J. F., 1959, *Manual of Surface Electromyography*, WADC Technical Report, No. 59-184.

Engel, B. T., Bickford, A. F., 1961, Response specificity, *Arch. Gen. Psychiat. 5:*82.

Foulkes, D., 1966, *The Psychology of Sleep*, Scribner, New York.

Folkow, B., and Neil, E., 1971, *Circulation*, Oxford University Press, New York.

Green, E., Green, A., and Walters, D., 1970, Voluntary control of internal states: Psychological and physiological, *J. Transpersonal Psychol. 1:*1.

Jacobson, E., 1938, *Progressive Relaxation*, University of Chicago Press, Chicago.

Jacobson, E., 1970, *Modern Treatment of Tense Patients*, Charles C. Thomas, Springfield, Illinois.

Lader, M. H., and Mathews, A. M., 1968, A physiological model of phobic anxiety and desensitization, *Behav. Res. Ther. 6:*411.

Luthe, W., 1963, Autogenic training: Method, research, and application in medicine, *Am. J. Psychother. 17:*174.

Luthe, W., 1965, ed., *Autogenic Training: Correlationes Psychosomaticae*, Grune & Stratton, New York.

Luthe, W., 1969, ed., *Autogenic Therapy*, (Vols. I–V), Grune & Stratton, New York.

Maley, M. J., 1967, Two-flash threshold, skin conductance and skin potential, *Psychon. Sci.* 9:361.

Malmo, R. B., 1966, Studies of anxiety: Some clinical origins of the activation concept, in *Anxiety and Behavior* (C. D. Spielberger, ed.), pp. 157–177, Academic Press, New York.

Malmo, R. B., and Shagass, C., 1952, Studies of blood pressure in psychiatric patients under stress, *Psychosom. Med. 14:*81.

Rechtshaffen, A., and Kales, A., 1968, *A Manual of Standardized Terminology, Techniques, and Scoring Systems for Sleep Stages of Human Subjects*, U.S. Dept. H.E.W., Bethesda, Maryland.

Rose, R. J., 1966, Anxiety and arousal: A study of two-flash fusion and skin conductance, *Psychon. Sci. 6:*81.

Sainsbury, P., and Gibson, J. F., 1954, Symptoms of anxiety and tension and the accompanying physiological changes in the muscular system, *J. Neurol. Neurosurg. Psychiat. 17:*216.

Shagass, C., and Malmo, R. B., 1954, Psychodynamic themes and localized muscular tension during psychotherapy, *Psychosom. Med. 16:*295.

Shapiro, D., Tursky, B., Gershon, E., and Stern, M., 1969, Effects of feedback and reinforcement on the control of human systolic blood pressure, *Science, 163:*588.

Sittenfeld, P., Budzynski, T. H., and Stoyva, J. M., 1972, Feedback control of the EEG theta rhythm, paper presented at the 1972 American Psychological Association meeting in Honolulu, Hawaii.

Sternbach, R. A., 1966, *Principles of Psychophysiology: An Introductory Text and Readings*, Academic Press, New York.

Venables, P. H., and Wing, J. K., 1962, Level of arousal and the subclassification of schizophrenia, *Arch. Gen. Psychiat. 7:*114.

Wallace, R. K., and Benson, H., 1972, The physiology of meditation, *Sci. Am. 226:*84.

Wenger, M. A., 1966, Studies of autonomic balance: A summary, *Psychophysiol. 2:*173.

Wolff, H. G., 1963, *Headache and Other Head Pain*, Oxford University Press, New York.

Wolff, H. G., 1968, *Harold G. Wolff's 'Stress and Disease'*, S. Wolf, ed., Charles C. Thomas, Springfield, Illinois.

Wolpe, J., 1958, *Psychotherapy by Reciprocal Inhibition*, Stanford University Press, Stanford.

Wolpe, J., and Lazarus, A. A., 1966 *Behavior Therapy Techniques*, Pergamon Press, New York.

CHAPTER 12

Sleep

M. B. Sterman

Neuropsychology Laboratory, Veterans Administration Hospital
Sepulveda, California
and
Department of Anatomy, University of California
Los Angeles, California

1. Introduction

Whenever I encounter an introductory textbook concerned in one way or another with *functional neuroanatomy*, I always turn first to the subject index and look up the term *sleep*. This topic is usually (but not always) listed in such texts these days, but one is almost always disappointed with the treatment it receives. I have yet to find more than two or three paragraphs devoted to the mysterious process which "ravels up the tattered sleeve of care" and consumes more than one-third of our existence. Most of what is written is often concerned, paradoxically, with such things as arousal functions of the midbrain reticular formation, mechanisms of thalamic recruiting responses, and even the neurophysiology of occlusion.

To be sure, the sleep literature has become extensive and a comprehensive picture is yet to emerge. However, there is much new information in this field which is worthy of consideration. It is now generally established that the brain works actively to initiate and maintain the state of sleep, and specific structures and pathways in the CNS have been associated with various aspects of this process. This chapter will attempt to untangle some of the facts relating to these developments and to focus on several issues which I feel have created the more difficult knots in this regard. I do not, however, intend to present an extensive review of the sleep mechanism literature; for this, the reader should refer to the recent comprehensive monograph by Moruzzi (1972) and the forthcoming text edited by Petre-Quadens and Schlag (1974).

A. AWAKE, ACTIVATED

LONGUS CAPITUS
EYES
LFT. FR. PAR CORTEX
RT. PAR. OCC. CORTEX
TRANS. OCC. CORTEX
OLFACT. BULB
LFT. BAS-MED. AMYGD
LFT. DORSAL HIPP.

B. DROWSY, SLOW WAVE

C. ASLEEP, SPINDLE BURST

D. ASLEEP, ACTIVATED

5 SECONDS

2.   The Measurement of Sleep

The behavior associated with sleep is more complex than it seems. McGinty (1972) has likened the sleep process to an active, appetitive behavior. In the adult the process usually consists of a sequence of phases, including selection of time and place, approached through appropriate preparatory acts and eventual consummation. The consummatory phase constitutes physiological sleep. However, while behavior provides an expanded perspective of the total sleep process, it is neither a valid nor a reliable measure of sleep. The objective measurement of physiological states became possible with the development of electroencephalography and the subsequent appreciation of composite polygraphic patterns. Most if not all physiological functions reflect the dichotomy between the states of wakefulness and sleep, as well as the occurrence of substates within these more general categories. The field has come to rely upon a few of these variables to provide a facile means of classification. These include EEG patterns, head and neck extensor tone (EMG), and ocular activity (EOG). Subcortical EEG patterns, as well as autonomic measures, are recorded in some studies to provide additional information. Overt variables such as posture, eyelid position, pupillary diameter, and respiration may also be easily monitored to aid in classification of the different stages of sleep. The perplexing thing about sleep, however, is the fact that none of these variables alone can provide a reliable measurement, with the exception of the EEG under strictly normal conditions. Thus, the covariance of a spectrum of variables·constitutes the only reliable basis for the quantification of state.

For both historical and practical reasons, and because of a strong similarity to man, the cat has been utilized as the primary subject in the neurophysiological study of sleep. In the cat, as in man, sleep consists of two general patterns which have been variously labeled, depending upon the criterion of interest. These include, among others, slow wave vs. activated sleep (with reference to the EEG), nonrapid-eye-movement (NREM) vs. rapid-eye-movement (REM) sleep (with reference to the EOG) and quiet vs. active sleep (with reference to behavior). The slow or quiet pattern

---

FIG. 1.   Compiled polygraphic patterns defining the four basic states of wakefulness and sleep in the cat. The terminology utilized here is somewhat outdated, since the slow wave designation today is usually associated with sleep pattern (c), characterized by both slow wave and spindle burst activity. The drowsy pattern is a substate within wakefulness, as indicated by a variety of neurophysiological findings. In this figure several traces indicate the changes in a number of limbic structures pertinent to this text. Note that the electrical activity of the olfactory bulb reflects respiration (slow undulations) in the awake and drowsy states, and that this relationship disappears during the two sleep states. (From Sterman *et al.*, 1965).

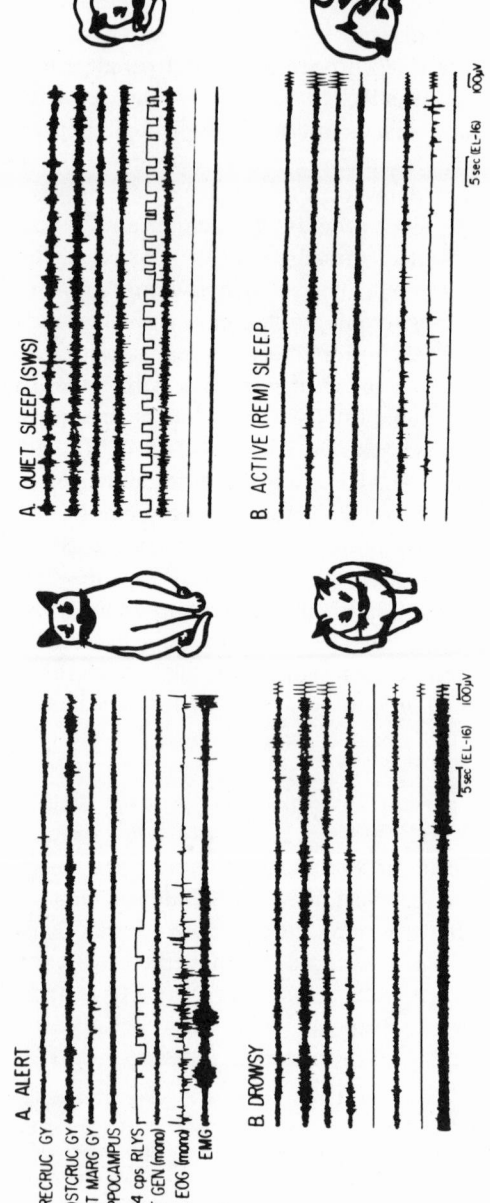

FIG. 2. Compiled polygraphic patterns of wakefulness and sleep in the cat are shown together with characteristic behavioral postures. State labels utilized here are consistent with present standards in our laboratory. Included in these polygrams are localized cortical recordings (in contrast to Fig. 1), lateral geniculate nucleus recordings (which reflect phasic discharge during REM) and automatic detection of sensorimotor cortex 12–14 cps spindle activity (of specific interest to our current studies). The diagram at lower right depicts method used to measure the period of the sleep–waking and REM cycles in the cat. Solid bars indicate REM periods on a baseline of sleep and open bars indicate alert periods on a baseline of waking. (From Lucas and Sterman, in preparation.)

contains several subphases and the activated or REM pattern is similarly divided into tonic and phasic subcategories. Examples of composite polygraphic state patterns in the cat are shown in Figs. 1 and 2. With the scoring of these states, it is possible to objectively evaluate pattern percentage, duration, and sequence and to employ statistical analysis. Normative data have been published for man (Agnew and Webb, 1966; Kahn and Fisher, 1969) and for the cat (Sterman *et al.*, 1965; Ursin, 1968). This quantitative approach provides also for assessment of the temporal organization of states, a more recent development in the field (see, for example, Figs. 2 and 3). Application of chronobiological techniques has disclosed systematic periodicities in this organization, which shed new light on brain mechanisms in addition to constituting yet another variable for standardized measurement (Aschoff, 1965; Webb, 1969; Globus, 1970; Sterman *et al.*, 1972; Sterman, 1972). At the present time, the sleep of some 20 mammalian species has been studied under more or less rigorous laboratory conditions (Allison and Van Twyver, 1970). These studies have disclosed a rather remarkable similarity in the physiological and temporal organization of sleep states in mammals, a fact which reflects the fundamental biological role of this process.

The objective measurement of sleep is a relatively new development requiring sophisticated recording and data reduction techniques. The pioneeers in this field did not have these tools available to them. Unfortunately, even today few neurophysiologists fully avail themselves of these ad-

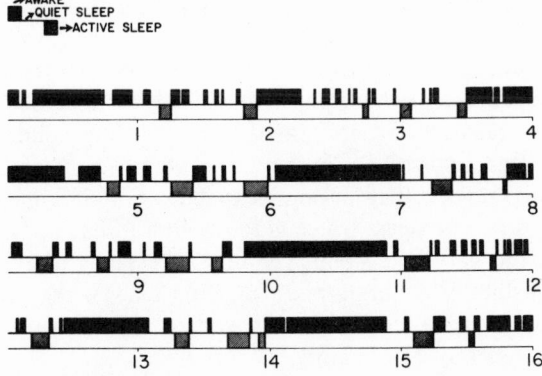

FIG. 3. Classification of polygraphic patterns of sleep and waking states allows for quantification and graphic display of these data. Such a display is shown here for a continuous 16-hour period of recording. Note that more or less sustained waking and sleep periods alternate in time resulting in a sleep–waking rhythm of about 100 minutes in this animal. Within sleep the recurrent REM state describes a cycle also, which averages to about 20 minutes. Sophisticated evaluation of the temporal organization of states can be obtained with computer analyses of such data.

vances. Distorted slow wave EEG patterns produced by drugs, lesions, or other significant CNS alterations are uncritically referred to as sleep. Some investigators do not even bother to monitor physiological activity but refer, instead, to postural reflexes or other unreliable behavioral manifestations. In some situations, such as in the newborn or decerebrate animal, the indices for state classification are either incomplete or absent. In these cases little attention has been directed to the problems of definition which these alterations create. I believe that this continuing failure to standardize definition and measurement has resulted in a confusing literature characterized, as we shall see, by contradiction. The physiologist has often failed to appreciate the problems of validity and reliability, whereas the behaviorist has failed to effectively utilize physiological measurement toward this end.

3. Perspectives: Past and Present

The earliest thinkers who concerned themselves with the problem of sleep were almost universally of the opinion that it was a state forced upon the organism. According to Kleitman (1963), the first sleep theory on record was proposed by a contemporary of Pythagoras in the 6th century, B.C., who felt that sleep resulted from a retreat of the blood into the veins. This idea can be listed as a forerunner of the *cerebral anemia* theories of sleep which were to evolve many years later. During this early period the importance of the central nervous system in these matters had not yet been established. However by the 19th century, great advances were made along these lines. Johannes Muller's *Elements of Physiology* (1843) presented a consolidated treatise on human physiology, and this included a chapter on sleep. Muller recognized the brain as the organ of the mind; and of sleep, he said, "The organic processes in the brain, which attend an active state of mind, gradually render that organ incapable of maintaining the mental action, and thus induce sleep, which is to the brain what bodily fatigue is to other parts of the nervous system." Muller, like many after him, believed that a changed state of the brain resulting from its own organic activity was responsible for sleep. A contemporary version of this early concept has been expressed recently by McGinty (1971).

Mauthner (1890) was one of the first investigators to anticipate later concepts by focusing attention on the midbrain, and more specifically on the area surrounding the nucleus of the third cranial nerve. He reported some observations on the pathology of an encephalitic condition called "nona", in which somnolence was a primary symptom. Postmortem examination indicated involvement of the central gray matter in the area of the oculomotor nucleus, and from the proximity of this area to the main sensory projections on their way to the thalamus, Mauthner concluded that sleep resulted from a break in these conduction pathways due to a "temporary cessation of function of the central gray." According to Mauthner, sleep resulted from a functional isolation of the cortex from the environment.

By 1935 it was apparent that the diencephalic–brainstem junction was important with regard to sleep and wakefulness. After performing a mesencephalic transection of the brainstem caudal to the nuclei of the third cranial nerve, Bremer (1935) reported that the functional condition of the diencephalon and of the cortex resembled the electrical and behavioral characteristics of sleep. He concluded, in agreement with Mauthner, that a sleeplike functional depression of the telencephalon and diencephalon resulted from suppression of the continuous flood of ascending impulses to the cerebral cortex.

This course of events had led to a dominating interest in wakefulness as the active state in the sleep–waking cycle. The ascendance of the concept of subcortical waking mechanisms was increasingly apparent from the literature, but the culmination of this trend came with the conceptualization of a diffuse arousal system in the brain stem by Moruzzi and Magoun (1949). These investigators observed that high-frequency electrical stimulation of the reticular formation in the brainstem, and its more rostral extensions into the diencephalon, produced an EEG and behavioral response similar to that normally seen in awakening. The wealth of afferent collaterals to the reticular formation from virtually every sensory pathway, together with descending projections from the cerebral cortex, provided for the realization of a system involved in the waking process, and potentially capable of important integrative functions (Magoun, 1963).

With so much attention diverted to wakefulness, one might think that sleep had been forgotten. On the contrary, during this same period in time an important sequence of discoveries was suggesting quite a different interpretation of the sleep phenomenon. At the turn of the century a strange encephalitic epidemic had spread through the city of Vienna, leaving a disruption of the sleep–waking rhythm in its victims as its primary symptom. During this period, von Economo, a pathologist, distinguished himself by a classic study of the central nervous system lesions involved (1918). By careful comparison of many clinical cases of encephalitis lethargica, von Economo described two symptomatic patterns of the disease associated with two localizations of inflammatory lesions in the nervous system. In those cases where somnolence and ophthalmoplegy were the distinguishing symptoms, the lesions were regularly found in the posterior wall of the third ventricle, continuing caudally to the level of the oculomotor nucleus.

In contrast to this, there were other cases in which insomnia and chorea were observed. The inflammation in these patients was associated with the rostral hypothalamus, the tuberal region, and adjacent portions of the striatum. From these observations, von Economo concluded that the affected areas must constitute a "Schlafsteurungszentrum" or "sleep regulating center" consisting of at least two parts: a rostral part (at the anterior end of the third ventricle), which, when appropriately excited, actively inhibits the thalamus and cerebral cortex and thus causes "brain sleep," and a more caudal part (in the posterior hypothalamus and rostral brain stem) which acts to decrease somatic and autonomic activity and thereby causes "body sleep."

The concept of an active sleep-inducing mechanism in the central nervous system achieved its most widespread attention through the pioneering work of Hess (1943, 1954). Hess had perfected a method of stimulating the brain in unanesthetized, unrestrained cats. Using low-frequency, low-voltage stimulation delivered through surgically placed electrodes, he reported sleeplike behavior obtained as a direct stimulation effect. Stimulation of a variety of points situated lateral to the ventral half of the massa intermedia in the thalamus resulted in a response which varied between drowsiness and a behavior that could not be distinguished from the cat's normal sleep.

More evidence suggesting that sleep was an actively induced state was forthcoming from the laboratory of Nauta. Seriously considering the earlier observations of von Economo, Nauta set forth to put them to an experimental test in rats (1946). He used a well-controlled surgical approach to make transections across the base of the brain at various frontal planes, and then observed the postoperative behavior of these experimental animals. As might be expected, transections placed in the posterior hypothalamus produced a state of persistent somnolence, and thus, led to the interpretation that the "waking center" had been separated from the rest of the forebrain. On the other hand, transections placed in the rostral half of the hypothalamus, particularly at a suprachiasmatic level, produced a complete insomnia uncomplicated by hypothermia or infection, and leading invariably to a state of lethal exhaustion. Sleepless behavior was only observed following bilateral and complete transections, and was found to be a continuation of relatively normal waking patterns rather than the onset of any bizarre motor activity. From these observations, Nauta concluded that "the rostral half of the hypothalamus, roughly conforming to the suprachiasmatic and preoptic areas, is the site of a nervous structure which is of specific importance for the capacity of sleeping." He disagreed with von Economo's interpretation of a thalamic or cerebral inhibition, suggesting, instead, a direct inhibition of the waking center in the posterior hypothalamus. Thus, the sleep cycle was thought to result from periodic decreases in the activity of the waking center, brought about by periodic increases in discharge from the sleep center in the rostral hypothalamus. Nauta also pointed out that several parasympathetic functions appear to be localized in the preoptic region. Since the transition from the waking to the sleeping state corresponds to a shift from sympathetic to parasympathetic predominance in the autonomic sphere, he suggested that the rostral parasympathetic area may similarly regulate the sympathetic discharge from more caudal hypothalamic levels. Nauta considered the possibility of an active inhibition of lower levels in the nervous system by a more rostral forebrain "center," this inhibition being reflected by the somatic, vegetative, and functional changes accompanying the onset of sleep.

As facts began to accumulate in favor of an active neural mediation of sleep, an ever-increasing effort was directed toward understanding this mediation. By the middle of the present century the pendulum had begun to swing in the opposite direction. Brain stimulation and recording techniques were well developed and contributed to this trend. Reports appeared which suggested that physiological sleep could be induced by stimulation* of a variety of nervous tissues, including: peripheral nerves (Pompeiano and Swett, 1962), caudal brainstem (Magnes et al., 1961a,b), rostral brainstem (Parmeggiani, 1962), midline and lateral thalamus (Hess et al., 1953; Mornier, 1950; Akimoto et al., 1956; Parmeggiani, 1962), the basal forebrain (Sterman and Clemente, 1962a,b; Hernandez-Peon, 1962), and the caudate nucleus (Buchwald et al., 1961). There emerged the concept of tonically active *hypnogenic* or *synchronogenic* brain areas, sometimes referred to, unfortunately, as *sleep centers*. Of course, this period in general was characterized by a tendency toward subcortical phrenology.

However, several consistent findings did develop from this flurry of activity. The group in Moruzzi's laboratory at Pisa, Italy, demonstrated a tonic EEG synchronizing influence originating in the lower brain stem. Midpontine pretrigeminal brainstem transections resulted in a sustained increase in EEG waking patterns above the level of transection (Batini et al., 1958, 1959). Favale et al. (1961) found that low-frequency electrical stimulation at certain sites in the pontine reticular formation elicited EEG slow waves and, after some delay, behavioral sleep. Working with encephale isole cat preparations, Magnes et al. (1961a,b) localized such effects to the tractus solitarius of the bulbopontine region, but found that the

---

* Findings derived from electrical stimulation studies have been the subject of much debate (Jouvet, 1967; Doty, 1969; Moruzzi, 1972). Electrical stimulation of the nervous system has provided an important tool in neurophysiology and, when properly utilized, still contributes to our knowledge in this area. The question of technique is very critical here, as it is with other sophisticated methods used to study the nervous system.

induced EEG synchronization was rather tenuous and dependent upon a background state of EEG drowsiness (behavioral assessment was impossible in these brain transected animals). When applied under proper conditions the induced EEG changes clearly outlasted the period of stimulation. The bulbopontine region thus was considered to possess neural mechanisms which contribute to the sleep process, most likely through mediation of protective reflexes related to systemic functions or of the soporific influence of a monotonous sensory milieu (Moruzzi, 1972).

In considering the question of central regulation in sleep a decade ago, we were impressed by the consistency of physiological findings in relation to a region at the base of the forebrain, including posterior orbital and paraolfactory cortex, the preoptic area, and anterior hypothalamus. This general region has since been termed the basal forebrain area (BFA). Nauta (1946) had suggested that this area was of particular importance in relation to sleep on the basis of the devastating insomnia resulting from transections just below this level in rats. Peripheral responses similar to those associated with the onset of sleep were typically elicited by stimulation of this same region. The preoptic area, in particular, was established as a site of parasympathetic integration on the basis of visceral responses elicited by electrical stimulation (Ranson et al., 1935; Hess, 1954). Behavioral inhibition also had been induced with electrical stimulation (Hess, 1954). Finally, appropriate endocrine changes, such as suppression of catecholamine and corticosteroid secretion, were produced by stimulation in these sites (von Euler and Folkow, 1958; Slusher and Hyde, 1961).

Because of Nauta's observations and those of von Economo before him, and this wealth of fragmentary data relating the basal forebrain area to the behavioral and physiological responses of sleep, we had good reason to explore the final link in the suggested association, the possibility that stimulation here could induce the EEG pattern of sleep. Electrical stimulation of this area in acute, unanesthetized cats elicited EEG synchronization and, additionally, proved capable of actively inducing EEG and behavioral manifestations of sleep in behaving cats (Sterman and Clemente, 1961, 1962a,b). These findings have been abundantly confirmed in other laboratories (Hernandez-Peon, 1962; Kaneko et al., 1962; Taylor and Branch, 1969; Bremer, 1970; Lineberry and Siegel, 1971). In view of the logic which first led us to explore this forebrain area in relation to sleep, it seems paradoxical today that several reviewers have interpreted its significance in this regard as being limited to the mediation of EEG synchronization (Jouvet, 1972; Moruzzi, 1972).

Be that as it may, several characteristics of the BFA distinguish it from other brain areas which had been related to sleep. Since Hess (1954), a number of studies have shown that electrical stimulation of the BFA can produce an almost immediate suppression of ongoing behavior (Sterman and Fairchild, 1966; Nielson and Davis, 1966). Moreover, if intermittent stimulation was continued, preceding behavior was terminated completely and the animal induced to sleep (Figs. 4 and 5). We have observed that pupillary myosis and relaxation of the nictitating membrane are frequent autonomic components of the response to stimulation here (Figure 5A), and that overt muscle relaxation and eye closure also may be elicited (Figure 5B).

It has been established that destruction of the BFA results in an acute and sustained disturbance of the sleep process. McGinty and Sterman (1968) found that large lesions placed bilaterally at the caudal borders of this area produced a marked suppression of sleep which lasted for 2–4 weeks, and which, in some animals, resulted in death during total insomnia. Sleep suppression persisted in surviving animals even after other physiological disturbances associated with lesions in this area had disappeared. Similar findings were reported by Madoz and Reinoso-Suarez (1968). In a more recent study we have confirmed the immediate onset of insomnia following BFA lesions in unanesthetized cats (Fig. 6), and found that relatively small lesions placed bilaterally in the center of this area were even more effective in producing a profound and long-lasting sleep disturbance (Lucas and Sterman, 1972). Interestingly, when a small lesion was placed

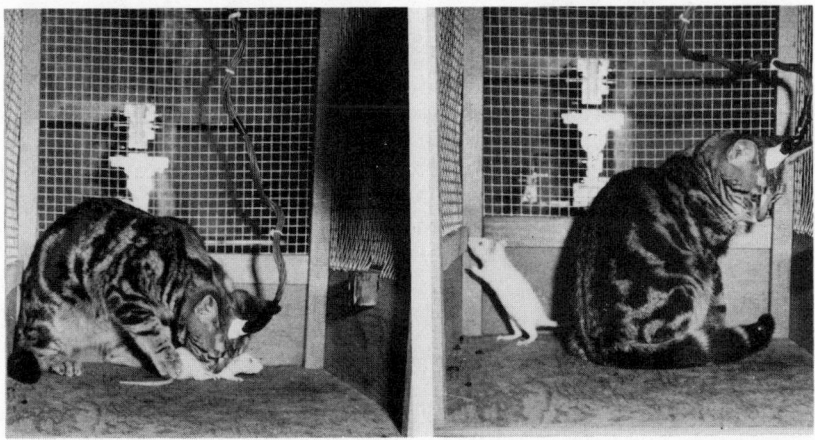

FIG. 4. These pictures show an aroused cat just prior to and 30 seconds after the onset of basal forebrain area stimulation. Exploratory and attack behavior were immediately terminated, the animal becoming drowsy and disinterested in the rat. Continued intermittent stimulation resulted in the onset of sleep. These results were obtained with both low- and high-frequency electrical stimulation. (From Sterman and Clemente, 1962b.)

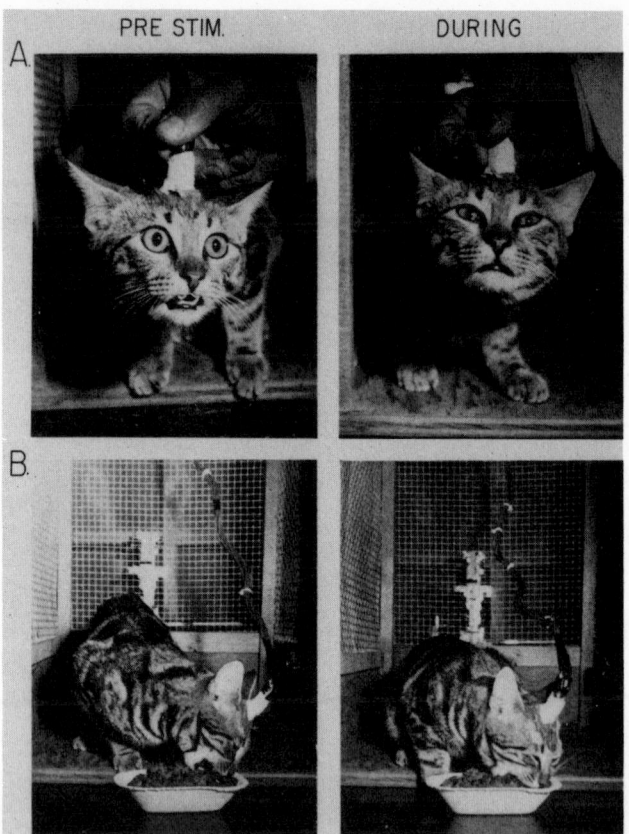

FIG. 5. Effects of basal forebrain area electrical stimulation on a variety of physiological manifestations are shown here in the cat. Sequence at A indicates induced pupillary myosis, relaxation of the nictitating membrane and change in muscle tone. At B, animal was eating prior to stimulation. Effects produced here included eye closure, postural relaxation, and, after removal of face from food dish, termination of feeding.

for therapeutic reasons in an homologous area of the human brain, a suppression of sleep similar to that obtained in cats was observed (Hauri and Hawkins, 1972).

The basal forebrain area receives a wealth of projections from the frontal cortex, thalamus, and limbic system (Nauta, 1958, 1964). In turn, fibers from the diffuse plexus of cells which make up the region project back upon these structures, and in addition descend into the hypothalamus and brain stem reticular formation (Clemente and Sterman, 1963, 1967; Scheibel and Scheibel, 1967; Mizuno et al., 1969). Bremer (1970) has indicated that these caudal projections effect a cephalic inhibition of arousal by inhibition of neurons in the brainstem reticular formation. More detailed considerations of possible mechanisms have been developed elsewhere (Sterman and Clemente, 1968, 1974; Moruzzi, 1972). In summary, we agree with Nauta (1946). The basal forebrain area, in its integration of neo-

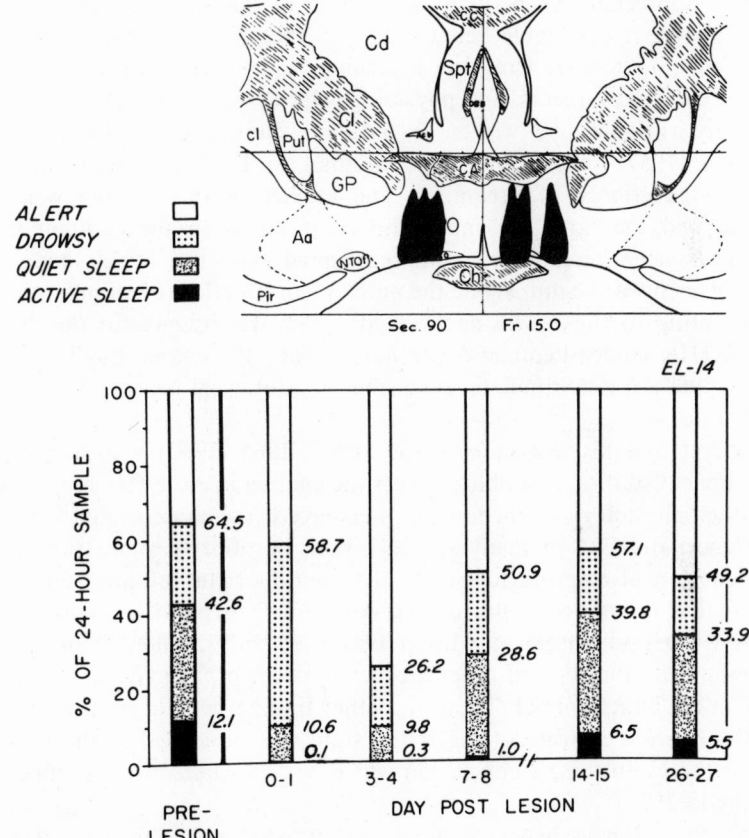

FIG. 6. The effects of bilateral basal forebrain area lesions on sleep and waking state percentages are shown here in the cat. The frontal section diagram at top shows a histological reconstruction of the actual lesion, and the graph below indicates pattern distributions in 24-hour samples obtained before and at the times indicated following placement of this lesion. The lesion was made in a behaving, unanesthetized animal. For approximately 12 hours immediately following tissue destruction this animal was continuously awake, pacing about the chamber in circles. No REM patterns were observed during the first week postlesion, and slow wave (quiet) sleep was reduced over 75% during the initial 24-hour period, as well as 3 days later. A total recovery of normal pattern distribution was never observed in this animal. (From Lucas and Sterman, 1972, and in preparation.)

cortical, limbic, and hypothalamic functions, does have "specific importance for the capacity of sleeping."

The study of the neural basis of sleep was to be directed along a parallel yet quite different line of investigation by the important contributions of Kleitman and his co-workers. In 1953 Aserinsky and Kleitman first drew the biological world's attention to the previously described rapid-eye-movement or REM state of sleep. Surprisingly, studies to that time had failed to appreciate the periodic occurrence of this state, which, as mentioned above, is detectable behaviorally by the appearance of gross body movements, twitching, irregular breathing, facial grimacing, and rapid, conjugate eye movements, and physiologically by significant changes in almost any variable one wishes to measure. Subsequently, Dement and Kleitman (1957) related this state in man to EEG activation and the cognitive experience of dreaming. The impact of this finding was immediate and, perhaps, the most important factor in the contemporary growth of sleep research. An unprecedented scientific attack upon the elusive dream was begun. While the outcome of his effort eventually proved disappointing to those who had sought a neural substrate for the dream process (Hernandez-Peon and Sterman, 1966; Pivik and Foulks, 1968; Berger, 1969), it did stimulate concurrent physiological investigation of the REM state.

Jouvet and his associates (1959, 1962, 1965, 1967) pioneered these physiological studies, describing in cats the characteristic EMG suppression and other physiological phenomena that have become associated with the occurrence of REM in many species. Also, he utilized brain transection techniques in attempting to isolate the neural origins of this state, and showed that the midcollicular or "cerveau isole" preparation continued to manifest a periodic atonic condition associated with rapid-eye-movements, autonomic instability, and other electrophysiologic phenomena similar to REM in the intact animal. These and other findings led Jouvet to conclude that the neural substrate of the REM state was organized at the pontine level of the brainstem, a conclusion which has now been widely supported (Zanchetti, 1967).

At first, Jouvet believed that the slow wave phase of sleep was an expression of corticofugal activity. He argued that this pattern was telencephalic in origin, in contrast to the rhombencephalic mediation of the REM or "paradoxical" sleep pattern (PS), as he termed it (1960, 1962, 1963). However, a growing interest in biochemical and neurochemical techniques was to alter this position substantially. The conclusions resulting from an extensive series of investigations in this new direction led Jouvet to propose a monoaminergic theory of the sleep–waking cycle, which placed the primary neural substrates for both sleep and wakefulness exclusively at the pontine and mesencephalic levels of the brain stem (Jouvet 1967a,b). According to Jouvet's most recent attempt at consolidation (1972), he proposes that slow wave sleep is initiated by the release of serotonin (5HT) at central serotoninergic synapses whose presynaptic elements arise within the anterior raphe nuclei of the brainstem. 5HT neurons located in the caudal raphe, on the other hand, "prime" REM sleep, and send terminals to the caudal two-thirds of the nucleus locus coeruleus. This latter nucleus is responsible for what he calls the "executive mechanism" of REM sleep.

Another important line of investigation in the neurophysiological study of sleep has developed from the brain transection technique introduced to this area by Bremer (1935). His classical findings in the *cerveau isole*, or intercollicular midbrain transected cat, characterized the acutely isolated forebrain as showing a pattern of sustained, high-voltage EEG synchronization, accompanied by pupillary myosis. At that time he concluded that sleep occurred passively in the forebrain upon the withdrawal of tonic activating input from sensory stimuli. His recent studies, carried out three decades later, have led to a reinterpretation, since he showed that stimulation of the basal forebrain area produced inhibition of cellular activity in the mesencephalic reticular formation (Bremer, 1970). As men-

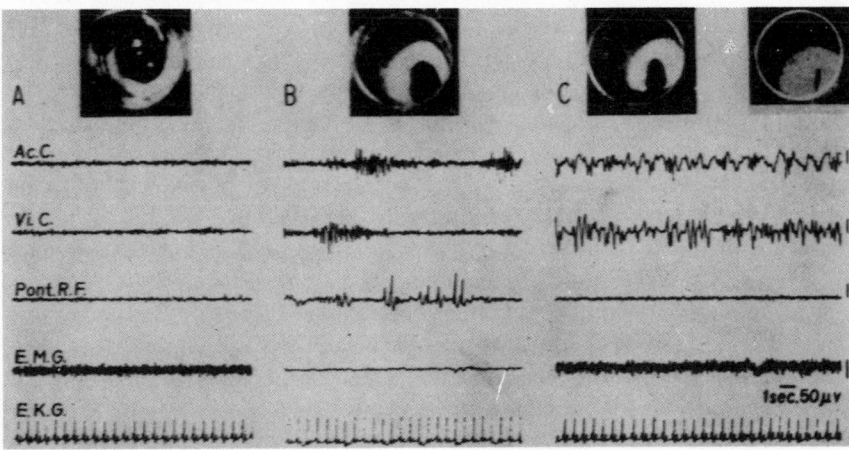

FIG. 7. Relationships between pupillary behavior, cortical EEG, pontine EEG, and peripheral measures in a chronic decerebrate cat preparation. At A, pupillary position and diameter as well as the cortical EEG pattern indicate a waking state in the isolated forebrain. A progression from early to later sleeplike patterns is shown in B and C from these forebrain measures. Note that the separated brainstem enters a REM state (as indicated by pontine spikes and neck EMG suppression) *during* this progression of sleep patterns in the forebrain. Such findings indicate that a complete dissociation of these states can be achieved by separating their neural substrates. (From Villablanca, 1966.)

tioned above, Bremer has suggested that descending forebrain influences may provide a means whereby higher centers can actively initiate sleep through a process of reticular deactivation.

In recent years the technique of brain transection has been significantly improved so that cat preparations can be maintained for long periods of time. As Moruzzi (1972) has pointed out, the state described after acute forebrain isolation by Bremer was probably one of coma. However, these more recent studies have demonstrated convincingly that the chronically isolated forebrain is, indeed, capable of showing alternating sleep and waking patterns as indicated by EEG, pupillary, and behavioral measures (Hobson, 1965; Villablanca, 1966; Slosarska and Zernicki, 1969). Villablanca (1966) described a consistent alternation between physiological patterns resembling sleep and wakefulness, in cats transected at a rostral midbrain level (Fig. 7). Slosarska and Zernicki (1969) utilized EEG criteria as well as orienting responses and conditioned olfactory and ocular reactions to demonstrate sleep and waking states in isolated midbrain and forebrain preparations. We also found recently that cats sustaining transection at a caudal diencephalic level still showed alternating EEG patterns (Fig. 8). The resulting synchronization–desynchronization cycle in the animal shown described a rather stable rhythm of approximately 3 hours. Additionally, the activity of variables controlled by the separated brainstem indicated a concurrent and completely independent REM cycle of approximately 40 minutes. It is interesting to note that these cycles were both altered in comparison with the intact animal by a factor of two. The normal cat shows a sleep–waking rhythm of approximately 1.5 hours and a REM cycle of about 20 minutes (Sterman et al., 1972; Lucas and Sterman, 1972). This suggests a continued temporal coupling of the sleep–waking and REM cycles even after separation of their neural substrates. As mentioned previously, many studies have shown that the REM cycle continues to be manifest in midbrain and high pontine preparations.

The implications of these findings are several. The fact that an animal devoid of the forebrain can still demonstrate all but the missing EEG criteria of the REM state cycle confirms the fact that the neural substrates for this phenomenon are organized in the brainstem. Conversely, the fact that the isolated forebrain can continue to manifest all obtainable signs of the sleep–waking cycle indicates that the primary neural substrates for this phenomenon are organized in the forebrain. As Moruzzi (1972) has pointed out, this conclusion creates complications for the humoral theory of sleep regulation proposed by Jouvet, since the regulatory elements in this model must originate in brainstem structures. We may conclude from these findings, also, that the origins of the REM cycle are more primitive than those of sleep and wakefulness, and that this mode of organization preceded sleep and wakefulness in phylogeny. In this case, ontogeny may

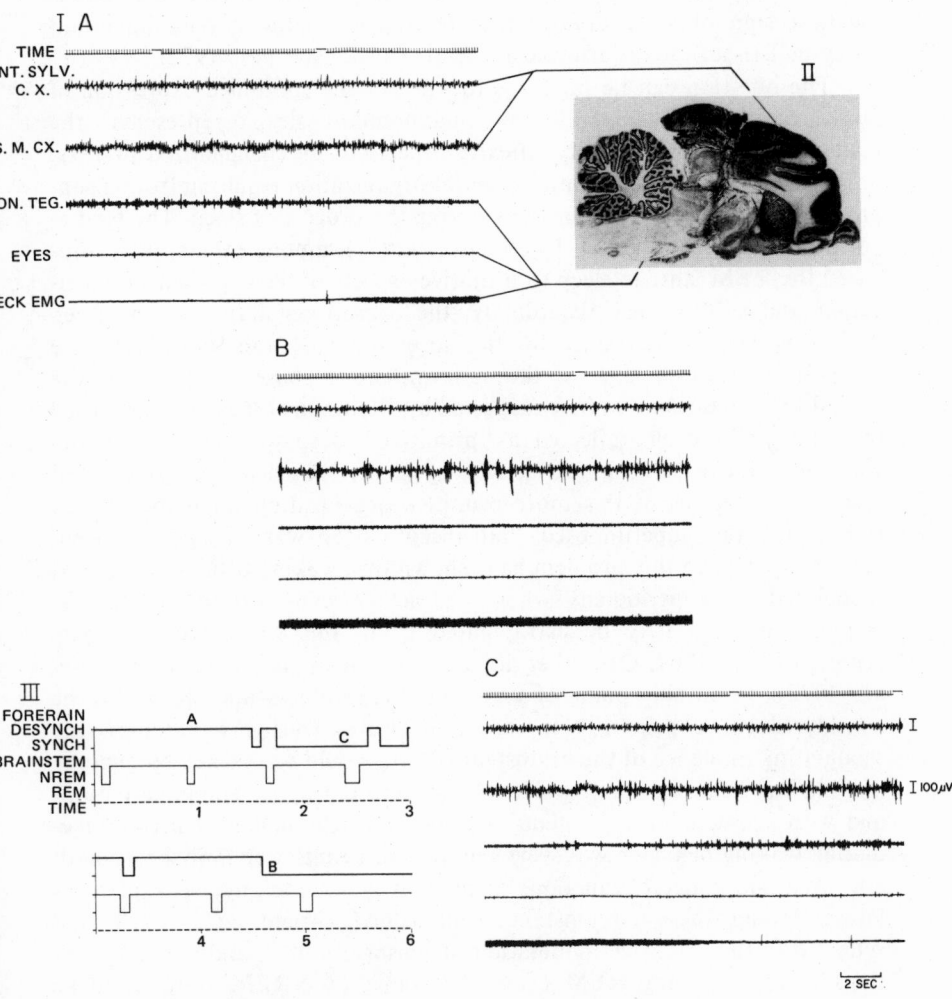

FIG. 8. Polygraphic records of forebrain and brainstem controlled variables are shown here at I. A–C, in a cat with brain transection achieved at a posterior diencephalic level in our laboratory. An alternating pattern of EEG desynchronization (low-voltage, fast activity) and synchronization (high-voltage spindles) was observed in continuous recordings from the isolated forebrain. The REM state pattern (as indicated by pontine spiking, eye movements, and EMG suppression) was recurrently noted in the separated brain stem (IA and IC) independently of the ongoing forebrain pattern. The actual transection is shown in II from a saggital histological section at L2-3. The temporal distribution of these state patterns from separated forebrain and brain stem substrates is shown at III from a continuous 6-hour recording. The points at which samples IA–C were taken are indicated here also. The characteristics of this temporal organization are discussed in the text.

indeed recapitulate phylogeny, since it is well known that the REM cycle is the first sign of state organization to appear in the developing infant (Dreyfus-Brisac, 1968; Parmelee and Stern, 1972; Sterman, 1972).

The question can be raised as to whether the continued expression of this primitive organization in mammalian sleep represents the manifestation of more basic, reflexive aspects of an encephalized process, or the release of a more primitive neural organization resulting from a suppression of certain higher functions during the process of sleep. The former position has been suggested by McGinty (1971), among others, who compared the REM state in sleep to primitive aspects of feeding such as mastication and swallowing. Accordingly, the overall regulation of the sleep drive has been taken over by the forebrain, but this more reflexive component is still a part of the consummatory phase. A basis for the second interpretation was first suggested by Kleitman (1963), who proposed that the REM cycle reflected a "primitive" sleep–waking organization which he termed the basic-rest-activity-cycle (BRAC). Kleitman speculated that manifestations of this more primitive organization might be present throughout the superimposed "advanced" sleep–waking cycle. Recent studies directed to this problem have shown that waking behavior is indeed modulated by a periodicity whose characteristically variable cycle corresponds to, and may be extrapolated from, the REM cycle of sleep (Othmer et al., 1969; Oswald et al., 1970; Globus et al., 1971; Sterman et al., 1972). From this point of view both wakefulness and sleep may be considered to be primarily forebrain functions. During wakefulness the modulating influence of the brainstem BRAC would be masked by ongoing and elicited behavior, and could only be detected under stable conditions and with sensitive measurements. During sleep the higher structures mediating waking behavior would be suppressed, resulting in a dissociation of cognitive and conative functions from sensory, motor, and visceral regulation. Under these circumstances the BRAC would be exposed, and reflected in the primitive modulation of sensory, motor, and visceral functions manifest as the REM cycle. The quiet or NREM state could be considered as the resting phase and the active or REM state as akin to wakefulness in this primitive functional organization. In support of this possibility, many neurophysiological measures obtained during the REM state show characteristics more similar to normal wakefulness than to slow wave sleep.

4.   Summary and Conclusions

In this chapter I have discussed several aspects of brain studies concerned with the neural basis of sleep. It was suggested that one of the main problems in this area has been the difficulty in achieving and then adopting strict criteria for definition and measurement of sleep. Sleep is viewed here as a specific physiological state of central nervous system integration which, at present, is impossible to measure directly. The expression of this state in a broad spectrum of physiological functions, themselves subject to idiosyncratic regulatory dynamics, provides the only means for reliable measurement. Thus, sleep can be measured by reference to composite polygraphic data, including primarily the EEG, tonic and phasic motor activity (i.e., EMG and EOG), and visceral activity. Relatively stable polygraphic patterns thus emerge, which can be quantified and subjected to statistical analysis. The temporal organization of these patterns provides an additional basis for assessment. Drugs and other manipulations of the CNS can alter these patterns and produce states which are functionally different from sleep (i.e., anesthesia and coma). These facts suggest that since we still do not know what sleep is we must attend to what it is not, and consider any seriously altered pattern as something different from sleep. This is not the case today and, as a result, pharmacologists still refer to anesthesia often as sleep, neurophysiologists frequently consider abnormal EEG slow wave patterns as indicative of sleep and also attribute this state to limp brain stem preparations, and behaviorists have been known to accept verbal reports of sleep or ascribe it to newborn infants who show grossly fragmented polygraphic patterns. Perhaps this approach would lead to a definition of sleep which would allow us to determine what it is, how it is derived, and how it is modified by pathology.

To date the study of the neural mediation of sleep has not been subject to such restrictions, and concepts have come and gone with the times. An attempt has been made here to present this historical perspective and to show that today we are burdened by the same kind of conceptual flux. A body of consistent data has developed, however, and these facts were stressed here. The neural substrates for the REM state cycle have been localized below the mesencephalon and continue to be active even in the absence of a forebrain. The mechanism for the sleep–waking rhythm, on the other hand, appears to involve an interaction between diffuse systems organized within mid- and forebrain structures.

Empirically, a system of fiber pathways and ill-defined nuclei which interconnect frontal neocortex with basal and mesial limbic structures, hypothalamic nuclei and midbrain core plays an essential role in the process of sleep in mammals. This system is not distinguished by a clear anatomic organization or the presence of well-defined neural structures. Its importance has been established because manipulations appropriately influenced all of the physiological indices described above as criteria for the definition of sleep. It was suggested that the emergence in mammals of a nonspecific mesodiencephalic arousal system modulated by this basal forebrain inhibitory system provided for the development in phylogeny of a more advanced neural organization, as manifest by the sleep–waking rhythm. Lower species, in this schema, are restricted to a more primitive modulation of sensory, motor, and visceral functions in the form of a basic rest–activity cycle organized at a brainstem level. This cycle continues to be manifest in mammals, and accounts for the modulation of arousal in the waking state and the alternation of REM and slow wave patterns during sleep.*

5. References

Agnew, H. W., Jr. and Webb, W. B., 1966, The first night effect: An EEG study of sleep, *Psychophysiol. 2:*263–266.

Allison, T., and Van Twyver, H., 1970, The evolution of sleep, *Nat. Hist. 79:*56–65.

Aschoff, J., 1965, *Circadian Clocks*, North-Holland Publ. Co., Amsterdam.

Aserinsky, E., and Kleitman, N., 1953, Regularly occurring periods of eye motility and concomitant phenomena during sleep, *Science 118:*273.

Batini, C., Moruzzi, G., Palestini, M., Rossi, G. F., and Zanchetti, A., 1958, Persistent patterns of wakefulness in the pretrigeminal mid-pontine preparation, *Science 128:*30.

Batini, C., Moruzzi, G., Palestini, M., Rossi, G. F., and Zanchetti, A., 1959, Effects of complete pontine transections on the sleep–wakefulness rhythm: the mid-pontine pretrigeminal preparation, *Arch. Ital. Biol. 97:*1–12.

Berger, R. J., 1969, The sleep and dream cycle, in *Sleep, Physiology and Pathology*, A. Kales ed., J. B. Lippincott Co., pp. 17–32.

Bremer, F., 1935, Cerveau isole et physiologie du sommeil, *Compt. Rend. Soc. Biol. 118:*1235–1241.

Bremer, F., 1970, Preoptic hypnogenic focus and mesencephalic reticular formation, *Brain Res. 21:*132–134.

Buchwald, N. A., Wyers, E. J., Okuma, T., and Heuser, G., 1961, The "caudate-spindle". I. Electrophysiological properties. *Electroenceph. Clin. Neurophysiol. 13:*509–518.

Clemente, C. D., and Sterman, M. B., 1963, Cortical synchronization and sleep patterns in acute restrained and chronic behaving cats induced by basal forebrain stimulation, *Electroenceph. Clin. Neurophysiol. 24:*172–187.

Clemente, C. D., and Sterman, M. B., 1967, Basal forebrain mechanisms for internal inhibition and sleep, In *Sleep and Altered States of Consciousness*, Ass. Res. Nerv. Ment. Dis. eds., Williams and Wilkins Co., Baltimore, p. 45.

Dement, W., and Kleitman, N., 1957, Cyclic variations in EEG during sleep and their relation to eye movements, body motility, and dreaming, *Electroenceph. Clin. Neurophysiol. 9:*673–690.

Doty, R. W., 1969, Electrical stimulation of the brain in behavioral context, *An. Rev. Psychol. 20:*289–320.

Dreyfus-Brisac, C., 1968, Sleep ontogenesis in early human prematurity from 24–27 weeks of conceptual age, *Develop. Psychobiol. 1:*162–169.

Economo, von C., 1918, *Die Encephalitis Lethargica.*, Deuticke, Wien.

* The research reported here from our laboratory was supported by the Veterans Administration and USPHS Grant MH 10083.

Euler, U. S., von, and B. Folkow., 1958, The effect of stimulation of autonomic areas in the cerebral cortex upon the adrenaline and noradrenaline secretion from the adrenal gland in the cat, *Acta Physiol. Scand. 42*:313–320.

Favale, E., Loeb, C., Rossi, G. F., and Sacco, G., 1961, EEG synchronization and behavioral signs of sleep following low frequency stimulation of the brain stem reticular formation, *Arch. Ital Biol. 99*:1–22.

Globus, G. G., 1970, Quantification of the sleep cycle as a rhythm, *Psychophysiol. 7*:248–253.

Globus, G. G., Phoebus, E., and Moore, C., 1971, REM "sleep" manifestations during waking, *Psychophysiol. 7*:308.

Hauri, P., and Hawkins, D. R., 1972, Human sleep after leucotomy, *Arch. Gen. Psychiat. 26*:469–473.

Hernandez-Peon, R., 1962, Sleep induced by localized electrical or chemical stimulation of the forebrain, *Electroenceph. Clin. Neurophysiol. 14*:423–424.

Hernandez-Peon, R., and Sterman, M. B., 1966, Brain functions, *An. Rev. Psychol. 17*:363–394.

Hess, W. R., 1943, Symptomatik des durch elektrischen reiz ausgelosten schlafes und die topographie des schlafzentrums, *Helv. Physiol. 1*:C61.

Hess, H. W., 1954, *Diencephalon–Autonomic and Extrapyramidal Functions*, Grune and Stratton, New York.

Hobson, J. A., 1965, The effects of chronic brain stem lesions on cortical and muscular activity during sleep and waking in the cat, *Electroenceph. Clin. Neurophysiol. 19*:41–62.

Jouvet, M., 1960, Telencephalic and rhombencephalic sleep in the cat, in *Nature of Sleep*, Ciba Foundation Symposium.

Jouvet, M., 1962, Recherches sur les structures nervouses et mechanismes responsibles des differents phases du sommeil physiologique, *Arch. Ital. Biol. 100*:125–206.

Jouvet, M., 1963, The rhombencephalic phase of sleep, *Brain Mechanisms*, in G. Moruzzi, A. Fessard, and H. H. Jasper, eds., Elsevier Publishing Co., Amsterdam, pp. 407–424.

Jouvet, M., 1965, Paradoxical sleep. A study of its nature and mechanisms, in *Sleep Mechanisms, Progress in Brain Research, Vol. 20*, W. A. Himwich, and J. P. Schade, eds., Elsevier Publishing Co., Amsterdam, p. 20.

Jouvet, M., 1967a, Neurophysiology of the states of sleep, in *The Neurosciences*, C. Quarton, T. Melnechuk, and F. O. Schmitt, eds., Rockefeller University Press, New York, pp. 529–544.

Jouvet, M.,1967b, Neurophysiology of the states of sleep, *Physiol. Rev. 47*(2):117–177.

Jouvet, M., 1972, The role of monoamines and acetylcholine-containing neurons in the regulation of the sleep-waking cycle, *Rev. Physiol. 64*:166–274.

Jouvet, M., and Michel, F., 1959, Correlations electromyographique du sommeil chez le chat decortique et mesencephalique chronique, *Compt. Rend. Seances Soc. Biol. 153*:422–425.

Kahn, E., and Fisher, C., 1969, The sleep characteristics of the normal aged male, *J. Nerv. Ment. Dis. 148*:477–494.

Kaneko, Z., Hishikawa, Y., Ueyama, M., Shimizu, A., and Ida, H., 1962, EEG synchronization induced by electrical stimulation of the hypothalamus, *Proceedings of XIth Annual Meeting of Japan EEG Society*, Tokyo.

Kleitman, N., 1963, *Sleep and Wakefulness*, University of Chicago Press, Chicago, pp. 552.

Lineberry, C., and Siegel, J., 1971, EEG synchronization, behavior inhibition and mesencephalic unit effects produced by stimulation of orbital cortex, basal forebrain and caudate nucleus, *Brain Res. 34*:143–161.

Lucas, E. A., and Sterman, M. B., 1972, Effects of performance and forebrain lesions on sleep-wake (S–W) and REM cycles in the cat, *Anat. Rec. 172*:357.

Madoz, P., and Reinoso-Suarez, F., 1968, Influence of lesions in preoptic region of the states of sleep and wakefulness, *Proc. Int. Union Physiol. Sci. 7*:276.

Magnes, J., Moruzzi, G., and Pompeiano, O., 1961a, Electroencephalogram-synchronizing structures in the lower brain stem, in *The Nature of Sleep*, G. E. W. Wolstenholme and M. O'Connor, eds., Churchill, London, p. 57–77.

Magnes, J., Moruzzi, G., and Pompeiano, O., 1961b, Synchronization of the EEG produced by low-frequency electrical stimulation of the region of the solitary tract, *Arch. Ital. Biol. 99:*33–67.

Magoun, W. W., 1963, *The Waking Brain*, Charles C Thomas, Springfield, Illinois.

Mauthner, L., 1890, Zur pathologie und physiologie des schlafes nebgst bemerkungen uber die "nona," *Wien, Med. Wschr. 40.*

McGinty, D. J., 1971, Encephalization and the neural control of sleep, in *Brain Development and Behavior,* M. B. Sterman, D. J. McGinty, and A. M. Adinolfi, eds., Academic Press, New York, pp. 335–357.

McGinty, D. J., 1972, Development of forebrain control of sleep, in *Sleep and the Maturing Nervous System,* C. Clemente, D. Purpura, and F. Mayer, eds., Academic Press, New York.

McGinty, D. J., and Sterman, M. B., 1968, Sleep suppression after basal forebrain lesions in the cat, *Science 160:*1253–1255.

Mizuno, N., Clemente, C., and Sauerland, E. K., 1969, Projections from the orbital gyrus in the cat. II. To telencephalic and diencephalic structures, *J. Comp. Neur. 136:*127–142.

Moruzzi, G., 1972, The sleep–waking cycle, *Rev. Physiol. 64:*165.

Moruzzi, G., and Magoun, H. W., 1949, Brain stem reticular formation and activation of the EEG, *Electroenceph. Clin. Neurophysiol. 1:*455–473.

Muller, J., 1843, *Elements of Physiology*, Lee and Blanchard, Philadelphia.

Nauta, W. J. H., 1946, Hypothalamic regulation of sleep in rats, *J. Neurophysiol. 9:*285–316.

Nauta, W. J. H., 1958, Hippocampal projections and related neural pathways to the midbrain in the cat, *Brain 81:*319–340.

Nauta, W. J. H., 1964, Some efferent connections of the prefrontal cortex in the monkey, in *The Frontal Granular Cortex and Behavior*, J. M. Warren and K. Akert, eds., McGraw-Hill, Inc., New York.

Nielson, H. C., and Davis, K. B., 1966, Effect of frontal ablation upon conditioned responses, *J. Comp. Physiol. Psychol. 61:*380–387.

Oswald, I., Merrington, J. and Lewis, H., 1970, Cyclical "on demand" oral intake by adults, *Nature 225:*959–960.

Othmer, E., Hayden, M. P., and Segelbaum, R., 1969, Encephalic cycles during sleep and wakefulness: 2 24-hour pattern, *Science 164:*447–449. .

Parmeggiani, P. L., 1962, Sleep behavior elicited by electrical stimulation of cortical and subcortical structures in the cat, *Helv. Physiol. Pharmacol. Acta 20:*347–367.

Parmelee, A. H., and Stern, E., 1972, Development of states in infants, in *Sleep and the Maturing Nervous System,* C. D. Clemente, D. Purpura, and F. E. Mayer, eds., Academic Press, New York.

Petre-Quadens, O., and Schlag, J., 1974, *Basic Sleep Mechanisms,* Academic Press, New York, 459 pp.

Pivak, T., and Foulkes, D., NREM mentation: Relation to personality, orientation time, and time of night, *J. Consult. Clin. Psychology, 33*(2):144–151.

Pompeiano, O., and Swett, J. E., 1962, EEG and behavioral manifestations of sleep induced by cutaneous nerve stimulation in normal cats, *Arch. Ital. Biol. 100:*311–342.

Ranson, S. W., Kabat, H., and Magoun, H. W., 1935, Autonomic responses to electrical stimulation of hypothalamus, preoptic region and septum, *A.M.A. Arch. Neurol. Psychiat. 33:*467–477.

Scheibel, M. E., and Scheibel, A. B., 1967, Structural organization of nonspecific thalamic nuclei and their projection toward cortex, *Brain Res. 6:*60–93.

Slosarska, M., and Zernicki, B., 1969, Synchronized sleep in the chronic pretrigeminal cat, *Acta Biol. Exptl. 29:*175–184.

Slusher, M. A., and Hyde, J. E., 1961, Effects of limbic stimulation on release of corticosteroids into the adrenal venous effluent of the cat, *Endocrinol. 69:*1080–1085.

Sterman, M. B., and Clemente, C. D., 1961, Cortical recruitment and behavioral sleep induced by basal forebrain stimulation, *Fed Proc. 20:*334.

Sterman, M. B., and Clemente, C. D., 1962a, Forebrain inhibitory mechanisms: Cortical synchronization induced by basal forebrain stimulation, *Exptl. Neurol. 6:*91–102.

Sterman, M. B., and Clemente, C. D., 1962b, Forebrain inhibitory mechanisms: Sleep patterns induced by basal forebrain stimulation in the behaving cat, *Exptl. Neurol. 6:*103–117.

Sterman, M. B., Knauss, B. A., Lehmann, D., and Clemente, C. D., 1965, Circadian sleep and waking patterns in the laboratory cat, *Electroenceph. Clin. Neurophysiol. 19:*509–517.

Sterman, M. B., and Fairchild, M. D., 1966, Modification of locomotor performance by reticular formation and basal forebrain stimulation in the cat: Evidence for reciprocal systems, *Brain Res. 2:*205–217.

Sterman, M. B., and Clemente, C. D., 1968, Basal forebrain structures and sleep, *Acta. Neurolog. Lat. Amer. 14:*228–249.

Sterman, M. B., 1972, The basic rest–activity cycle and sleep: Developmental considerations in man and cats, in *Sleep and the Maturing Nervous System*, C. D. Clemente, D. Purpura and F. E. Mayer, eds., Academic Press, New York.

Sterman, M. B., Lucas, E. A., and Macdonald, L. R., 1972, Periodicity within sleep and operant performance in the cat, *Brain Res. 38:*327–341.

Sterman, M. B., and Clemente, C. D., 1974, Forebrain mechanisms for the onset of sleep, in *Basic Sleep Mechanisms*, O. Petre-Quadens and J. Schlag, eds., Academic Press, New York.

Taylor, A. N., and Branch, B. J., 1969, Interactions of forebrain and bulbar inhibitory mechanisms with the reticular activating system in the control of ACTH release, *Fed. Proc. 28:*438.

Ursin, R., 1968, The two stages of slow wave sleep in the cat and their relation to REM sleep, *Brain Res. 11:*347–356.

Villablanca, J., 1966, Behavioral and polygraphic study of "sleep" and "wakefulness" in chronic decerebrate cats, *Electroenceph. Clin. Neurophysiol. 21:*562–577.

Webb, W. B., 1969, Twenty-four-hour sleep cycling, in *Sleep: Physiology and Pathology*, A. Kales, ed., J. B. Lippincott Co., Philadelphia and Toronto, pp. 53–65.

Zanchetti, A., 1967, Brain stem mechanisms of sleep, *Anesthesiol. 28:*81–99.

Index